Searching Eyes

CALIFORNIA/MILBANK BOOKS ON HEALTH AND THE PUBLIC

Searching Eyes

Privacy, the State,
and Disease Surveillance
in America

Amy L. Fairchild
Ronald Bayer
James Colgrove

with Daniel Wolfe

⊞

UNIVERSITY OF CALIFORNIA PRESS
Berkeley   Los Angeles   London

MILBANK MEMORIAL FUND
New York

The Milbank Memorial Fund is an endowed operating foundation
that engages in nonpartisan analysis, study, research, and communication on significant issues in health policy. In the Fund's own publi-
cations, in reports or books it publishes with other organizations, and
in articles it commissions for publication by other organizations, the
Fund endeavors to maintain the highest standards for accuracy and
fairness. Statements by individual authors, however, do not necessarily
reflect opinions or factual determinations of the Fund. For more
information, visit www.milbank.org.

University of California Press, one of the most distinguished university
presses in the United States, enriches lives around the world by
advancing scholarship in the humanities, social sciences, and natural
sciences. Its activities are supported by the UC Press Foundation
and by philanthropic contributions from individuals and institutions.
For more information, visit www.ucpress.edu.

University of California Press
Berkeley and Los Angeles, California

University of California Press, Ltd.
London, England

Library of Congress Cataloging-in-Publication Data
Fairchild, Amy L.

   Searching eyes : privacy, the state, and disease surveillance in
America / Amy L. Fairchild, Ronald Bayer, James Colgrove ; with
Daniel Wolfe.
      p.   cm.   (California/Milbank books on health and the public)
   Includes bibliographical references and index.
   ISBN: 978–0–520-25202-8 (cloth : alk. paper)
   ISBN: 978–0–520-25325-4 (pbk. : alk. paper)
   1. Public health surveillance.   2. Privacy, Right of.   I. Bayer,
Ronald.   II. Colgrove, James Keith.   III. Wolfe, Daniel, 1960–
IV. Title.   V. Series.
   [DNLM: 1. Population Surveillance—United States.
2. Confidentiality—United States.   3. Health Policy—history—
United States.   4. Privacy—United States.   5. Public Health
Practice—history—United States.   WA 105 F165s 2007]
   RA652.2.P82F35   2007
   362.10973—dc22   2007001053

Manufactured in the United States of America

16   15   14   13   12   11   10   09   08   07
10   9   8   7   6   5   4   3   2   1
This book is printed on Natures Book, which contains 50% post-
consumer waste and meets the minimum requirements of ANSI/NISO
Z39.48–1992 (R 1997) (*Permanence of Paper*).

For Allan Rosenfield
Dean, Mailman School of Public Health, Columbia University

CONTENTS

ILLUSTRATIONS

ABBREVIATIONS

AACC	Association for the Aid of Crippled Children
AALL	American Association for Labor Legislation
ABLES	Adult Blood Lead Epidemiological Survey Program
ACLU	American Civil Liberties Union
ACoS	American College of Surgeons
AICP	Association for the Improvement of the Condition of the Poor
AMA	American Medical Association
APHA	American Public Health Association
ASCC	American Society for the Control of Cancer
ASTHO	Association of State and Territorial Health Officers
BLS	Bureau of Labor Statistics
CCHC	Citizens' Council on Health Care
CDC	Communicable Disease Center; subsequently Center for Disease Control; then Centers for Disease Control and Prevention
CIFS	Childhood Immunization Follow-Up System
CSS	Community Service Society
CSTE	Council of State and Territorial Epidemiologists
DHEW	Department of Health, Education, and Welfare
DHHS	Department of Health and Human Services
FAC	Federation of Associations of Cripples
FDA	Food and Drug Administration
FERPA	Family Educational Rights and Privacy Act
HIPAA	Health Insurance Portability and Accountability Act
IOM	Institute of Medicine
MOD	March of Dimes
NARA	National Archives and Records Administration
NCI	National Cancer Institute

NEDSS   National Electronic Disease Surveillance System
NFIP   National Foundation for Infantile Paralysis
NIH   National Institutes of Health
NIOSH   National Institute for Occupational Safety and Health
OCAW   Oil, Chemical and Atomic Workers Union
OSH   Occupational Safety and Health
OSHA   Occupational Safety and Health Administration
PANIC   Prevent AIDS Now Initiative Committee
PHS   Public Health Service
PLAC   Privacy Law Advisory Committee
PROVE   Parents Requesting Open Vaccine Education
RODS   Real Time Outbreak and Disease Surveillance System
RWJ   The Robert Wood Johnson Foundation
SEER   Surveillance, Epidemiology, and End Results Program
SENSOR   Sentinel Event Notification System for Occupational Risks
SHE(O)s   Sentinel Health Events (Occupational)
UNITE   Union of Needletrades, Industrial and Textile Employees

FOREWORD

The Milbank Memorial Fund is an endowed operating foundation that works to improve health by helping decision makers in the public and private sectors acquire and use the best available evidence to inform policy for health care and population health. The Fund has engaged in nonpartisan analysis, study, research, and communication since its inception in 1905.

Searching Eyes: Privacy, the State, and Disease Surveillance in America is the eighteenth of the California/Milbank Books on Health and the Public. The publishing partnership between the Fund and the University of California Press seeks to encourage the synthesis and communication of findings from research that could contribute to more effective health policy.

The authors of *Searching Eyes* offer a new approach to surveillance policy. They analyze surveillance as an issue in the politics of policy making for public health, which it has been for more than a century.

Fairchild, Bayer, and Colgrove, with a significant contribution from Daniel Wolfe, describe the practical tension between privacy and the welfare of society since the nineteenth century. Their extensive research in primary sources reveals how difficult it has been to make and implement surveillance policy. The book begins in the late nineteenth century when, as a result of advances in scientific knowledge, "public health officials moved," the authors write, "to pull chronic infectious disease into the ambit of public health surveillance." Next the authors describe significant occasions during the twentieth century when "many people with illness [for example, occupational disease, cancer, and birth defects] would demand the right to be counted so that the extent of their afflictions could serve as a prod for . . . ameliorative legislation." This aspect of the history of surveillance, the authors find, "democratized" privacy as "different constituencies balanced privacy against what they perceived to be their own greater interests."

The era of "democratic privacy" is likely to continue indefinitely as new issues of surveillance policy arise. One such issue is the tension between policy to create immunization registries and the privacy of parents and children. Another is likely to be whether and how to use information about routine laboratory testing of the blood of persons with diabetes to improve the quality of care for individual patients.

Daniel M. Fox
President

Samuel L. Milbank
Chairman

Disease provokes enormous fear. Dread of sickness and death is often matched by anxiety about the loss of privacy, which can place one's reputation, resources, and even autonomy and liberty at risk. These two deeply rooted apprehensions come together as the state seeks to monitor diseases in the name of the public's health.

For more than two decades, beginning in the mid-1980s, the world of American public health was roiled by a bitter controversy over whether the names of people infected with Human Immunodeficiency Virus (HIV) should be reported to state public health registries. Pitted against each other were gay rights and privacy advocates on the one hand and public health officials on the other. Name reporting, the former argued, would threaten harm to those most at risk for HIV and would be counterproductive from the point of view of public health, driving the AIDS epidemic underground. Most public health officials asserted in response that disease notification was a long-established and essential feature of public health practice, permitting the monitoring of an epidemic's course. Many were incredulous that their efforts to protect the public health would generate skepticism, even hostility. Further, they were troubled that concerns about privacy seemed to all but ignore what they felt to be the profession's exemplary history of protecting surveillance records.

The extended and often bitter conflict—repeated in many states— posed questions of when the needs of public health could justify intrusions into the confidentiality of the doctor-patient relationship. At its broadest level, then, the encounter represented a clash over how to negotiate the contested terrain of privacy in America.

In retrospect, what was most striking about the contours of the encounter over HIV reporting was the extent to which men and women with or at risk for infection had sought to define the appropriate balance between the claims of privacy and those of public health. They had, in fact, democratized a dispute that in earlier eras might have involved only physicians and public health officials in an intra-professional battle that, though not shrouded from view, would have been largely immune to popular influence.

The AIDS struggle captured our attention and set the stage for undertaking a broad study of public health surveillance in the United States. We were drawn to a set of political and ethical questions that had received only episodic attention: When and why did the practice of reporting the names of those with diseases to public health authorities begin? What impulse or anxiety, either implicit or explicit, informed the efforts of public health officials as they first undertook surveillance activities and subsequently sought to extend the scope of such efforts? Did such efforts always produce conflicts like those that surrounded HIV? When there were such conflicts, who was brought to the fray and what arguments did they make? How did physicians view reporting? As an invasion of the sanctity of the doctor-patient relationship? As an intrusion into their professional domain? As a conscription into the service of public health? As a responsibility reflecting the broader mission of medicine? Were there occasions when the potential subjects of surveillance appeared to accept such efforts? When they did so, was it because they believed they could not win a struggle against those who put such proposals forward? Were their own interests served by surveillance? Might reporting enable the delivery of needed services or state protections from threats to their well-being? Were there times when the potential subjects of surveillance became its most ardent proponents? How have race and class shaped the politics of surveillance?

As we considered this set of questions, we came to believe that a history of public health surveillance in the United States could best be told against the backdrop of the changing role and importance of privacy—what the constitutional law scholar Lawrence Tribe has described as "nothing less than society's limiting principle"—in American life.[1] In 1957, in the context of cold war intrusions into the privacy of the home, Supreme Court justice William O. Douglas warned against "the searching eyes of government."[2] In so doing, he touched upon a recurrent concern in American society: the sanctity of a private realm, marked by a boundary between the state and the individual. What is necessary, as Tribe has written, is to specify the "substance of what is being protected, . . . the character of the choices or the information we are to classify as special."[3] We frame public health surveillance as a social practice that is embedded within particular contexts rather than as a purely technical undertaking that is insulated from politics and society. Thus reactions to disease reporting have often been colored by more general attitudes toward other types of state surveillance and intrusion into personal privacy.

Public opinion surveys since the early 1990s, when more than 80 percent of Americans expressed concern about privacy,[4] have underscored a generalized state of anxiety about the ability to prevent others from "seeing, hearing, and knowing."[5] People especially feared the degree to which their medical information could be shared or viewed by others, placing them at risk for discrimination. A Lou Harris poll in 1992 found that more than 25 percent of Americans believed that their medical information had been improperly disclosed. In 1996 another poll noted that almost three-quarters of those surveyed were troubled by the prospect that their medical records would be used for research without their consent.[6] Three years later, one-quarter of Americans surveyed for the California Health Care Foundation said that they trusted neither health plans nor government programs such as Medicare to keep their information confidential. In the same survey, one in seven said that they had taken steps to avoid embarrassment, stigma, or the threat of discrimination: they had been less than candid with their doctors or had even decided to forego care. Finally, in 2004 a poll found that more than a third had very little trust that government would use personal information about individuals appropriately. The relevance of these polls to disease reporting is not straightforward. We do not know for certain whether health departments are viewed with the same degree of suspicion as other government entities.

Nevertheless, a broader sense of disquiet cannot but shape the climate within which public health surveillance occurs. The act of surveillance, as one scholar recently explained, is Janus faced: it is "as vital to the maintenance of our welfare and freedom" as it is to "a policy of rounding up undesirable minorities."[7] If public health practitioners and their allies have stressed the first function, those influenced by the work of Michel Foucault have generally stressed the second, viewing surveillance as a threatening prelude to social control.[8]

Ironically, both appropriate the vision of the eighteenth-century utilitarian Jeremy Bentham. His proposal for a model prison, a panopticon, was an exemplar of watchfulness and would serve as an inspiration for those who fashioned disease surveillance systems in the nineteenth century. For Foucault, the panopticon represented a "striking emblem of everything he detested about modern society."[9]

Over the course of the twentieth century, privacy achieved the status of a constitutionally protected right. It is in the shadows of this sweeping, conflict-punctuated narrative of the politics of privacy that the politics of surveillance plays out, as individual disease notification became an activity central to the protection of the public's health. Our focus, in this examination of the more than century-long history of privacy and public health surveillance in the United States, is on the ongoing, name-based reporting of cases of disease to state and local health departments, which historically triggered interventions to control disease, such as contact investigation.[10] Over time, its meaning expanded to include program planning, implementation, and

evaluation.[11] Some health professionals ascribe to an even broader definition of disease surveillance that encompasses epidemiological studies,
whether conducted by state agencies or academic researchers; inspections
of hazardous workplace or environmental conditions, including dangers
that might be posed by contaminated food and water; and screening efforts,
whether conducted at the workplace or in clinical settings.[12] What constitutes surveillance has evolved and been the subject of dispute over the
course of the twentieth century.[13] As he reflected on the change he had witnessed, Alexander Langmuir, who did more than any other figure in public
health to define surveillance, found himself "utterly frustrated." On the one
hand, he had tired of "repetitive dialogues" with federal officials who would
try to narrowly define "The Science of Surveillance." On the other, he was
equally dismayed "with the explosion of the use of the term."[14] Yet the year
before his death, Langmuir reminded himself, "surveillance must be flexi-
ble and adapt to current needs."[15] Regardless, then, of how it is defined,
every effort to understand the patterns of disease and mortality contributes
to the goals of surveillance. To the extent that these investigations shaped
the direction of government-based disease reporting efforts or revealed
their limits, they became part of the complex account we present in the following chapters.

Not all acts of surveillance elicit public controversy. For example, the
"shoe leather epidemiology" involved in investigating outbreaks of acute
communicable diseases such as meningitis or common-source outbreaks
such as salmonella inevitably requires the collection of names and the follow-up of cases.[16] This vital part of the day-to-day practice of public health
surveillance has almost never provoked concerns about privacy.[17] In part
this is true because of a widespread acknowledgment that such clear and
present dangers to the public health necessitate identification of the threat's
source. We were drawn not to such well-accepted staples of surveillance but
to extended controversies involving the expansion of public health reporting that could illuminate the contested terrain where public health surveillance meets the claims of privacy.

Searching Eyes is, then, a history of both privacy, a value central to American democratic life, and public health surveillance, an activity essential for
protecting the welfare of society. We begin, in part 1, in the late nineteenth
century as public health officials moved to pull chronic infectious disease
into the ambit of public health surveillance. It was an era punctuated by
furious and extended conflicts that pitted doctors, who sought to defend a
notion of privacy that was bound up with their professional authority,
against public health officials. It was in the context of highly stigmatized illnesses linked to social status or personal behavior—tuberculosis and venereal diseases—that these battles over what we will call "paternalistic privacy"
unfolded.

But the prospect of disease surveillance has not always been the occasion for expressions of alarm or an enterprise to be negotiated exclusively among professionals, as we make clear in part 2, which deals with occupational disease reporting, cancer registries, and birth defects surveillance. Indeed, over the course of the twentieth century, many people with illness would demand the right to be counted so that the extent of their afflictions could serve as a prod for social reform and ameliorative legislation. In the eight-decade saga over the notification of occupational disease, workers and their representatives challenged employers, who invoked the language of privacy in a dogged effort to resist state intervention and regulation. The call for surveillance could also reflect the belief that only official enumeration could open the way to understanding the causes and possible prevention of diseases with elusive etiologies and to providing needed services. Disability and birth defects, as well as cancer notification, exemplified the extent to which different constituencies balanced privacy against what they perceived to be their own greater interests. The battles over privacy in these encounters would be democratized as those with or at risk of disease or disability gave voice to their own needs. It is this dynamic that we characterize as "democratic privacy."

In part 3 we turn to conflicts that would unfold almost entirely in the new era of democratic privacy, characterized by popular participation in the struggles over the scope and functions of surveillance. The extraordinary two-decade battle that erupted over AIDS exemplified the new political landscape. The history of immunization registries underscores the complex forces called into play as efforts were made to extend surveillance from the monitoring of disease or disability to the enforcement of health. Child health advocates confronted opponents concerned about interference with parental autonomy, an issue that mirrored early anxieties about clinical authority. In the final chapter of this section, we turn to a new era of conflicting imperatives: to extend disease surveillance on the one hand and to curtail such efforts on the other as concerns about privacy reached a new zenith. It is within this context that the boundaries of public health are both tested and strained. These efforts at extending surveillance involved areas as diverse as child health, bioterrorism, and the clinical treatment of diabetes and HIV. In each of these cases, public health officials would have to address the centrality of privacy as a social and political value, as exemplified by passage of the Health Insurance Portability and Accountability Act (HIPAA).

As we begin a new century of disease surveillance, it is clear that we are at a very different place at the beginning of the twenty-first century than we were at the end of the nineteenth. When the modern era of disease surveillance began, it was doctors who protected privacy as an instrumental value. In the current era, patients, their advocates, and concerned citizens more generally are all actively engaged in defining the benefits and limits of privacy.

ACKNOWLEDGMENTS

During the course of this project, which we first imagined in the early 1990s and began in earnest more than five years ago, we accumulated more debts than we can acknowledge, but we shall do our best. The first goes to our colleague Daniel Wolfe, who provided incisive comments on many aspects of the book and was the primary researcher and author of the occupational disease chapter. We could not have completed the book without him.

The book could not have been undertaken without the support of the National Cancer Institute and the Robert Wood Johnson Foundation's Investigator Awards in Health Policy Research Program. It would have been all too easy for any agency or foundation to see only one particular slice of this work as being relevant to its mission, so we are grateful for the vision of these two organizations. We particularly thank Brenda Edwards, our program officer at the National Cancer Institute, and David Mechanic and Lynn Rogut, who served as our shepherds at RWJ.

Numerous colleagues generously read this volume in whole or part and gave us critical advice regarding sources and interpretation. Chief among them, we thank our colleagues in the Center for the History and Ethics of Public Health at Columbia's Mailman School of Public Health: David Rosner, Gerald Markowitz, Gerald Oppenheimer, and Barron Lerner. In the Department of Sociomedical Sciences, our academic home, we thank Jennifer Hirsch, who organized an interdisciplinary group of faculty and students who commented on our work. Connie Nathanson, Eugene Litwak, Carole Vance, Ben Meier, Nadav Davidovitch, Kathrine Meyers, and others whose contributions extended even beyond that discussion all helped us to see our topic through the eyes of sociology, anthropology, and law.

Numerous talks also provided an opportunity for receiving vital feedback. Early in the project an opportunity to collaborate with staff at the

Centers for Disease Control and Prevention, which included Patricia Sweeney and Patricia Fleming, and Larry Gostin and Lance Gable at the Georgetown University Law Center, inspired us to begin framing the early history of surveillance. Given his involvement in much of the history that we recount, Larry in particular informed our project in insightful ways. As our work progressed, Ted Brown provided a warm welcome during a wintry month at the University of Rochester. John Harley Warner, Naomi Rogers, Cindy Connelly, and others among their colleagues and students gave critical advice at Yale. John Warner, David Rosner, Georgina Feldberg, and Allan Brandt organized a conference honoring Barbara Rosenkrantz and her vision of public health and the state, which provided yet another chance to test our analyses. Students and faculty in the History of Medicine Program at Johns Hopkins twice read chapters from the book and provided the opportunity for us to learn about Randy Packard's unexpected connection to this work. We thank Nathaniel Comfort and Harry Marks for facilitating those discussions, the second of which provided the occasion to gain the invaluable perspectives of Graham Mooney, who was working on his own history of surveillance in England. Chris Warren at the New York Academy of Medicine, as part of the organization's annual Sauter Lecture, allowed us to present portions of our work to the medical community. The Robert Wood Johnson Foundation provided not only funding but also a chance to present our work plan to a group of investigators who offered many valuable comments. As evidence of the kind of ongoing intellectual support they provided, involvement in a book project edited by Rosemary Stevens, Charles Rosenberg, and Lawton Burns helped to crystallize the central argument of *Searching Eyes.*

If our work was made richer by our colleagues at both Columbia and other universities, it was truly made possible by our exceptional graduate students. Martina Lynch and Elizabeth Robilotti helped us in the opening phases of this project. Erin Simpson and Valeri Keisig generously undertook research trips to Chicago and Atlanta, respectively. Marian Moser Jones is a research wonder. She not only thoroughly plumbed any archive into which we sent her, but she also organized and summarized all of the documents she retrieved. Likewise, Alison Bateman-House and Ava Alkon provided superior research support and needed administrative oversight in pulling the manuscript into final order. To them we extend thanks beyond thanks.

Substantively, we are utterly indebted and forever grateful to the dozens of people who allowed us to interview them, sometimes for hours on end, about the history of surveillance and privacy in their fields. This book quite simply could not have been written without the memories and cooperation of those who have been intimately involved in and committed to establishing or combating the development of public health surveillance in America.

Many of them are cited in the text; countless others provided a kind of deep background that helped us draw the connections between different types of surveillance initiatives. Some will agree with both our specific and broad analyses; others, no doubt, would have had us write a different history. We value the time, energy, and perspective that each one contributed.

We were also reliant on the wonderful staffs of archives around the country. David Rose at the March of Dimes not only keeps records in meticulous order, which he knows inside and out, but can also appropriately quote Lewis Carroll at the drop of a hat. At the Municipal Archives of New York City, we thank Leonora Gidlund. Access to the Alexander D. Langmuir Papers at Johns Hopkins University's Alan Mason Chesney Medical Archives would seemingly have been impossible—ironically, on the grounds of privacy—had it not been for Andrew Harrison and Gerard Shorb, who helped us navigate that institution's access requirements. As always, staff at the National Archives and Records Administration was superb, both in Atlanta and College Park. Likewise, librarians at the New Jersey State Library gave their considerate attention. Laura L. Carroll at the American Medical Association Archives in Chicago and Stephen Greenberg at the National Library of Medicine were unfailingly helpful. Finally, we would like to thank the staff at Columbia's own Special Collections in Butler Library and in the interlibrary loan offices on both the Morningside and Washington Heights campuses.

As we were drawing our research and writing to a close, Dan Fox at the Milbank Memorial Fund brought the book into the foundation's series with the University of California Press. We appreciate both his encouragement and financial support, which allowed us to hire a research assistant in the final leg of our journey. Dan introduced us not only to Lynne Withey's editorial acumen but also to an exacting book review process that involved a remarkable two-day discussion with reviewers from academia, public health, and the world of politics. Gus Birkhead, Janlori Goldman, Kay Johnson, Gerald Markowitz, Gene Matthews, Nelson Sabatini, and Stephen Thacker gave the manuscript a thorough reading. They identified important errors of fact and, more critically, gave us insight into how professionals understood the central argument we were making. This provided us with an unprecedented opportunity to clarify and refine our central themes. Once the book was at the press, Hannah Love and Marilyn Schwartz oversaw the final polishing with goodwill and patience. We thank them, too, for selecting Jimmée Greco as our meticulous copyeditor.

Although not always pleased by the time involved in the making of this book, Amy's own little privacy snatchers, Max and Georgia, showed remarkable enthusiasm in the publication process for two so young. Amy also thanks her husband, Jerry Carrino, and her parents and in-laws for trying their best to keep up with them in order to give her a modicum of extra time. Ron thanks Emily Yeong-Ae Kim Stapleford and Ella Maeve Stapleford Barth. In time they will know why. James thanks Robert Sember for his unwavering support and love.

Finally, we thank Allan Rosenfield, the dean of the Mailman School of Public Health, to whom we dedicate this book, and Richard Parker, chair of the Department of Sociomedical Sciences. Allan made the Mailman School a place where it was possible for faculty to pursue books as well as grants. Richard made Allan's vision flourish.

Introduction

Surveillance and the Landscape of Privacy in Twentieth-Century America

The discovery that cases of paralytic polio in 1955 were caused by a singl
manufacturer of Salk vaccine, the linkage of toxic shock syndrome to tam
pons in 1979, the identification of the sentinel cases of AIDS on the Ea
and West Coasts in the early 1980s, the recognition of West Nile virus, SAR!
and avian flu at the turn of the twenty-first century—all were the result (
surveillance systems, through which alert and troubled physicians cou!
communicate with public health officials. In each instance, it was such vij
lance that permitted the recognition of new threats and the initiation
measures that could limit the human toll.

Surveillance serves as the eyes of public health. It has provided the fou
dation for planning, intervention, and disease prevention and has been c
ical for epidemiological research into patterns of morbidity and mortality
a wide variety of diseases and conditions. Registries have been essential
tracking individuals and their conditions over time. Surveillance has a
served to trigger the imposition of public health control measures, such
contact tracing, mandatory treatment, and quarantine. The threat of s
intervention and long-term monitoring has provoked alarm and rende
surveillance suspect for those concerned about the unwarranted exercis
state authority in the name of public health. Thus the history of surveilla
has been bounded by a promise of disease control and a specter of intrus

THE PROMISE OF DISEASE SURVEILLANCE

The idea of disease reporting in America is an old one, dating back t(
colonial era. Rhode Island, for example, required tavern keepers to re
infectious diseases to local officials as early as 1741. Early surveil!
statutes typically conceived of disease reporting as a sporadic, public re

sibility in two broad respects. First, reporting was not the exclusive domain of the physician: lodging house proprietors, owners or operators of ships, and family members were obliged to report. The conditions of concern were acute infectious diseases: cholera, yellow fever, smallpox. Second, reporting was public in the sense that there existed no permanent public health bodies in the United States prior to the mid-nineteenth century, so reports were made to local officials, often mayors.[1] As late as 1884, the Massachusetts legislature required both family members and physicians to report "small-pox, diphtheria, scarlet fever or any other disease dangerous to the public health" either to local politicians or, if one existed in a community, the local board of health.[2] The intent was to warn about possible epidemics and establish temporary health boards to undertake epidemic control measures.[3]

The context of early disease surveillance was a preindustrial one in which life was not segmented along the lines of home and work.[4] Conducting business (which often included housing boarders) in homes with relatively few rooms put family life in the public sphere.[5] In the case of artisans, tavern owners, innkeepers, and shopkeepers, often the business was also the home.[6] While the idea that a man's home is his castle is an ancient one, the presence of servants and lodgers within the home—particularly during colonial era America, when living in isolation was suspect—further shaped expectations about privacy.[7] But above all a "communal spirit" created a kind of intimacy of daily life. Although it would shift over time, particularly with the decline of Puritan values, colonial and preindustrial life in America was characterized by interdependence.[8] People knew one other, were aware of one another's personal lives, and engaged in a kind of "brotherly surveillance."[9] The expectations for tracking disease were embedded in a culture where people broadly monitored and controlled entry into and behavior within the community.[10]

The lack of stable public health structures for monitoring disease reflected not only the expectation that communities themselves could perform such functions, but also the belief that infectious disease represented an episodic threat. Thus New York State law in 1858 specified that physicians only need report disease "at such times, and in such forms as said Board may prescribe." Regular reporting was required only of lodging house owners and the "master, owners, or consignee of a vessel lying at wharf"—it was such individuals who transported and housed immigrants and so were thought to be the first contact with "foreign" sources of infection.[11]

As disease notification began to emerge as a tool for epidemic control, it was bolstered by the more well-established reporting of vital statistics, the registration of births, marriages, and deaths. But while vital statistics were treated as a reform tool capable of exposing the damage that urbanization wrought on health,[12] disease notification was a tool for direct intervention

with individuals.[13] The first attempt at an ongoing survey of infectious diseases in a defined area was initiated in Massachusetts, where in 1874 Henry Bowditch and other members of the state board of health asked a select group of physicians to undertake weekly reporting of infectious diseases in their area. To those physicians he invited to participate, Bowditch described the plan as "the first practical attempt in any part of the world to make a systematic weekly registration of diseases."[14]

In the latter half of the nineteenth century, Louis Pasteur, Robert Koch, and others laid the foundations for understanding that some diseases were caused by germs, microbes too small to see with the human eye but capable of spreading from person to person. The new conception of disease as germ-borne and hence controllable by health departments brought professionalism to disease control. While many states would continue to limit reporting to the traditional epidemic diseases through the first two decades of the twentieth century and would maintain reporting as a broad public responsibility, the rising prominence of bacteriology signaled the importance of laboratory diagnosis and consequently the decline, though not elimination, of a lay role in reporting.[15] The rise of bacteriology coincided with accelerating industrialization in America and the subsequent emergence of the home as a distinctly private sphere as work became centered in factories and women increasingly withdrew from paid employment.[16]

Bacteriology also heightened a sense of authority over disease on the part of a new cadre of public health practitioners. Prior to the twentieth century, public health in the United States was largely the domain of the sanitarians, social reformers, and occasionally physicians devoted to eliminating the filth and squalor believed to cause disease through miasmas. Although reformers and sanitarians maintained a presence in the public health movement after the bacteriological revolution, the field was increasingly dominated by a new set of professionals, many educated in northeastern medical schools and further trained in European laboratories.[17]

An emerging group of public health professionals embraced bacteriology because of the control over disease it promised and the status and authority it consequently conveyed. By the same token, bacteriology became one of the foundations for medical advances in a society that held enormous faith in the promise of science to resolve social problems.[18] By the 1880s and 1890s, medical schools began to incorporate bacteriology and basic science into their curricula as a means of transforming medical education and increasing the status of the medical profession, whose ranks in the mid-nineteenth century included hydropathic, homeopathic, and eclectic physicians.[19] Adopting the accouterments of scientific medicine paved a road to status and reputation for physicians in an intensely competitive environment.[20]

Disease detection and control thus shifted to professionals who commanded new diagnostic technologies.[21] Indicative of the shift that was occurring, the 1902 Health Officers' Manual for New York State made no mention of the duties of any but physicians to report and specified that he who failed to report "is guilty of criminal neglect and should be punished with the extreme penalty."[22] "A Model State Law for Morbidity Reports," endorsed by the State and Territorial Health Authorities in conjunction with the U.S. Public Health Service (PHS), recommended reporting only by physicians and schoolteachers.[23] In 1914 a volume on public health administration observed that because "the great mass of the people can not" detect disease, the duty to report "is generally imposed upon physicians."[24] While requirements for lay reporting lingered—primarily "to guard against any possibility of omission"—health officials increasingly embraced the position that "it is idle to require, indeed it would be dangerous to accept, this service from those who can not see or do not know. The burden is made to rest upon every member of the only class which is in a condition to contribute anything to the accomplishment of the purpose" of reporting: the physician.[25]

In a few locales like New York City, the establishment of a permanent public health infrastructure preceded the bacteriological revolution. In most, however, bacteriology provided the rationale for the creation of permanent health departments. Bacteriology gave force to public health strategies such as isolation, contact tracing, and house-to-house inspection as measures to control disease in the population on a day-to-day basis. Surveillance was the foundation on which the new public health was built, not only in the United States but also in Europe.[26]

Notification of infectious diseases by name in Europe followed a period of public protest over compulsory or coercive health policies. In Great Britain, from the mid-nineteenth century through the beginning of the twentieth, the antivivisection and antivaccination movements challenged the authority of scientific medicine and asserted the rights of the individual against the public health policies of the state.[27] Of particular note were the protests that surrounded the British Contagious Diseases Acts of the 1860s, which allowed the compulsory testing of suspected or known prostitutes for venereal disease. The acts granted officials broad authority to confine and forcibly treat women for up to nine months. In the wake of an emerging women's suffrage movement, a cross-class alliance of middle-class women, working-class men, and, to some extent, prostitutes persistently campaigned until the 1886 repeal of the acts.[28] While protest movements would largely curb the authority of public health practitioners on the Continent, these social movements were never as powerful or widespread in the United States.

To be sure, there were antivaccination and antivivisection movements in this country.[29] There were also public protests over coercive public health interventions. Cities such as Milwaukee endured riots over vaccination in 1894, and the New York City health department encountered resistance on the part of tenement dwellers to mandatory quarantine during the polio epidemic of 1916.[30] In the instance of disease surveillance, however, neither patients nor the public were at the forefront of efforts to resist the authority of public health. What conflict there was involved encounters, in the last decade of the nineteenth century and first two decades of the twentieth, between public health authorities and physicians regarding reporting, particularly for tuberculosis and venereal disease.

Surveillance was crucial in the encounter with threatening pathogens. Over the course of the twentieth century, public health officials reiterated the importance of surveillance, arguing that without the name and location of diseased individuals they worked "in the darkness of ignorance" and might "as well hunt birds by shooting into every green bush."[31] It was the prospect of what surveillance might offer that raised hopes—for the delivery of services, for lifesaving knowledge, and for protection of individuals and communities. Hermann Biggs, a titanic figure in the history of public health and perhaps the most important late-nineteenth- and early-twentieth-century architect and philosopher of public health surveillance, made it clear that names of the diseased were never collected "in order to keep clerks or adding machines busy."[32] Toward the end of the twentieth century, Surgeon General David Satcher would state the value of surveillance as plainly as had Biggs: "In public health, we can't do anything without surveillance . . . that's where public health begins."[33] When surveillance opened the doors to vital services and knowledge, as we shall see in part 2 of this book, its subjects could well become among its most ardent advocates, thus underscoring a politics that went beyond the politics of privacy.

THE SPECTER OF DISEASE SURVEILLANCE

The constitutional basis for the control of disease through the control of persons and personal property had its foundations in the 1850s, when Lemuel Shattuck described a public realm in a landmark Sanitary Commission report to the Massachusetts state legislature. It was during this era that Chief Justice John Marshall coined the term "police power" in reference to the state's authority to regulate for the benefit of the public health and safety.[34] Indeed, in the 1851 case of *Commonwealth v. Alger,* the Supreme Court not only affirmed the police powers of the state but broadened those powers: what one observer called the "commonwealth ideal" was expanded "from a case-by-case investigation of whether each citizen had harmed the interest of another, to a broad instrument for the control of property potentially injurious to the interests of the community."[35]

Officials drew explicitly and frequently on this commonwealth doctrine in justifying new levels of intrusion into the private sphere.[36] The dictum *Salus populi est suprema lex*—the health of the people is the supreme law—

captured the worldview of the most forceful proponents of the new public health.[37] In a late-nineteenth-century treatise on the law of public health, the force of this view was unambiguous: "Persons may be seized and restrained of their liberty or ordered to leave the State; private houses may be converted into hospitals and made subject to hospital regulations; buildings may be broken open and infected articles seized and destroyed, and many other things done, which, under ordinary circumstances, would be considered a gross outrage upon the rights of persons and property."[38] One legal commentator stressed the "humanitarian impulses" of the state and that its "power to confine by force to medical treatment those who are afflicted with a contagious or infectious disease, rests upon the danger to the public."[39]

The progressive era, the decades from roughly the 1890s through the First World War, were characterized both by profound anxiety regarding changes in the social and economic fabric of rapidly industrializing America as well as heady confidence in science as a tool for social and democratic reform. It was in this context that Hermann Biggs made the case for surveillance,[40] giving full expression to the moral foundations of public health: "The government of the United States is democratic, but the sanitary measures adopted are sometimes autocratic, and the functions performed by sanitary authorities paternal in character. We are prepared, when necessary, to introduce and enforce, and the people are ready to accept, measures which might seem radical and arbitrary, if they were not plainly designed for the public good, and evidently beneficent in their effects."[41] Assistant Surgeon General John Trask stated the case in a somewhat less muscular fashion: "The health officer is the servant of the community. He is the one employed by the people to look after their health interests, taken in the aggregate. It is no more rational to employ a health officer and then not give him every facility and assistance for accomplishing the things for which he has been employed than it would be to hire a gardener and then not supply him with tools."[42]

It was not always "plain," however, that invasions of privacy were "beneficent in their effects," particularly in the case of highly stigmatized diseases. The extension of surveillance, with its duties falling squarely on physicians, would neither be smooth nor direct, as will become clear in our discussion of the early conflicts over notification of tuberculosis and venereal diseases in chapters 2 and 3. In part, these battles revolved around the contested terrain created by scientific advance: "The bacteriological laboratory," argued one medical editorialist, "is invading the former domain of the clinical practitioners."[43] But the battles between clinicians and health officials were not simply turf wars. As important as claims to authority were, it was the issue of the privacy of the clinical relationship that typically provided the justification for physicians' resistance to reporting the names of their patients.[44]

Tuberculosis and venereal disease were not, after all, just two more contagious diseases, but conditions to which tremendous moral opprobrium was attached. The consequences of disclosure could be devastating: loss of social standing, housing, employment, and death benefits. Although rarely imposed, quarantine threatened the liberty of those with both VD and TB. How the tensions over surveillance would play out over the twentieth century and the forms such tensions would take reflected transformations in the conceptions and roles of medical confidentiality and of privacy itself.[45]

PATERNALISTIC PRIVACY

The invocation of privacy in contemporary public debates suggests a timeless individual right, almost always under siege, requiring vigilance to prevent the imposition of tyranny (fig. 1). But it was only in the nineteenth century that privacy began to take on dimensions of a right inherent to persons.[46] It was in 1890, for example, that there was public protest against census questions related to infectious diseases.[47] In the context of public health, privacy would take a shape that we might hardly regard as privacy today. The idea of privacy in the late nineteenth and early twentieth centuries had little to do with prohibitions against sharing information, much to do with the sanctity of the home, and everything to do with clinical authority.

With the ascendancy of the new scientific medicine,[48] the relationship between doctor and patient became characterized by deference to clinical authority.[49] To the extent that privacy concerns were acknowledged, they were embedded in a medical and public health culture that was both highly paternalistic and authoritarian. The prevailing conception of privacy yoked the patient's well-being to the physician's authority: physicians represented the gatekeepers to patients and protected them from the intrusions of others. As public health surveillance took shape in the late nineteenth century, the first battles over tuberculosis and then venereal disease surveillance would throw this conception of paternalistic privacy into bold relief and shape the nature of surveillance for nearly half a century.

The effort to craft a surveillance system for tuberculosis took place in the years after the legal scholars Samuel Warren and Louis Brandeis famously framed privacy as the "right to be let alone." Warren and Brandeis were centrally concerned with the way in which "instantaneous photographs and newspaper enterprise have invaded the sacred precincts of private and domestic life." Such invasions of privacy involved a clash in a realm governed by tort and the common law. But in a seminal 1890 article, Warren and Brandeis also provided the foundations for thinking of privacy as a kind of "sanctuary," a protection from "seeing, hearing, and knowing" grounded in Fourth Amendment protections against unreasonable searches and seizures.[50] In so doing, they built on the thinking of Thomas Cooley, a con-

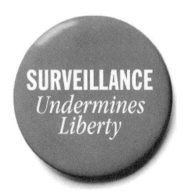

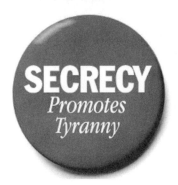

Figure 1. Buttons from *The Nation,* 2005. Buttons designed by Milton Glaser for www.nationmart.com. ©2001. Reproduced with permission from *The Nation.*

stitutional lawyer who, earlier in the nineteenth century, invoked the Fourth Amendment to argue that "a man's house is his castle," that he should be protected "in his home against the prying eyes of the government."[51]

However important the concept of privacy, the "medical secret" was not absolute. For Warren and Brandeis, the "difficult task" was to determine the "line at which the dignity and convenience of the individual must yield to the demands of the public welfare."[52] In the latter part of the nineteenth century, as public health surveillance took form, drawing that line would indeed be difficult and would provide the context for intense, sometimes acrimonious conflicts between doctors in private practice and public health officials. In those encounters, privacy emerged as not so much a right of the patient, but rather as a feature of the clinical relationship. It was the doctor who controlled the terms of privacy in an instrumental way, that is, in a fashion that contributed to good medicine (and that protected medical authority).[53] And good medical practice could sometime require disclosure of personal information.

The American Medical Association (AMA) code of ethics had long acknowledged that "peculiar circumstances" always tempered protection of "secrecy and delicacy."[54] In making decisions about divulging medical secrets, as in making decisions more generally about the patient's welfare, it was the physician's "own judgment" that was of paramount importance.[55] Such revelations could be guided by a doctor's obligations to the patient's family and household. The responsible physician felt ethically bound, for example, to report a case of syphilis in a prospective groom to the bride's father or a case in a domestic servant to the master of the household.[56] The patient, like a child, was in the "caring custody" of the physician, who, like the patriarch, made decisions in the best interests of all.[57] An AMA pamphlet on medical ethics, sized to be carried in a shirt or jacket pocket, gave voice to that view: "A physician should act as he would desire another to act toward one of his own family under like circumstances."[58] In the early twentieth century, the AMA ethical code broadened to acknowledge the physician's duty to the community in general. In 1903 the AMA code of ethics yielded to the law, explicitly allowing exceptions to strict confidentiality when "imperatively required by the laws of the state."[59] The 1912 version of the AMA code of ethics explained, "A physician may not reveal the confidences entrusted to him in the course of medical attendance, or the deficiencies he may observe in the character of patients, unless he is required to do so by law or unless it becomes necessary in order to protect the welfare of the individual or the community."[60]

As health departments extended the scope of compulsory disease surveillance, those medical organizations that endorsed the practice did so in a way that preserved this paternalistic conception of privacy, in which access to the patient was mediated by the physician. Public health officers like Hermann Biggs accordingly accommodated physician demands to determine when health officials might intervene with those they served—a concession that typically protected "respectable" middle-class or wealthy private patients, granting them the right to be let alone in the shelter of their homes.[61]

As the recipients of disease reports, public health officials were mindful of both the importance of privacy and the stigma associated with both tuberculosis and venereal diseases. Officials thus stressed the importance of protecting disease registries from unwarranted exposure. They felt bound by the same clinical and ethical norms that governed privacy within the clinical relationship and defined it as something essential to good medical care and public health. The rise of yellow journalism and an explosion of highly personal newspaper coverage with little respect for boundaries, particularly in matters of sex and vice, heightened public health concerns about privacy.[62] In 1913, as if to distinguish them from prying journalists,[63] Biggs explained that health officials were "all medical men and well versed in medical ethics."[64] And like the private physician, the health department was widely counted on to use its "wise discretion . . . to determine what safeguards and regulations should protect the privacy of its records."[65]

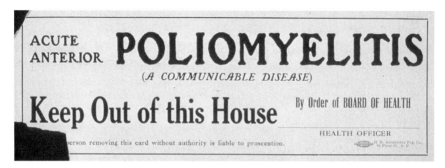

Figure 2. Isolation placard for poliomyelitis. Courtesy of the National Library of Medicine.

But here too there were limits. Just as doctors might disclose information to protect family and community, so too might health departments. When deemed appropriate, health officials broadcast the names and addresses of those with contagious diseases in order to fulfill a duty to warn the public. In the instances of acute infectious diseases like diphtheria and smallpox, officials placarded the homes of the infected (fig. 2). During epidemics, health officials would publish a daily list in local newspapers of the names and addresses of individuals who were infectious.[66] But if the rapidly expanding muckraking press was seen as a threat to individual privacy, the transformation of American journalism was also central to the creation of an informed, democratic community.[67] Thus what might, on first blush, seem like a sensational disclosure was a vital means for communal self-protection.[68]

For instance, during the 1916 New York City polio epidemic, surveillance became a public affair. The city's health commissioner published a daily tally of new cases and deaths by name and street address in local newspapers (fig. 3).[69] These measures elicited no objection from physicians or the private patients they served. Polio bore no moral taint, and the middle classes did not have to fear the threat of quarantine. Children of those who lived in tenements or other types of multifamily dwelling, however, were taken, sometimes by force, to public hospitals. As a consequence, resistance to reporting and the interventions that followed has been documented only among poor, working-class, or immigrant families. In 1916 one mother warned that she and her child would disappear by morning if her doctor reported the case to health authorities. A nurse assigned to inspect tenements received a letter, threatening, "If you report any more of our babies to the Board of Health we will kill you and nobody will know what happened to you. Keep off our streets and don't report our homes and we will do you no harm."[70]

Likewise, in 1928 New York City health officials freely disclosed the name

Names and Addresses of Those Stricken with Paralysis.

The following is a list of the names and addresses of the new cases of infantile paralysis and deaths in the city yesterday:

NEW CASES—BOROUGH OF MANHATTAN.

Morris Katz, 208 E. 7th St.
Bella Cohen, 647 E. 11th St.
Charles Barisch, 502 E. 16th St.
David Shapiro, 241 E. 25th St.
Rose Sciascia, 228 Chrystie St.
Muriel Weiss, 308 Broome St.
Caroline Vilini, 218 Bowery.
Giuseppe LaRocca, 119 Elizabeth St.
Nathan Holneck, 33 Henry St.
Stephen Milianosky, 58 Monroe St.
Jenny Serrelese, 359 W. 53d St.
William Soles, 458 W. 166th St.
Carl Thornihlin, 731 Tenth Av.
Bennie Katz, 57-59 E. 112th St.
Madeline Schuman, 188 Eighth Av.
Nicoletta Volnini, 414 E. 120th St.

DEATHS—BOROUGH OF MANHATTAN.

David Shapiro, 241 E. 25th St.
Carmelo Cirrincini, 346 E. Houston St.
Giuseppe LaRocca, 119 Elizabeth St.
Bennie Katz, 57-59 E. 112th St.
Sam Greenberg, 206, E. 6th St.
Bella Cohen, 647 E. 11th St.

Figure 3. Names of new cases and deaths from poliomyelitis with addresses. *New York Times,* July 22, 1916. New York Times Co.

of a six-year-old Puerto Rican boy with leprosy before transferring him to an isolation facility in Carville, Louisiana. Not only did they name the boy and provide his address, but they also named his guardian, an uncle who served as a ship's cook.[71] By the 1940s, as effective therapies for leprosy became available and the city developed an outpatient treatment program, health officials began withholding the identity of patients from reporters, stating that this was in the best interests of the patient.[72] Likewise, as the city developed a system for monitoring healthy carriers of typhoid, it refused to make public the names of those in the registry. Once in the registry, a case had "to conform to the rules on typhoid carriers, which include[d] regular supervision by the Health Department and the prohibition against taking part in any cooking or food serving on penalty of isolation."[73] In short, it became inappropriate to warn the public about threats from specific individuals as public health developed the means to protect the community through long-term monitoring or treatment of infectious patients.

COMPLIANCE, RESISTANCE, AND THE COURTS

Despite the limits of infectious disease notification and the compromises made to accommodate physicians in private practice, by the 1920s disease reporting had become a core feature of what public health departments believed was essential to their work. Hence there emerged a new emphasis on the importance of reporting for all diseases.[74]

The imposition of the duty to report met with resistance and indifference. Reporting rates for different diseases varied widely.[75] For example, a 1921 report found that while only 20 percent of diphtheria cases in the United States went unreported, 84 percent of puerperal septicemia went unreported. For venereal diseases, which were so morally laden, reporting varied considerably by state.[76] The sustained effort of public health officers to persuade physicians of their duties spoke to the ongoing problem of physician resistance, if not active opposition, to reporting. In 1920 Dr. J. L. Bowman, a Public Health Service (PHS) epidemiologist stationed in Alabama, lamented that "physicians and surgeons in general have failed to study the subject sufficiently to understand why this extra burden of reporting should be placed on them and why they owe such reports to the public and to the profession." Bowman recognized that a rigid enforcement of the law would only create antagonism between doctors and public health practitioners. He sought, therefore, to show "that these reports [were] necessary for the welfare of the public and the advancement of science" and believed this would encourage "the great majority of the medical profession [to] report without an application of the law."[77]

While Bowman offered a carrot, others demanded a stick. For example, Dr. William Edler, a PHS officer and director of the Bureau of Venereal Diseases in Louisiana, derided the notion of polite persuasion and put forth the argument for a draconian approach: "State and city boards of health need a law enforcement division for physicians, rather than an educational department. The physician *knows;* he simply does not consider the reporting of communicable diseases a part of his professional duties; and until such time when he is punished for law violations the same as any other individual, until such time as he is impressed with license revocations varying in time with the degree of his offense, not until then will reporting of disease reach any degree of accuracy. One or two prosecutions of this kind in a community, with ample publicity, will produce more communicable disease reports in a week than will years of propaganda."[78] The reality was that, nationwide, between 1887 and 1932, very few physicians were ever prosecuted for failure to comply with notification requirements.

When state courts did confront such cases, there was a broad legal consensus that physicians could be required to report. Neither claims of privacy nor the burden of such efforts could justify refusals to follow the dictates of state law or regulation. In 1913, for example, a Vermont physician was convicted of neglecting to report a case of diphtheria. In *State v. Pierce* the court ruled that it was inconceivable that he could not have known his patient had diphtheria, as claimed. The village was in the throes of a diphtheria epidemic, and there were numerous placards in the vicinity warning of the threat. The court accepted evidence that he had correctly diagnosed the disease in the past and found him guilty of failure to alert the public health authorities.[79]

Whereas Pierce pleaded ignorance, refusals to report more typically turned on the time and effort required for reporting, a burden that physicians viewed as a demand for unpaid labor and hence a deprivation of liberty and property. In 1888, early in the history of reporting, the Connecticut Supreme Court rejected such claims. In *State v. Wordin* the court embraced an expansive view of the right of the state to protect its citizens from fatal and contagious diseases: "Of absolute necessity this power inheres in every organized community; otherwise there would be only organized suicide." Given such overriding necessity, the protection of the community "takes unwritten precedence over all provisions for the protection of rights of property and includes the right to require as much of the services or property of each as may be necessary to the preservation of the lives of all, without provision for payment therefor."[80] But there were limits to what could be expected. In 1911 Ohio overturned a state requirement for the reporting of births and deaths because the statute imposed upon medical professionals the duty to answer questions that "would not necessarily or naturally come with the knowledge of the attending physician or midwife." Such efforts, the Ohio Supreme Court declared in *State v. Boone*, violated the constitutional protection against "draft[ing] a citizen into particular service without substantial compensation."[81] (As one editorial in the *Journal of the American Medical Association* snidely queried, "Does anyone ever see a lawyer doing any of this charity work for the good of the general public? . . . It is time the doctor took a little more business-like view of his calling.")[82] In the only other recorded case in which a physician won a victory against the imperative to report, the court determined that, in fact, the patient had not been in the clinician's charge.[83] The overarching trajectory of rulings upheld reporting mandates.

Laypersons also won civil suits involving physician failure to report. In *Jones v. Stanko* an Ohio appeals court ruled, in 1928, in favor of the widow of Stephen Stanko. Mrs. Stanko claimed that the physician was liable for the death of her husband from smallpox. The physician had been attending a sick neighbor and, in response to Stephen Stanko's query, told him that the neighbor did not have a communicable disease. On the basis of this assurance, Stanko continued to care for the neighbor during his illness and then helped with the funeral and burial. The Ohio Supreme Court ruled that because the physician also failed to report the case to the health department, preventing authorities from issuing proper warnings, he could be held liable for Stanko's subsequent death from smallpox.[84]

When the courts were presented with cases that touched on the privileged nature of communications between doctors and their patients, they also uniformly upheld mandatory reporting. In a case involving tuberculosis, the Supreme Court of Michigan held in 1902 that a patient's concerns about privacy did not override the state's interest in controlling threats to the public health. Patients with infectious diseases might object to reporting, but "it would hardly be contended that the physician could excuse his noncompliance with the requirements of [reporting] statutes by showing a dissent in the particular case or generally."[85]

While patient objections were invoked in the Michigan case, it is important to underscore that all of the legal encounters over surveillance pitted physicians against health officials. More striking than the legal consensus regarding the legitimacy of surveillance was that never did a citizen challenge disease reporting. It would be more than seven decades before the Supreme Court would finally address the issues of privacy posed by mandatory reporting, upholding the authority of the state to require physician disclosure to public health registries. When the court did so, it was in a case brought by the subjects of surveillance.

By the 1920s both the political and legal challenges to reporting had largely ceased. Debate centered upon making the process easier, more efficient, and less demanding. Dr. Hibbert Hill, author of the 1916 book *The New Public Health*, for example, insisted, "The health department should not ask a physician to answer a thousand fool questions on the report about the epidemiology of the case. . . . All you want from the physicians is the patient's name and address so that you can go to the house."[86] In 1921 Indiana determined that the information required in physician reports (which included color, nativity or race, sex, age, marital condition, occupation, stage of disease, source of infection, when contracted, date of infection, and diagnosis) was too extensive and thus not systematically reported, making "much of the data . . . of doubtful value" or even "worthless." The forms used for collecting the required data, the state argued, tried to turn the physician into an "epidemiologist and social enumerator" without giving him the requisite special training. Health officials called, therefore, for strictly limiting physician reporting to name, age, color, source of infection, and diagnosis.[87] Such simplification was all the more important as the number of diseases declared notifiable expanded.

The extension of public health surveillance took place against a backdrop of wartime and postwar repression. World War I inspired new attacks (and reinvigorated old ones) on civil liberties: censorship of the press, self-censorship in the movie industry, prohibition, raids against those deemed to be politically subversive, immigration restriction, book bans, and limits on distributing supposedly obscene materials through the mails. These kinds of intrusions in private life stood in marked contrast to state deference to business: "Liberty of contract has been made the be-all and end-all of personal freedom; . . . the domain of business has been defended against control from without in the name of freedom," declared the economist Walton H. Hamilton.[88] This disjunction, argues one historian, "opened the door to a new appreciation of civil liberties—rights an individual may assert even against democratic majorities—as essential elements of American freedom. Building on prewar struggles for freedom of expression by labor unions, socialists, and birth-control advocates, some reformers now developed a greater appreciation of the necessity of vibrant, unrestricted political debate."[89] Thus in 1917 the Civil Liberties Bureau was born, which by 1920 would become the American Civil Liberties Union.[90]

It was also a period in which the right to privacy was being put forth as a constitutional norm governing the relationship between individuals and the state.[91] As a Supreme Court justice, Louis Brandeis would elaborate on the Fourth Amendment foundations to the right to privacy in his 1928 dissent in *Olmstead v. United States,* a case involving telephone wiretapping. The Constitution, Brandeis argued in that case, had to take cognizance of the ever-expanding ability to invade the private realm: "Subtler and more far-reaching means of invading privacy have become available to the government. Discovery and invention have made it possible for the Government, by means far more effective than stretching upon the rack, to obtain disclosure in court of what is whispered in the closet."[92] He proclaimed the "right to be let alone . . . the most comprehensive of rights and the right most valued by civilized men."[93] Brandeis's dissent in *Olmstead* was part of an emerging challenge to infringements on civil liberties as the Supreme Court began to hear a number of cases centering on the question of free speech. By the late 1920s the tide began to slowly turn toward recognition of the rights of the individual.[94] It would, however, be more than three decades before the Supreme Court gave the right to privacy a constitutional imprimatur.

COLD WAR PRIVACY

With the onset of the cold war and the domestic crusade against subversion, concerns about privacy and the threat of the "surveillance state" took on new vitality. In 1947 the House Un-American Activities Committee launched its intensive investigatory efforts to find communists within government and private industry. As the demand to name names provoked anxiety and fear-inspired protest, so too did intrusions on the sanctuary of the private home, which was increasingly viewed as standing at the center of American democracy.[95] These encounters would ultimately have a profound impact on the emergence of a broadened conception of privacy that would shape responses to a wide array of invasive government measures.[96]

It was at this juncture that long-established and unchallenged public health measures, though not specifically disease surveillance, would become the subject of judicial concern. In 1959 the Supreme Court upheld the right of the health department to arrest and fine a homeowner who refused a search for rat infestation because the health inspector had no warrant. Writing for the majority of the court in *Frank v. Maryland,* Justice Felix Frankfurter recognized the right of privacy, particularly against "arbitrary" search and seizures, as being "fundamental to a free society." But he was impressed by the "safeguards designed to make the least possible demand on the individual occupant," which caused "only the slightest restriction in his claims on privacy," and concluded that the "particular context and. . . . social need" legitimated the public health law.[97]

In his dissent, William O. Douglas, joined by Chief Justice Earl Warren and Justices Hugo Black and William Brennan—the core of what would become the famously liberal Warren Court—remarked that "health inspections are important," but "many today would think that the search for subversives was even more important than the search for unsanitary conditions. It would seem that the public interest in protecting privacy is equally as great in one case as in another." Even when inspection presented "only the slightest restriction in [the individual's] claims on privacy," Douglas rejected the "official's measure of his own need" as not "squar[ing] with the Bill of Rights" in "an era 'when politically controlled officials have grown powerful through an ever increasing series of minor infractions of civil liberties.'"[98] Forcing the state to obtain a court order, moreover, was not going to bring the public health system to its knees. Most people, Douglas argued, would continue to respond to requests on the part of health officials when they wished to inspect a residence. Citing William Whyte's widely read description of the increasingly homogenous nature of American society in *The Organization Man,* the dissent concluded, "One rebel a year is not too great a price to pay for maintaining our guarantee of civil rights in full vigor."[99] Indicative of the way in which concerns about privacy in one domain would be brought to bear on others was that Douglas drew upon a case involving the House Un-American Activities Committee in which particular attention was given to government interventions that would subject individuals to "public stigma, scorn and obloquy."[100]

While Douglas lost the day in *Frank,* he had begun to articulate a critique of official rationalizations for the erosion of privacy.[101] By grounding his arguments in the Fourth Amendment, he sought to deny the state an "open sesame" that would diminish protections against unreasonable searches and seizures "to the vanishing point."[102] Douglas thus emerged as heir to

Brandeis, who had made his trenchant claims for privacy thirty years earlier in the *Olmstead* dissent. But while the foundations were being laid for a jurisprudence of privacy that would attempt to secure the individual within the home, disease surveillance—especially the reporting of names to public health departments—remained unchallenged legally. Public health reporting requirements were insulated from judicial and political scrutiny by the still-central belief that the threat of infectious disease necessitated notification and that physicians would protect their patients against what they viewed as unjustifiable intrusions.

Indeed, cold war concerns about biological warfare provided the impetus to expand disease surveillance efforts at the federal level. Alexander Langmuir, a preeminent figure in American epidemiology and public health, described the atmosphere of acute "emotional tension about BW [biowarfare]" that arose when, only six months into the Korean War, Chinese propaganda about the American reliance on biological weapons—along with the implication that retaliation in kind would be appropriate—began to circulate.[103] Langmuir drew on these anxieties to justify the creation of the Epidemic Intelligence Service (EIS) at the Communicable Disease Center (later the Centers for Disease Control and Prevention).[104] For Langumuir, "Epidemiology means getting out to the scene to see what's happening. We ring doorbells. We pound the pavements. We go to the patients instead of waiting for the patients to come to us."[105] The EIS did not lead to the creation of centralized CDC databanks, but it did lead to greater interaction of federal officials with individuals with infectious disease in the states. It also represented a moment in which the CDC would begin to play a greater coordinating and funding role in state public health surveillance.

PRIVACY GOES PUBLIC

The sharp reaction against the legacy of Joseph McCarthy and the ascendancy of the liberal majority on the Warren court in the 1960s assured that concerns about the erosion of privacy would be given greater attention. Emblematic of the shift that was occurring was the 1967 Supreme Court decision in *Camara v. the City and County of San Francisco,* which overturned its own eight-year-old holding in *Frank v. Maryland.* "When the right of privacy must reasonably yield to the right of search," wrote the court, "is, as a rule, to be decided by a judicial officer, not by a policeman or government enforcement agency."[106]

Fueling concerns about privacy were technological developments that were laying the groundwork for the transformation of the social organization and control of the most intimate information about individuals. The allure of computerization and the promise of efficiencies that could be achieved through the centralization of vast networks of data were most dra-

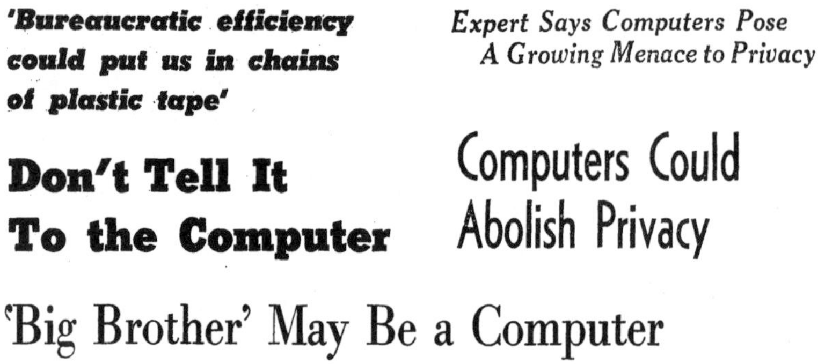

'Bureaucratic efficiency could put us in chains of plastic tape'

Expert Says Computers Pose A Growing Menace to Privacy

Don't Tell It To the Computer

Computers Could Abolish Privacy

'Big Brother' May Be a Computer

Figure 4. Press coverage of the proposed National Data Center and concerns about privacy in *New York Times* headlines, January 8 and September 18, 1967 (©1967, New York Times Co.), and the *Los Angeles Times*, October 8, 1967, and December 13, 1965 (©1967 and 1965, Los Angeles Times).

matically illustrated by a 1966 proposal to create a National Data Center, which would have brought together vast amounts of federal information regarding population, housing, wages, jobs, education, health, and taxes into a single database. The national outcry it provoked was of sufficient magnitude to scuttle that project, though other aggregation efforts would continue.[107] In response to mounting concerns about such data collection, Justice Douglas, who had emerged as privacy's tribune, would declare, "We are rapidly entering the age of no privacy, where everyone is open to surveillance at all times; where there are no secrets from government." More ominously, citizen dossiers were now "being put on computers so that by pressing one button all the miserable, the sick, the suspect, the unpopular, the offbeat people of the nation can be instantly identified."[108] Thus computers came to symbolize the Frankenstein of the emerging technological era (figs. 4 and 5).

In his 1964 sociological classic, *The Naked Society,* Vance Packard asserted that computers—"giant memory machines"—were ominous not only because they represented centralization of government data relating to all aspect of an individual's life, but also because they were "producing pressures that intrude upon most of us where we live, work, shop, go to school, or seek solitude."[109] These anxieties were echoed in Myron Breton's widely read exposé of the apparatus of surveillance. "Big Brother in his civilian clothes" was the focus of Breton's attack. "Our private lives," he wrote in *The Privacy Invaders,* "are becoming other people's commercial property—in the marketplace, on the job, and around the community," making "intrusion a way of everyday life."[110] It was, then, not only government intrusions that

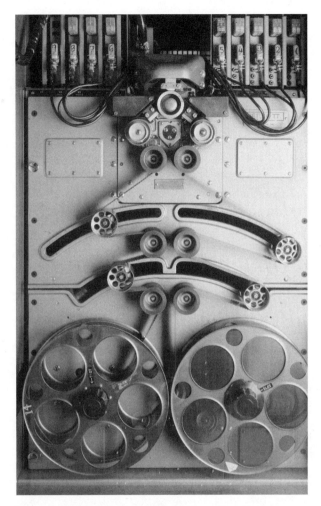

Figure 5. Elliott 803 computer with magnetic tape.
Courtesy of the National Museum of Photography, Film,
and Television/Science and Society Picture Library.

were of concern, but also the "widespread use of polygraph and personality tests, as well as over-the-counter sales of electronic eavesdropping devices."[111] In the era of the electronic database, the very existence of centralized lists—both governmental and commercial—and not simply potential government action based on those lists created profound cultural anxiety.[112]

It was the potential threat of such abuse that, beginning in 1965, fueled congressional debates about what personal information to protect and how best to protect it.[113] The 92nd and 93rd Congresses witnessed the introduction of nearly three hundred bills focused on access to and dissemination of personal data.[114] Reflecting the principle set out in *Camara,* that proper consent was required for inspection of the home under public health law, policy and lawmakers flirted with the notion of obtaining consent from individuals when it came to obtaining or using personally identifiable records.[115] They were responding to the growing sense that "mile after mile, acre after acre, in metal cabinets and on computer tapes, the confidential files of Uncle Sam grow steadily and, some say, ominously"[116] (fig. 6). Indeed, a 1966 Senate judiciary subcommittee survey found that the federal government had amassed, without meaningful confidentiality safeguards, "more than 3 billion records on citizens, nearly half of which were retrievable by computer, including 27.2 billion names, 2.3 billion present and past addresses, 264 million criminal histories, 280 million mental health records, 916 million profiles on alcohol and drug addiction, and over 1.2 billion financial records."[117] "If knowledge is power," exclaimed Maryland Republican senator Charles Mathias, "this encyclopedic knowledge gives Government the raw materials of tyranny."[118]

While many saw the new capacity for and utilization of surveillance as a grave threat requiring radical responses, others sought to reframe the question. By the late 1960s, as politicians and a range of federal agencies had become engaged in a discussion of what to do, Alan Westin, a Columbia University professor who was at the forefront of debates about privacy, argued that "surveillance is obviously a fundamental means of social control" in his probing analysis *Privacy and Freedom.* Without surveillance, he continued, "society could not enforce its norms or protect its citizens, and an era of ever increasing speed of communication, mobility of persons, and coordination of conspiracies requires that the means of protecting society keep pace with the technology of crime."[119] The challenge, in his view, was to determine the limits of surveillance.

Whatever the effort to determine such limits across a range of policy domains, public health disease reporting continued to enjoy a privileged status, shielded from scrutiny by assumptions about its traditions. In the view of both Westin and Packard, professional codes of medical ethics and their strong precedents for protecting intimate health information provided adequate sanctuary from the broader assault on privacy.[120] Even the harshest critiques of modern life and computerization assumed that a well-honed, time-tested system of normative constraints provided sufficient protection for privacy in the medical and public health arenas.[121]

That public health professionals seemed to respond to the growing sensitivity about matters of privacy contributed to the sense that the self-governing norms of doctors and public health officials provided sufficient protection. For example, health departments brought to an end the con-

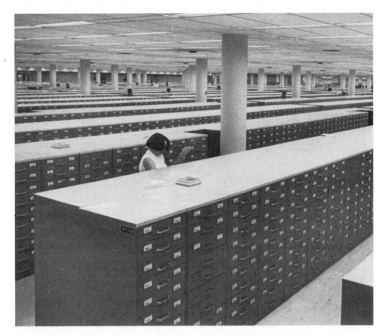

Figure 6. The Social Security Administration filing cabinets. "Somewhere in this maze is the original social security application of everyone who has ever received a card." Vance Packard, "Don't Tell It to the Computer." *New York Times.* January 8, 1967, 44. George Tames/ New York Times Co./Redux Pictures.

vention of routinely providing newspapers the names and addresses of individuals diagnosed with dangerous contagious diseases. Although practices in smaller suburban and rural areas may have varied, a review of the *New York Times, Los Angeles Times, Washington Post,* and *Chicago Tribune* indicates that this practice had ended by 1961. As much as such moves represented a nod to mounting privacy concerns, they were also undoubtedly facilitated by the perception that infectious diseases posed a declining threat to the public's health.

Another factor that shielded public health from mounting concerns about the computer menace was that health departments were decidedly behind the technological curve. Indeed, in 1962 National Institutes of Health and PHS officials called for "fully exploit[ing]" the potential of computers, particularly when it came to registries of chronic diseases, including tuberculosis and cancer. Health officials continued to manage registry data kept on filing cards by hand, with the assistance of clerks or punch card systems. For sizeable registries, matching data, eliminating duplicates, and abstracting and summarizing data was a daunting task. "These problems," federal health officials concluded, "have contributed to the limited research use of registries to date," allowing for little more than tracking the grossest changes in incidence over time.[122]

Closer scrutiny of the extent of data collection and the adequacy of individual privacy protections ultimately posed challenges to the "ancient and predominantly honorable traditions" of medical record keeping. Yet the most significant critiques related to public health in the new information age came from within the field itself. In 1964, for example, Arthur Kraus, chief of the Division of Statistical Research within the Maryland Department of Public Health, called for "more discriminating use of statistical activities." In language that echoed the position of the CDC's Alexander Langmuir, who had stressed the role of surveillance as a call to action, Kraus decried the publication of reams of undigested statistics "without an accompanying analysis of patterns or significant relationships. Agencies have a responsibility to interpret the data they produce."[123]

But increasingly there were concerns about privacy as well. In 1973 the secretary of the Department of Health, Education, and Welfare's (DHEW) Advisory Committee on Automated Personal Data Systems noted that it was "not prepared for the discovery that," even when intended only for reporting or research, "the data are often totally vulnerable to disclosure."[124] While building on the growing imperative to protect the subjects of research that, in the shadow of the DHS's Tuskegee Syphilis Study and other revelations of research abuses, would lead to the National Research Act of 1974, the DHEW committee did not recommend that the subjects who were "asked to provide data for statistical reporting and research" give their consent. Nor did it suggest independent oversight of this process, such as an institutional review board or the judiciary body, as demanded by the Supreme Court in its 1967 decision in *Camara*. Instead, the committee insisted that individuals be aware that collection efforts were taking place. Additionally, it sought to protect those records from disclosure as part of its proposed Code of Fair Information Practices.[125]

As the scandal of Tuskegee had fueled a searching investigation of research practices, the Watergate revelations animated congressional debate about how to address the misuse of personal information.[126] The resultant 1974 Privacy Act was a subdued response to what a 369-page *Michigan Law Review* critique described as the emergence of a "dossier society."[127] The act took an important symbolic step, however, embracing the language of the nearly decade-old Supreme Court decision in *Griswold v. Connecticut*, which overturned a statute that prohibited physicians from prescribing birth control for married couples. The Privacy Act declared, "Congress finds that the right of privacy is a personal and fundamental right protected by the Constitution of the United States."[128] Yet it merely codified the DHEW's 1973 Code of Fair Information Practices, which had stipulated that there must be "no personal data record-keeping systems whose very existence is secret," required transparency in record keeping involving "personally identifiable" data, gave individuals access to their records, and limited secondary disclosures of data.[129] Nevertheless, the act left public health surveillance untouched. Further, the act noted that agencies may take "take any appropriate action otherwise prohibited" if "the public health or public safety may be adversely affected or significantly threatened."[130]

Given the Privacy Act's focus on the appropriate uses of data already in hand, it is remarkable that the study commission that it mandated posed challenges to conventional assumptions that surrounded disease surveillance activities.[131] At last, concerns about privacy pierced the shield that had protected such efforts from challenge. Drawing on growing calls to limit or perhaps prohibit altogether data acquisition in the absence of a compelling state interest, the study commissioners were skeptical about the necessity of reporting names of diseased people.[132] Noting that over half of the states provided no statutory confidentiality protections—indeed, one allowed for the possibility of "public inspection," and another gave "citizens the right to examine public records" of disease—the commission called for new privacy regulations. But the commission went further: such reform "would still not preclude the possibility that subsequent contact by agents of authorities to whom the information is properly reported will startle or embarrass an individual unnecessarily, particularly if the individual is not aware that a report was made." In a radical departure, it recommended that when any kind of reporting occurred "pursuant to a statute. . . . the *individual* [be] notified of each such disclosure" (emphasis added).[133] While the proposals would have no immediate impact on the practice of surveillance, broader political and social changes in American cultural and political life would set the stage for the first constitutional challenge to disease reporting.

THE CONSTITUTIONAL CHALLENGE
TO PUBLIC HEALTH SURVEILLANCE

By the late 1960s, patients' rights, feminist, and consumer activist movements all galvanized challenges to medical paternalism and physician authority.[134] In 1969, for example, the Boston Women's Health Collective proclaimed in its classic work of self-assertion, *Our Bodies, Ourselves,* "We had all experienced similar feelings of frustration and anger toward specific doctors and the medical maze in general, and initially we wanted to do something about those doctors who were condescending, paternalistic, judgmental and non-informative."[135] As they shattered the "myth" that doctor and patient "meet one another as parent and child," the collective championed autonomy: "We want you to be more alert to our responsibility in the relationship, just as you would in any other adult relationship where you are purchasing services. . . . Don't let yourself be stampeded into any sudden decisions or forced to accept any medications or procedures you don't understand or want. It's your body."[136] As one historian observed, "The rules for patients had changed: docile obedience was to give way to wary consumerism."[137] The forces that gave birth to such changes provided the context for and were in turn energized by the new bioethics, which had as its lodestar a commitment to patient self-determination and a rejection of medical paternalism.

Within this climate, the Supreme Court, at last, forcefully articulated a constitutional right to privacy. From *Griswold v. Connecticut* in 1965, the decision about married couples' use of birth control, to *Roe v. Wade* and *Doe v. Bolton* in 1973, which upheld the right of a woman to make decisions about terminating her pregnancy, the Supreme Court charted a new course on privacy. In commenting on the robust notion of privacy that emerged, Lawrence Tribe wrote that such rights "have been located in the 'liberty' protected by the due process clauses of the fifth and fourteenth amendments. They have been cut from the cloth of the ninth amendment—conceived as a rule against cramped construction—or from the privileges and immunities clauses of article IV and of the fourteenth amendment. Encompassing rights to shape one's inner life and rights to control the face one presents to the world, they have materialized from the 'emanations' and 'penumbras'—most recently dubbed simply the 'shadows'—of the first, third, fourth, and fifth amendments. They elaborate the 'blessings of liberty' promised in the Preamble, and have been held implicit in the eighth amendment's prohibition against cruel and unusual punishments. Wherever located, they have inspired among the most moving appeals to be found in the judicial lexicon."[138]

The cultural embrace of an invigorated conception of privacy and the emergence of the patients' rights movement would ultimately set the stage for a constitutional challenge to surveillance by public health departments in the 1977 case of *Whalen v. Roe.* Although it involved the reporting of prescriptions, not illness, it had direct bearing on disease notification. For the first time in the seven decades since surveillance had become a centerpiece of public health activity, individuals who were the subjects of reporting relied upon the claims of privacy to resist the authority of the state to collect names. In a series of cases, the federal courts were compelled to address the constitutional dimensions of surveillance in light of the new jurisprudence of privacy.

In 1972 New York State modified its public health law, requiring the state department of health to keep a computerized record of the names and addresses of anyone prescribed a Schedule II drug. Drugs in this category, under a new classification created by President Richard Nixon's 1969 Comprehensive Drug Abuse Prevention and Control Act,[139] were considered to have a high potential for abuse but also acceptable medical uses. They included opium and its derivatives, methadone, amphetamines, and methaqualone, which were used to treat conditions like epilepsy, narcolepsy, hyperkinesias, migraine headaches, and schizo-affective disorders.

The purpose of the computerized surveillance file—which built on earlier efforts to monitor people who had become addicted to opiates in the course of medical treatment—was to enable health officials to conduct systematic queries of the database so that they could identify individuals obtaining prescriptions from multiple doctors or receiving more than a thirty-day prescription per month. They also sought to identify doctors who over- or misprescribed potentially addictive drugs. Some forty-one health department employees had access to the newly centralized files and were authorized to look into cases of potential abuse. Records were to be kept for five years in a secure system before being destroyed. Security measures included a locked wire fence and alarm system for the room receiving state copies of the prescriptions by mail. Computer tapes were kept in a locked cabinet and run on a computer that was inaccessible from other terminals.[140] Unauthorized disclosure of personal identities carried fines of up to $2,000 or one year in prison.[141] Two cases were investigated within the first twenty months of the act.[142]

Although the surveillance effort predated more punitive approaches to drug use, New York governor Nelson Rockefeller's "get tough" approach to the problem—which would involve "sweeping the streets" of all drug dealers and, indeed, drug users—cast a dark shadow upon the public health reporting effort.[143] Immediately before implementation of the new surveillance system, a small group of patients and physicians challenged the state reporting requirements. The judge in the U.S. district court in New York who first heard the case found the question of whether the law violated emergent conceptions of the right to privacy particularly challenging, although he noted it was not a wholesale "invasion" and "publication" of one's entire medical history that was at stake.[144] Indeed, District Judge Robert L. Carter wrote, "Even the illness for which a Schedule II drug is prescribed need not be revealed." The only distinguishing feature of the new legislation was that the records were now computerized: "The only difference is that now the state has developed the means to make effective use of that basic power *which remains unchallenged*" (emphasis added). While Carter sympathized with those concerned about the "over-zealous data collection and instant data retrieval," he could not take "seriously" the fundamental assertion "that governmental use of this new technology is constitutionally impermissible."[145]

A U.S. Second Circuit Court of Appeals, however, sent the case back to the district court on the grounds that the U.S. Supreme Court had ruled that a single judge could not dismiss a complaint on questions of constitutionality. In remanding the case, the appeals court suggested that while the right to privacy was certainly not absolute, it might impose broad limits on the ability of the state to collect information. "If there is anything 'obvious' about the constitutional right to privacy at the present time," wrote Chief Judge Henry Friendly, "it is that its limits remain to be worked out in future cases. Should the constitutionally protected zone of privacy be extended. . . . the individual's interest in keeping to himself the existence of his physical ailments and his doctor's prescriptions for them would lie rather close to the continuum."[146] Thus any effort to centralize record collection might potentially be called into question.

When the case was heard again by a panel of three judges in a federal district court, Judge Carter again wrote the opinion. But this time he reasoned that the injury to the plaintiffs was "sufficiently serious to overcome any competing state interest." One mother, whose child had been treated for hyperkinesias with Ritalin, argued that having her child's name in a central file was stigmatizing. She took him off the drug, arguing that though he "is not doing well without the medication," the alternative "is to have him branded for life." Another plaintiff feared being "labeled a drug addict." Others, expressing concerns for confidentiality at a time in which discussions of drug abuse had achieved "unparalleled . . . national prominence,"[147] described how they discontinued taking medications for migraines and severe pain.[148] Physicians affirmed the perspective that the law harmed patients. One refused to prescribe Schedule II drugs because of the reporting requirements. In short, mounting efforts to define and criminalize drug abuse intersected with the growing concerns about the power of computers to expose people in new ways.

Referring to *Roe v. Wade*, the district court maintained that "the doctor-patient relationship is one of the zones of privacy accorded constitutional protection. Justice Douglas has described the expectation of privacy in the doctor-patient relationship as being exceeded only by that expectation in the relationship of a penitent to his priest." Thus the court concluded, "An individual's physical ills and disabilities, the medication he takes, the frequency of his medical consultation are among the most sensitive of personal and psychological sensibilities. One does not normally expect to be required to have to reveal to a government source, at least in our society, these facets of one's life." While the district court, like the appeals court, agreed that the right to privacy had its limits and that reporting represented a "legitimate government function," in this case the reporting had resulted in finding only one case of prescription abuse on the part of a patient in the more than twenty months the law had been in effect. Thus the district court concluded, "The diminution of a constitutionally guaranteed freedom is too great a price to pay for such a small governmental yield." It further rejected the state's argument that it was doing no more than it had already done under the old regulations by requiring pharmacists to keep records of names: "A name on a prescription in the files of one of many thousands of pharmacists in the state of New York is entirely different from one's name on a form in Albany which is transferred to computerized records and stored for instant retrieval."[149]

Despite the new course it had charted on privacy in the arena of reproductive rights, in 1977 the U.S. Supreme Court unanimously reversed the opinion of the lower court, holding that the failure to prove the necessity of reporting was not a sufficient reason for ruling that the law was unconstitutional. Indeed, the court determined that the law was "manifestly the product of an orderly and rational legislative decision" and that the state's interests in policing drug abuse "would support a decision to experiment with new techniques for control." It was up to the legislature to determine whether this endeavor amounted to "the foolish expenditure of funds to acquire a mountain of useless information."[150]

Further, it ruled that because the state did, in fact, safeguard confidentiality and limit access, privacy was not invaded or abridged. In short, the computer storage of records did not of itself represent a violation of privacy. While "broad dissemination" of intimate personal information would constitute an invasion of privacy, even this, Justice Brennan added in his concurring opinion, could be justified by "compelling state interests." The court, however, found no evidence that the law would not be properly administered or enforced. Although it was possible that the record might be subpoenaed and made part of a court record, the court concluded that this remote possibility "is surely not a sufficient reason for invalidating the entire patient-identification program."[151]

The decision rejected the notion that a single chink in the armor of privacy would threaten the clinical relationship. The statute did not, therefore, represent state interference in medical decision making. While patients might refuse needed medications based on concerns about potential disclosures, the law neither deprived patients of access to Schedule II drugs nor prohibited physicians from prescribing them. Indeed, the court noted that the state had processed one hundred thousand prescriptions per month without inciting any other patient objections.[152] Disclosure of private patient information not only to the state health agencies but to doctors, hospital personnel, and insurance companies might be "unpleasant," but it was "an essential part of modern medical practice," even when such "disclosure may reflect unfavorably on the character of the patient." And then, critically, the court gave its imprimatur to surveillance more generally, citing venereal disease, child abuse, deadly weapons injuries, and fetal death reports, including abortion records, as "familiar examples" of legitimate public health reporting.[153]

In ruling in favor of New York State, however, the court did express sympathy for those who had raised concerns about privacy: "We are not unaware of the threat . . . implicit in the accumulation of vast amounts of personal information in computerized data banks or other massive government files," wrote Justice Stevens for the court. In a concurring opinion, Justice Brennan affirmed that "most troubling" in this case was the issue of computer storage. While a new technology did not invalidate otherwise legitimate data collection and storage, he argued, "The central storage and easy accessibility of computerized data vastly increase the potential for abuse of that information, and I am not prepared to say that future developments will not demonstrate the necessity of some curb on such technology." In this particular instance, however, such a curb was not necessary because of the state's "carefully designed program" of "numerous safeguards."[154]

Thus, in the first—and still only—public health surveillance case considered by the U.S. Supreme Court, the tribunal turned back a challenge to the constitutionality of such efforts. But the politics of surveillance would not be resolved so easily. In the last decades of the twentieth century, the potential subjects of surveillance moved beyond the status of plaintiffs to become active participants in the process of policy making, empowered by a new democratic ethos.

THE DEMOCRATIZATION OF PRIVACY

Whalen was decided just before the first cases of AIDS were reported by the CDC in 1981. It was in the context of that epidemic threat, which we describe in chapter 7, that the ideal of democratic privacy would reach its fullest expression, as AIDS activists, gay community organizations, and their liberal political allies joined in the struggle against state health departments that sought to make HIV a reportable condition. Most remarkably, although physicians played a role in this struggle, the movement to assure that patient voices were heard was one that was essentially driven by those who were asserting claims on their own behalf. The case being made was no longer that privacy was instrumental to the clinical relationship, but rather that respecting patient desires was instrumental to the public health enterprise.

Democratic privacy, then, entails a displacement of the physician as the mediator between patients and public health officials. It reflects the desire and ability of the subjects of surveillance to dictate the terms of privacy for themselves. It would be a mistake, however, to conflate democratic privacy with resistance to disease surveillance. Without denying the importance of privacy, people have also demanded the right to be counted, rejecting privacy as a value that trumps all others. Most important, it was those affected

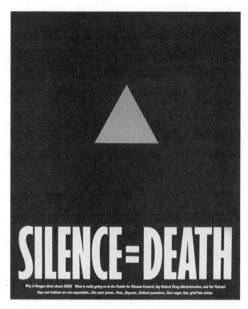

Figure 7. *Silence=Death.* A familiar ACT UP image underscoring that achieving the promise of democratic privacy in the context of the early AIDS epidemic required relinquishing anonymity. www.actupny.org.

who sought to define the relative weight that should be accorded to privacy. But whenever they entered the public forum as advocates for or against surveillance, newly empowered constituencies had to shed the anonymity afforded by the old paternalistic privacy. There was no alternative to coming out in the political process (fig. 7).

PART I

The Rise of Surveillance and the Politics of Resistance

Opening Battles

Tuberculosis and the Foundations of Surveillance

It was with tuberculosis that the extensive, systematic, and contested surveillance of disease began in the United States. This effort was triggered by the bacteriological revolution and informed by the juridical and ideological articulation of the state's authority to intervene to protect the communal well-being. Although historians have typically, although not uniformly,[1] been concerned about the more extraordinary measures that health officials might take—especially isolation and quarantine—it was not such liberty-limiting measures that were primarily at stake.[2] At issue was who was responsible for monitoring and controlling the health of the patient—physician or health official? The often pitched battles between physicians and health officials would be cast in the language of paternalistic privacy.

FIRST FORAYS

A number of states and municipalities began to discuss the notification of tuberculosis (TB) in the early 1890s. Michigan passed legislation requiring TB reporting in 1893.[3] The following year William Osler—the towering Johns Hopkins physician whose textbooks and curriculum marked a new direction in American medicine—strongly supported Philadelphia's efforts to require name reporting for TB.[4] The result was a bitter and contentious battle within the College of Physicians and Surgeons of Philadelphia, where a majority took great exception to the measure. As Dr. Frank Woodbury argued, "Registration would eventually divide physicians into two classes—those who reported their consumptive patients and those who did not. The physicians having the reputation of not reporting their cases would naturally have a larger clientele than others." This would not only be patently unfair but would defeat the objective of reporting.[5]

Others centered their opposition to surveillance on claims about its potential utility. Dr. James B. Walker, citing the example of typhoid, asserted that reporting had never lowered mortality. In his mind, it was with physicians themselves that the responsibility for the protection of the public health rightfully rested: "The physician," he insisted, "is capable of doing all that the Board of Health can, without the manifold evils and annoyances of public registration."[6] But others doubted that much could be done to control the disease among the "poorer classes" because of the sheer scale of the problem, limited resources, and inadequate understanding of effective measures: "If it were possible by systematic notification for the Board of Health to locate a considerable number of these infected houses, what steps would it take to purify them? How would it deal with those of the poorer classes who are affected with this disease, and with the furniture, bedding and rooms?"[7]

Lawrence Flick, Philadelphia's chief proponent of notification, suggested that the city's leading medical men failed to understand the demographics of this disease: "I grant that it may be hard," he argued, "for wealthy people to be recorded as suffering from tuberculosis, but this is a disease of the poor; the vast majority of consumptives are very poor, and the necessities of the poor so demand registration that it should outweigh the sensitiveness of the rich." Responding to the sensitivities of the rich, he proposed to register only the *houses* of the infected rather than infected individuals themselves.[8]

For others, the opposition to reporting hinged on the continuing belief in a hereditary predisposition to the disease and in its lack of contagiousness.[9] Fear and stigma would be the only result. Dr. Owen J. Wister imagined that notification "may lash the whole community into a panic" and create "a feeling of hostility" toward "the unfortunate victims," encouraging their treatment "as criminals guilty of consumption."[10] Wister was joined by Dr. J. M. Da Costa, who asked, "Why fix the brand of leper on the poor unfortunate because he has consumption? . . . Why have him pursued from house to house, why have him a marked man?"[11]

Deep suspicions about the contagious nature of tuberculosis and its stigma carried the day in Philadelphia. The College of Physicians and Surgeons resolved that "the attempt to register consumptives and to treat them as the subjects of contagious disease would be adding hardship to the lives of these unfortunates, stamping them as outcasts of society. In view of the chronic character of the malady, it could not lead to any measures of real value not otherwise attainable."[12] It was a decision that protected the privacy of the poor but also denied them any resources that might have been provided by the health department. For better or worse, Philadelphia's tubercular would have to rely on what physicians could offer. But if in Philadelphia paternalistic privacy worked to shield both the wealthy and the poor from the intrusions—benevolent or punitive, welcomed or opposed—

of health officials, in other locales it would allow the public health and medical communities to chart a very different course. In New York City, after a protracted controversy that revolved around the relative authority of private physicians and the department of health, municipal authorities embraced notification.

THE "JEALOUS" EYES OF MEDICINE

The prospect of TB reporting had been discussed in New York City as early as 1868. Stephen Smith put it simply: "When a Commissioner of Health from 1868 to 1875, I endeavored to have tuberculosis reported as contagious, but failed."[13] Efforts in 1889 likewise failed to bear fruit after the health commissioner wrote to "twenty-four of the most prominent and influential physicians of the city" to solicit their opinions about the "necessity" of reporting. The very few physicians who even bothered to reply to the health commissioner indicated that the medical professional would not offer "cordial support."[14]

It would take almost three decades from Smith's 1868 effort before notification would be mandated. Although the climate of medical opinion had hardly become any warmer, the Board of Health was ready to wager on a new consensus regarding the danger and the imperative to act: "The communicability of pulmonary tuberculosis has been so thoroughly established . . . that the time has arrived when active steps should be taken looking towards its prevention in this city."[15] In 1893 Hermann M. Biggs—in his capacity as chief inspector of the Division of Pathology, Bacteriology, and Disinfection—recommended that public institutions be required to report the names of the infected. "It was not deemed wise, however, in the beginning, to make it obligatory for physicians to report cases, especially as it was comparatively easy to obtain reports from public institutions, which would give the most numerous classes of patients and those whom it was most important to instruct." The Board of Health merely sent out a circular requesting private physicians and institutions to report cases of TB.[16]

Although it was clear that the city planned to investigate cases and that reporting was intended as a means of allowing direct health department intervention, every effort was made to assuage the fears of physicians regarding encroachments upon their professional authority. Biggs thus stated that "this information will be solely for the use of the Department, and in no case will visits be made to such persons by the Inspectors of the Department, nor will the Department assume any sanitary surveillance of such patients, unless the person resides in a tenement-house, boarding-house or hotel, or unless the attending physician requests that an inspection of the premises be made." Even then, "in no case where the person resides in" multifamily or multiperson residences "will any action be taken if the physician requests that no visits be made by Inspectors and is willing himself to deliver" information circulars regarding the spread of TB and how to prevent its transmission.[17]

In 1894 the department of health acceded to Biggs's request for mandatory notification on the part of public institutions.[18] The TB registry not only contained the name of the infected and tracked all changes in address but also recorded every public health action taken in the case until the patient's death or recovery. Individual case records were only destroyed following a patient's death.[19] The *Sun*, in New York, predicted that compulsory notification "will come later on. It is the only thing that remains to be done, to put the worst of all contagious diseases into the column where it properly belongs."[20]

The *Sun* was prescient. In 1897 Biggs recommended and the Board adopted "more comprehensive and radical measures": compulsory notification for all cases.[21] Biggs's full report regarding mandatory notification was reprinted in the *Medical News,* which described it as "one of the most important reports it ha[d] ever received."[22] While the health department's careful observation of the rights of private physicians and their patients garnered Biggs and the department some medical support regarding compulsory notification,[23] the overall medical response was decidedly hostile.[24] This was not, of course, a test case for notification. Systems of reporting were already in place for conditions like smallpox and typhoid. They had elicited no controversy. When reporting was extended to polio in the early decades of the twentieth century, it too would provoke no backlash from the medical community. Indeed, the medical community had expressed outright support for such reporting.[25]

Tuberculosis—the "white plague"—was different. Mortality from tuberculosis began to decline in a continuous fashion in the United States in the 1860s and 1870s. Nonetheless, the "grim monster" remained the most significant scourge of progressive era America.[26] The overall annual mortality rate from tuberculosis was, in 1900, approximately 200 per 100,000 in the white population. Among blacks, the rate was 400 per 100,000.[27] Urban areas suffered the most. In New York City, for example, the overall mortality rate was 428 per 100,000 in 1870 and 256 per 100,000 in 1890. The New York City mortality rate varied from 49 per 100,000 on the Upper West Side to 776 per 100,000 in the tenement district of lower Manhattan.[28]

Compounding this high death rate, TB was also chronic. Measures that had become standard for the control of epidemic infections—vaccination, isolation, and quarantine—would have marginal relevance in the instance of tuberculosis. New York City's health commissioner, George Fowler, sought to assuage the medical community by stressing that his department had not declared tuberculosis to be a *contagious* disease requiring immediate intervention, but "had [instead] declared it to be among the infectious and *communicable* diseases, dangerous to the public health."[29] But this assurance did little to comfort physicians, because there was no "clear-cut idea" about what these terms meant.[30] To the extent that there was a general understanding that by "communicable," the department meant that transmission required prolonged exposure to infection,[31] some retorted that "there was high authority against the positive statement that tuberculosis was infectious and communicable."[32] In Philadelphia, where conflict over how the disease was spread also raged, Lawrence Flick felt certain that once the distinction was made clear, the feeling that TB surveillance represented "unnecessary espionage" would dissipate.[33] But the classification of TB as a communicable disease was offensive even for those who felt no confusion because surveillance for this class of disease represented an extension of notification into new terrain.[34]

Biggs would later comment, "I have always felt that much harm has been done by calling tuberculosis a contagious disease; it produces confusion in the minds of both the laity and the medical profession, because the conception of a contagious disease is always related to such diseases as scarlet fever, smallpox, etc., in which very limited contact or even simple proximity may result in their transmission. Every intelligent person knows that tuberculosis is different in nature from these diseases, and I believe that this distinction should be made and kept clear and definite. Tuberculosis is communicable, but not contagious."[35] It was precisely because the city had "always drawn a very sharp distinction between tuberculosis and the other infectious diseases which sanitary authorities *ordinarily deal with*" that notification was so threatening.[36] It was unprecedented for the health department to require reporting when there was no clear course to prevent the spread of a disease. If the traditional interventions were unlikely to stem transmission and avert or contain an epidemic, some believed the health department should stay its hand. John Shaw Billings proclaimed, "If we knew of some way by which we could prevent the spread of pneumonia, the compulsory notification of such cases would be the first steps taken toward that end."[37] Given that health officials were not going to be able to approach TB as they did other contagious threats, how did they intend to act on case reports?

To the medical community, it seemed obvious that this was an effort to usurp physician authority over cases. *Medical Record* editor George Shrady, who had explicitly supported notification for conditions like typhoid and even advocated for small physician remuneration for such services,[38] complained, "The compulsory step taken is a mistaken, untimely, irrational, and unwise one. . . . The real obnoxiousness of this amendment to the sanitary code is its offensively dictatorial and defiantly compulsory character. It places the Board in the rather equivocal position of dictating to the profession and of creating a suspicion of an extra bid for public applause by unduly magnifying the importance of its bacteriological department." Already, he continued, "The profession as a whole has watched with jealous eye the encroachments of the Board upon many of the previously well-recognized privileges of the medical attendant."[39]

Surveillance raised the question of who would be making decisions on behalf of the patient. As another clinical combatant explained, "If the sanitary code of the present city should become that of the greater city . . . the health board would be given practically the treatment of all infectious diseases, and it had only to declare a disease infectious in order to take charge of it."[40] The medical community thus claimed, "There is no objection to the reports of pulmonary cases for statistical purposes" but objected stringently to "the extra missionary work assumed by the board which is the ominous and threatening quantity in the equation—the desire to assume official control of the cases after they have been reported, thus not only, by means of alarming bacteriological edicts, directly interfering with the physician in the diagnosis and treatment of the patient, but in the end, by creation of a public suspicion of his ignorance, possibly depriving him of one of the means of a legitimate livelihood."[41]

Thus the medical community insisted that reporting entail "no direct or indirect interference between patient and physician, either in the way of official inspections, bacteriological diagnosis, forced isolation, suggestions for treatment, or presumptuous instructions to the patient regarding hygienic precaution."[42] In fact, the Standing Committee on Hygiene of the Medical Society of the county of New York endorsed the reporting measure with only the proviso that lay at the heart of notions of paternalistic privacy: "Inspectors are forbidden to visit or have any communication with the patient without the consent of the attending physician, believing that the attending physician is capable of giving all the necessary instruction."[43] If health officials had no access to the patient, then the authority of physicians remained unchallenged, and they too could enjoy the "right to be let alone."

Other medical groups remained hostile to any form of notification. The New York and Kings County Medical Societies had bills introduced into the state legislature that would have rescinded those portions of the New York City charter giving the health department its authority to deal with tuberculosis as a communicable disease. C.-E. A. Winslow, a notable public health figure and Biggs's biographer, spun a dramatic tale about how, with considerable effort and negotiation by Biggs, who reportedly spent the winter in Albany during the legislature's 1898 and 1899 sessions, the health department blocked passage of the bills.[44]

Medical opposition, however, remained staunch. Even the New York Academy of Medicine—where Biggs had influential health department colleagues supportive of the initiative, including Drs. Edward G. Janeway, T. Mitchell Prudden, and William Park—rejected the idea of compulsory notification as "inexpedient and unwise,"[45] causing the *Medical Record* to retort to Biggs, "It would now appear that the time has come for the health board to rescind the obnoxious regulation, in order that it may, as formerly, work in harmony with the wishes of the profession."[46]

In the encounter with the medical community, Biggs underscored his conviction about the central and preeminent role the health department had to play in protecting the public health. It was an understanding that raised the question of who truly served the best interests of the patient and that stressed the ultimate subordination of the individual to the public good. Physicians, he asserted, objected to making TB a notifiable condition because they wished to protect patients from knowledge of their infection. Biggs rejected such misdirected benevolence: "How frequently have I heard patients complain most bitterly of their physicians, for not having informed them of the nature of their disease." That fact aside, however, Biggs emphasized, "One of the fixed principles in the organization of society is that, if necessary, the welfare of the individual must be sacrificed to the welfare of the community."[47] This was not, therefore, a matter of who could best care for the individual patient; rather, it was about who could best decide for the community. Only the health department had the knowledge and perspective to make decisions for *all*.

Not all public health officials shared the enthusiasm of Hermann Biggs for tuberculosis surveillance. Some believed the tool that Biggs so forcefully promoted would, in fact, impose impediments on the effective response to tuberculosis and would rend relations between physicians and public health departments. Arthur R. Reynolds, Chicago's commissioner of health, wrote, "I have never been able to convince myself that tuberculosis should be a notifiable disease. . . . The only object to be gained by notification would be to enable health officials to warn the sufferer of the danger in his sputum and to placard the house to warn off approaching visitors. It is my belief, based on practical experience with other contagious diseases, that these results may be better obtained through the voluntary cooperation of the profession." TB notification, he continued, "had not only been a demonstrated failure, but the tactless efforts to enforce the provision had alienated a most valuable ally of any health department."[48] The notion of a partnership between physicians and public health officials would become the great, unrealized dream on the part of proponents of public health throughout the century.[49]

In New York, even though state health officials were pleased with their unexpected success in introducing notification, they shied away from following the monitoring path charted by the city. The state's health commissioner, for example, readily instituted free sputum testing and a system of lab-based reporting. Yet, he wondered, "after that, what shall be the next step for the State Department to undertake? In connection with the State government I do not think it would be justifiable to carry out such an elaborate system as that now practiced in New York city; it would perhaps partake too much of paternalism to be justified."[50]

The battle over TB reporting, while primarily engaging only physicians and health officials, was not confined to the medical press. The public was well aware of the furious struggle. When they sought to rally the public, physicians invoked the specter of "government paternalism."[51] One physician wrote in the *New York Times,* "I think it can confidently be said that one of the horrors added to the dread of the 'great white plague' is fear of official registration, with its accompanying inspection and the resulting greater or less surveillance."[52] But although they warned the public of the dangers to their own liberty, physicians chose to emphasize that the health department was guilty of "robbing the physician of his legitimate work, and his bread and butter."[53]

But the mainstream press was unmoved. The *New York Times* charged physicians with "Crippling the Board of Health." "Certain doctors," noted the *Times,* "have drawn fanciful pictures of the invasion of the homes of their private patients by Health Inspectors; they have seen in fancy their earnings dwindle under the machinations of the board; they have prattled of espionage and grown almost tearful under the threatened horrors of paternalism, and altogether have worked themselves into an attitude of panic almost pitiful—if it were real." The *Times* concluded, "Surely a department which requires from all simply a notification of the existence of each case of tuberculosis, but which deals officially only with those neglected by everybody else cannot be regarded as a serious menace to the rights of the laity or the emoluments of the medical profession."[54]

The extent to which "the more intelligent part of the population" embraced tuberculosis notification no doubt turned on the degree to which the health department had successfully convinced them that it would focus its efforts "among the more ignorant, and for the most part, foreign-born population," where, to date, "the department has been powerless to interfere."[55]

A FAR-REACHING PROGRAM

In the 1890s, before the surveillance plan hit its full stride, George Fowler, the New York City health commissioner, sought to quell physician opposition. He addressed members of New York Medical Society and suggested that physicians had misinterpreted the new directive as compulsory *inspection* of suspected cases rather than compulsory *notification.*[56] But it was clearly far more than mere notification. For Biggs, as for many other health officials, if surveillance was anything at all, it was a call to action. As John Fulton, his counterpart in Baltimore, explained, "A registration law merely for the accumulation of information would be a very feeble measure."[57] Indeed, in almost every instance in which health departments moved to TB registration, the intent of state laws was to enable officials to monitor cases.[58] A 1905–6 survey demonstrated that in most cities the purpose of the law was to allow public health investigations. Argued one locale: "The warfare must be waged in the individual case."[59] Thus, when New York City launched its tuberculosis reporting program in 1897, it made clear that its aim was to investigate cases and that reporting was intended as a means of allowing direct health department intervention.

The most dramatic measure that the department might take was compulsory isolation of the infected. But it was not the most important element of TB control.[60] Health officials themselves expressed skepticism about linking surveillance to coercive measures. When state health officials endorsed TB surveillance, they explicitly rejected using it as the basis for isolation and quarantine, measures "which would excite such resentment."[61] When the president of the American Congress of Tuberculosis endorsed notification at an international conference, he warned against linking it to quarantine.[62] But if the ambitions of departments of health were far less punitive, they were also grander. The surveillance system was intended as a far-reaching program of sanitary inspection and monitoring of all cases.[63]

The city's inspection plan amounted to a system of active surveillance in which health officials did not merely receive and catalog reports, but hired a team of investigators to seek out reports and keep information on patients up to date. In addition to collecting reports, the New York City health department also had the authority to inspect suspected cases of TB, typically reported by the laity, nurses, or charity organizations throughout the city.[64] The city was divided into districts to which a nurse was assigned. Each had a TB clinic. Each day the nurse in charge visited her district clinic, collected the names of all new and discharged cases, and reported these names to the local borough health office by telephone. When she made this call, she would also receive the names of all newly reported cases in her district. The expectation was that the nurses would visit each newly reported case and conduct a monthly follow-up visit unless it was a report that came from a private physician. In this case she kept a record "for information only." But this exception did not amount to a total absence of surveillance. Although the nurse would not actually contact the patients, she would visit the locality "to ascertain if there is a house at the address given, and its character—i.e., private, one family house, tenement, etc."[65] Although only minimal information—name, address, and diagnosis—was required in the initial physician report, elaborate patient records were created as a result of the monitoring process (figs. 8 through 11). The city's TB registration card, for example, made clear that surveillance amounted to more than the creation of a record. It also required an inspection of the home. Nurses assessed aspects of both the patient's and the family's lives, including cleanliness, air space, sleeping space, patient income, expectoration arrangements, and nutrition.

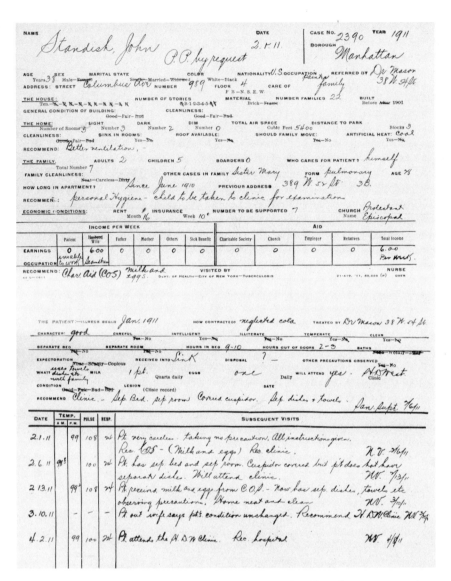

Figure 8. A New York City tuberculosis registry form detailing the extent of information recorded on each case and household. This patient was visited five times in three months. John Shaw Billings, "The Registration and Sanitary Supervision of Pulmonary Tuberculosis in New York City," *Department of Health of the City of New York Monograph Series* 1. New York, 1912. Courtesy of the New York Academy of Medicine.

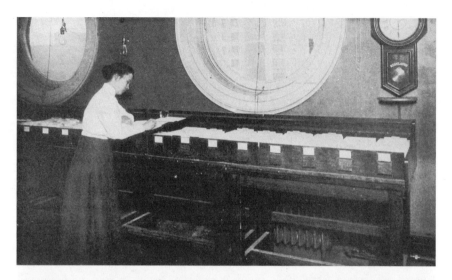

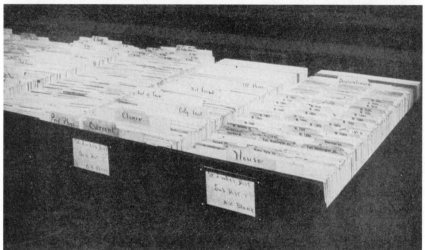

Figures 9 and 10. The New York City tuberculosis registry. John Shaw Billings, "The Registration and Sanitary Supervision of Pulmonary Tuberculosis in New York City," *Department of Health of the City of New York Monograph Series* 1. New York, 1912. Courtesy of the New York Academy of Medicine.

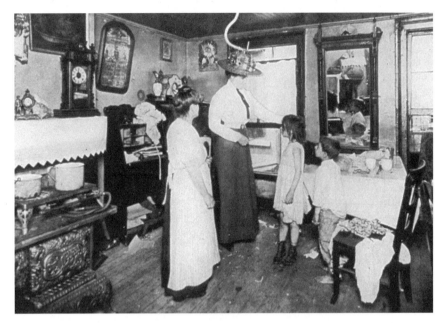

Figure 11. A home nursing visit. National Library of Medicine.

This created not only a caring opportunity, but also a tutelary one, particularly in the case of immigrant families who were perceived to be in need of a kind of indoctrination into American standards of hygiene.

While New York City regulations formally required this extensive level of supervision, limited financial resources, in fact, drastically restricted the number of inspections that nurses could perform. There had been seven nurses on duty in Manhattan (sixteen on duty throughout New York City) in 1908—a number the department deemed "ridiculously inadequate." In 1909 the budgets were slashed, and only eight nurses remained on duty in the entire city, meaning that they "could do but little more than make one visit to each new case reported."[66] In 1910, however, appropriations for communicable disease control increased dramatically. Eight new clinics were opened and one hundred fifty-five nurses employed. By 1912 there were twenty-one department clinics in Manhattan, two in the Bronx, six in Brooklyn, and one each in Queens and Richmond.[67] While the percentage of TB cases under department supervision—patients being cared for in a city hospital or clinic and those monitored by visiting nurses within their homes—remained relatively stable over time, the number of home inspections almost quintupled in 1910, when nurses made nearly two hundred fifty thousand home visits.

By 1911 health officials had sufficient resources to observe the "cardinal point" of assessing all TB cases in the city once a month, "oftener if necessary."[68] After 1911 nurses from the sanitary inspection program made more frequent visits to a subset of cases, as the department began to focus on the noncompliant or recalcitrant TB patient.[69] Such a focus was part of a restructuring of the TB program made, at least in part, in response to both "physicians and patients," who objected to monthly visits as being "needlessly annoy[ing]."[70] The city began to classify as "under periodic observation only" those cases in which the condition of the patient's household was found to be satisfactory and adequate precautions for disease transmission were observed. Physicians were required to file a monthly report updating the health department on the address of such patients.[71] These "at home" cases might receive a nursing visit only once every two months. In sharp contrast, in instances where public health nurses were not satisfied, cases were classified as being "under close sanitary supervision," and patients were visited "every two or three days until the faulty conditions were corrected, or the case terminated by recovery, death or removal."[72] In 1912 the city required not only supervising nurses but also the attending physicians at all city clinics to call on the "very ill" and "delinquent . . . cases at their homes."[73]

Both the burdens and the benefits of such attention, then, accrued to only some members of the community. Indeed, that had been the intent from the outset. As early as 1904, it was clear that the health department was primarily concerned with preventing the spread of tuberculosis among the poor. The closest supervision and compulsory measures were enforced against the "homeless, friendless, dependent, dissipated and vicious consumptives" who were "most likely to be dangerous to the community."[74] These classes of individuals were not to be found among the English-speaking inhabitants of the slum districts, but among "the non-English-speaking inhabitants of the poorest tenement-house districts, recruited as they continually are by fresh supplies of the most filthy and ignorant classes from all parts of Europe."[75] But if, on the one hand, popular prejudices about the tubercular fueled sanitary surveillance efforts in New York City, the success of those efforts could also unravel insidious assumptions. Many years later, President Franklin Roosevelt's secretary of labor, Frances Perkins, explained when she had been a tenement house inspector on the city's Lower East Side, it was the "happy practice" of reformers to "console [themselves] with the thought that the residents of that district were entirely of Irish extraction, and the Irish . . . were the 'seedbed' of tuberculosis." Yet the success of the public health campaign against the disease caused her to give up such a narrow conception of disease causation, bringing her and others "to the conclusion that it was something in the environment that had made it favorable for the growth of whatever seeds might be planted anywhere in the human body," and not something inherent in the peoples who succumbed to tuberculosis or any other disease.[76]

The practice of surveillance did not necessarily work to change understandings of the links between class and race and disease. In southern locales, it was the black population that became the chief target of surveillance. Baltimore was one of the first major urban centers to require the compulsory notification of TB in 1896. As in New York, the focus of surveillance was on the poor residing in tenement-type dwellings unless private physicians provided a written exemption for their patients. For wealthy patients, the onus was on physicians to actually request sanitary supervision. Thus the two-tiered approach to TB control was more pronounced in Baltimore, where some classes and races could, by design, avoid notification altogether.

Because the percentage of cases reported by physicians was unimpressive, health officials advanced more expansive surveillance, which included enlisting whites in the surveillance of blacks.[77] The effort involved a control campaign focused almost exclusively on African American homes.[78] The interventions were shaped by prevailing beliefs regarding the inevitability of "black extinction"—TB was just one of the predictable consequences of emancipation.[79]

In Jim Crow–era Atlanta, a containment campaign focused on "Negro servants," washerwomen in particular, who were believed to represent the critical vector of infection from the poor black slums into the respectable white neighborhoods. Slavery, reasoned southern physicians, had had an ameliorating "quarantine effect" that was lost in the postbellum decades.[80] Blurring any boundary between public health and law enforcement, the city merged the "criminal justice and public health objectives of registration" and attempted to erect a bimonthly system of physical examinations and health certifications for laundresses.[81] Such efforts reinforced deeply held fears about emancipation and determination to maintain a color line. Just as significant, however, was the cross-class, cross-racial alliance of black servants and middle-class white women who depended on their services, which successfully resisted such harsh surveillance initiatives. Here, a broader kind of politics involving labor and its control framed the politics of privacy and surveillance.[82]

In San Francisco, public health surveillance also involved questions of race, labor, and citizenship. Here it was the Chinese laundries that drew the attention of Board of Health members, who attempted to bring them under "sanitary surveillance" with the intention of closing them down altogether. Dr. H. Hart in particular sounded the alarm about the "loathsome" Chinese practice, which he claimed was pervasive among the "coolie" laundry workers, of spraying tubercular water from the mouth onto clothing in preparation for ironing. Although the "consumptive Chinese" and his "dangerous mouth spray" was the focus of this campaign, this practice was also linked to syphilis and infections of the skin.[83]

In Los Angeles, government obligations to control tuberculosis were likewise racialized and, during the Depression era, dovetailed with repatriation efforts targeted at Mexicans and Filipinos. Yet the role of the state as a kind of purger or purifier did not mean that the TB control program lacked important care-giving aspects. The politics of exclusion, rather, gave those efforts a particular shape. Thus even when acting in their capacity as providers, municipal health authorities always premised the delivery of care on the economic potential of the immigrant and hence focused on "transforming as many patients as possible into productive workers."[84] Health officials sought to deport those beyond "transformation."

APPLYING "CONTINUOUS PRESSURE"

After the turn of the century, New York City's upheavals over TB reporting began to subside. Biggs would claim victory. "The experimental state of registration for tuberculosis is past," he announced. "The practice has proved successful wherever tried."[85] Bearing him out, opinion in the medical press had softened.[86] In 1903 the AMA, without making any direct mention of disease reporting, endorsed the collection of vital statistics, stressing the significance of timely death notification as one of the obligations of the modern practitioner.[87] More predictably, the following year the Association of State and Territorial Health Officers (ASTHO) strongly endorsed name-based TB reporting.[88] Practitioners in New York were likewise receptive. A writer in the *New York State Journal of Medicine* assured readers in 1904 that departmental procedure protected private patients from unwarranted intrusion and, indeed, reasoned that "the very fact [of] notification by the attending physician has the greatest educational value and justifies the assumption, in those instances in which the case is under the supervision of a private physician, that reasonable and necessary precautions for the protection of others will be taken." In other words, notification signaled physician control of the case.[89]

By 1910 the New York City Board of Health claimed that 90 percent of all TB cases were registered with the city.[90] The free diagnosis of sputum— which required that the "name, address, age and sex of such person, and the name and address of the attending physician, accompany the specimens of sputa for record" if it was to be examined[91]—was doubtless instrumental in the success of the system.[92] Indeed, Biggs noted that while many physicians refused to report tuberculosis cases, they "would regularly send specimens of sputum for examination, with all the necessary data regarding the patient." In response to New York's success, a public health official in Baltimore would deduce that the roots of medical opposition "are not . . .

made fast, as physicians usually say, to the principle of medical confidence. If that were so, the free examination of sputa at public laboratories would have aroused the same opposition. . . . Medical opinion is . . . very sensitive, and may be easily be misguided by considerations of apparently trivial nature."[93]

The New York City Department of Health emphasized cooperation and downplayed the need for punitive measures designed to achieve physician compliance. "It is true," wrote Biggs, "that the department of health has not endeavored to enforce strictly the regulations. It was not the intention to do so when they were enacted. It has not prosecuted physicians who have failed to report cases; the board is well aware of the fact that large numbers of cases are not reported; but still a constant advance is being made."[94] In sharp contrast, in Boston, prosecuting physicians seemed to increase tuberculosis reporting: in 1910 physicians failed to report some 328 cases of tuberculosis, as determined by an examination of death certifications, but by 1911, following a prosecutorial campaign, the department of health found only 63 unreported cases and only 14 in 1912.[95]

Despite the less aggressive posture taken by New York City officials, the health department did not simply rely on the goodwill of physicians; it took decided steps to ensure that physicians reported cases and then kept the department updated on the progress of those patients.[96] In 1907 the department began sending out an annual letter to the attending physician of each "'private' case," requesting "information as to the outcome of the case." If the physician failed to reply, "the original address of the case is visited by a Department Inspector." If the individual was found, the case was brought "under the supervision of the department."[97] In short, if reporting signaled physician control of a case, the failure to keep the department informed about the condition of that case represented delinquency.

To pressure physicians to initiate reporting, the department of health systematically compared the TB and death registries. When TB was noted as a cause of death but the case had not been reported, the responsible physician's name would be placed on a blacklist.[98] The department would then send letters to physicians reminding them of the requirements of the sanitary code and asking "for an explanation for the failure to report the case." Biggs remarked, "A second letter has been rarely required."[99] Indeed, from 1894 to 1907 physicians were fined anywhere from $50 to $200 in only about six instances.[100] The aim was to apply "continuous pressure . . . on all sides to secure increased accuracy in the reports."[101] This system of using death certificates to monitor physician reporting continued until at least 1918.[102]

Department of health TB inspectors—who received reports of "suspected cases" from landlords, charity organizations, dispensaries, and even private citizens who filed complaints—also served as a double check on

physicians. If while on a routine visit or in response to a report of a suspected case, an inspector made a diagnosis of TB and was told that that a
physician had attended the case, the inspector would visit the physician,
inquire as to why the case had not been reported, and then assure that it was
entered into the city's registry.[103] John Shaw Billings, the physician who managed the city's TB registry, thus described the department as having
achieved "excellent control over [physicians]."[104]

Nonetheless, health department officials complained that even physicians who reported cases and who requested that their patients not be visited by any health department personnel failed to exercise adequate supervision over their patients. A department study conducted in 1918 found
that 80 percent of 70 physicians in the city's Chelsea district were unable to
report any information regarding the home conditions of and behavioral
precautions taken by their TB patients, such as use of separate plates and
separate bedrooms. The department concluded, "Without infringing upon
rights or prerogatives of private physicians in control of their cases, we
should require them to render an accounting at stated intervals with respect
to home conditions observed by them, so that we may be assured that there
is no relaxation in measures for prevention of the spread of tuberculosis."[105]

Other locales that experienced similar physician inattention to the living
conditions of the poor would also require that physicians record data that
went far beyond name, address, and diagnosis. For example, in Maryland
the initial case report included information about the patient's occupation,
work capacity, and earning power as indicators of his or her economic condition. In addition to data about the size and habits of the family (for example, Does the patient "habitually kiss other persons on the mouth?" share
tableware and napkins? spit on the floor?), records also required information on the condition of the patient's habitat, covering size of dwelling, the
degree to which it was tidied, and number of beds per occupant, which
reflected on the practice of bed sharing.[106] But if, in Maryland, the initial
case report required considerable detail, it was far surpassed by the information ultimately recorded by New York City health inspectors.

THE PLACE OF PRIVACY

As it sought to consolidate its program of tuberculosis notification, the New
York City health department placed great emphasis on the confidentiality of
the registry it was creating. Health officials framed notification in terms of
the "rights of both physicians and patients," with physicians receiving priority.[107] Concern for confidentiality had multiple sources. First, the city
health department, like others, feared that if it did not protect records,
physicians would intensify their opposition to reporting. But it was also
widely understood, especially in the context of both tuberculosis and vene-

real disease, that a failure to protect records could injure patients. In the instance of tuberculosis, a visit from a city health inspector could result in loss of housing if a landlord suspected the condition.[108] Recognizing this risk, the city's department of health stipulated that "in tracing cases on first visit or, if unable to obtain admission, when making a revisit, no messages are left with neighbors. The reason for the nurse's visit (i.e., that there is a consumptive on the premises) is only to be given to the family."[109] Patients were admonished to carefully guard knowledge of their condition: "Do not talk to anyone about your disease, except your physician," the department warned patients in its standard, widely distributed informational circular published in a number of languages and given to all patients registered with TB.[110] In invoking privacy, the department of health reconfirmed and reinforced the medical guardianship of patients.

With regard to its central records, officials clearly stated from the very outset that the registry was intended "solely for the use of the department."[111] Indeed Biggs made plain that reporting to the health department did not involve "notification to the community at large."[112] Echoing this position, New York State in 1913 enacted legislation specifying that the TB registry "shall not be open to inspection by any person other than the health authorities of the State and of the said city, town, or village; and said health authorities shall not permit any such report or record to be divulged so as to disclose the identity of the person to whom it relates, except as may be authorized in the sanitary code."[113]

In Maryland, where TB surveillance was so shaped by racial politics, it was not unusual for physicians to inquire with the registry about whether a case had been previously reported by a colleague. But even here, health officials felt impelled to say that "privacy is secured in express and unequivocal terms." Physicians who thus tried to solicit information from health officials were informed that officials "are forbidden to divulge information of this sort. . . . The physician realizes in a moment the impropriety of his inquiry, and sees that the confidential character implied by the terms of the law is secured in its practical operation."[114]

While placarding tenements or hotels to indicate the presence of an acute infectious disease like cholera or polio was common practice throughout the United States,[115] in the instance of TB, placarding occurred only when rooms once occupied by a patient with tuberculosis who had died or left the premises were not properly disinfected by landlords.[116] Placards read: "NOTICE: Consumption is a communicable disease. This apartment has been occupied by a consumptive and may have become infected. It must not be occupied by persons other than those now residing here until an order of the Board of Health, directing that the apartment being cleansed and renovated, has been complied with." A placard listed the name of the former tenant and indicated which apartment he or she had occupied. Placards could not be removed until compliance with department renovation orders. Sanitary policemen ensured that the warnings remained in place.[117]

THE INFORMAL STATE

Health department activities were complemented by those inspired by charitable callings. During the period of progressive era TB control, charity societies—groups interested in mother and child health and welfare in particular—formed around the cause of identifying and aiding crippled children, up to 90 percent of whom were tubercular.[118] New York City's Association for the Aid of Crippled Children represented a group of upper-class women who, beginning in 1907, raised funds to transport children suffering primarily from tuberculosis of the bone to public schools so that they might become "self-supporting useful men and women."[119] The Federation of Associations for Cripples—organized by the wife of a prominent New York City surgeon and the wives of local businessmen—sought to create a registry of such children in order "to form a basis for an accurate working knowledge of the extent of the cripple problem and to discover how adequately existing agencies are dealing with the question of proper care and physical care and education for cripples."[120] As with other charity organizations in the United States, the key to initiating such "community action" was "fact-finding."[121]

Shelby Harrison, a prominent progressive era social worker, argued that the collection and distribution of information related to social problems was "a means to better democracy by informing the community upon community matters," which "provided a basis for intelligent public opinion."[122] It was part of a larger, oft-expressed desire for greater individual and community participation in democracy through decentralization.[123] Indeed, the movement grew out of the progressive tradition of social reform, particularly after the turn of the century, when commission governments and initiative and referendum movements sought to ensure, in Teddy Roosevelt's words, "the right of the people to rule."[124] TB, within this framework, was the great "social disease" that demanded a "new social conscience" and a powerful civic movement that went beyond the efforts of health officials and physicians to ensure its eradication.[125] The public sentiment was "We need to establish a small antituberculosis society in every social, fraternal, and business organization which can be reached."[126]

While the charity movement extended beyond the state, it was, at the same time, viewed as part of public health activities directed by the state. In its extensive 1912 report, *The Registration and Sanitary Supervision of Pulmonary Tuberculosis*, the New York City Department of Health included a diagram that illustrated the organizational approach to TB control (fig. 12). The department itself was, of course, the hub of this effort. While not

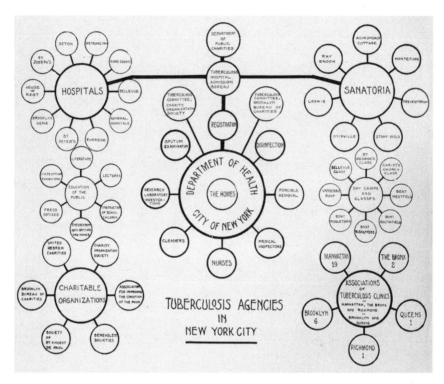

Figure 12. The organization of the New York City tuberculosis program. While the health department shows no direct links to the charitable organizations, they are seen in the far left-hand corner. These organizations were clearly viewed as part of the network and as part of the working relationships of the department. John Shaw Billings, "The Registration and Sanitary Supervision of Pulmonary Tuberculosis in New York City," *Department of Health of the City of New York Monograph Series* 1 (New York, 1912).

directly linked to its activities, the broad range of charitable organizations was clearly viewed as a vital part of the landscape of TB control. Indeed, the health department referred nearly three thousand patients to charity organizations between 1908 and 1911, and these organizations, in turn, reported "suspected" cases to health officials.[127]

The New York Charity Organization Society, for example, worked almost hand in hand with the health department and were ardent advocates for client adherence to its hygienic, nutrition, and household maintenance recommendations. The society provided prescriptive health standards and material relief, such as food, fuel, towels, and bedding. It could use the withdrawal of relief or the threat of health department compulsion to assure compliance. And, like the department of health's nursing corps, charity workers conducted their own, sometimes unannounced, household inspections.[128] As a consequence of these kinds of interactions, community-based initiatives often ended up leading to the creation of state bureaucracies as the efforts of local reformers became institutionalized within state agencies. This held true not only for TB but also for a number of reform efforts.[129]

But whatever the organizational consequences, the intent, as one social theorist described it, was to transform the "private into public" by extending the realm of community life.[130] The purpose of documenting the extent of social problems like childhood tuberculosis was to "draw in the general public" and establish opportunities for consistent interaction between the needy and the educated or affluent, which motivated local initiatives such as the "friendly visit."[131]

The quest for community participation in and control of social problems did not mean, however, that registries of the needy were a matter for the public record. Charity organizations relied on case histories to appeal and galvanize the community through newspaper human interest stories and articles in popular and professional journals. But "identifying data" was always removed, and agency records remained "carefully guarded."[132] Observation of strict norms of confidentiality did not, however, represent a bar to the sharing of information among the fold of citizens' organizations that were recognized within a local community. In Boston, for example, charities exchanged their information freely. Reformers established a central registry of families—known as a central social service exchange or "confidential exchange"—so that different agencies might determine what relief a family had received. In this way various agencies both avoided duplication of effort and connected individuals or families to the network of services more effectively.[133]

Not all communities had a formal confidential exchange, but the clear expectation was that information might be shared.[134] There was also a mutual understanding of the rules of sharing that was guided by notions of paternalistic privacy. Just as the clinician's authority over the patient demanded respect, the interests of the "parent" charity organization, which acted as the guardian or steward of the child or family, had to be acknowledged. Thus the reformers who undertook the census of New York City cripples in 1914 assured the organizations whose data they sought that "we will take no action in regard to any case which you refer to us without your consent."[135] The Association for the Improvement of the Condition of the Poor, at least, was more than happy to oblige, responding, "We can surely give you the names, ages and addresses of all cripples now under our care in tenement families."[136] The New York Charity Society opened its records to public schools, the police, the courts, newspapers, as well as employment bureaus and city agencies.[137]

TB SURVEILLANCE TAKES HOLD

The New York City experience blazed a path for the extension of reporting in other major cities. The city had always been the public health vanguard for the nation. "The eyes of the world," observed prominent social reformer Florence J. Harriman in 1912, "are upon New York" and its notification program.[138] Just as the city's careful documentation of its conquest of infectious disease shaped social, health, and urban policy in cities and states, the nation would look to the experience of New York City in extending surveillance to tuberculosis.[139]

As of 1901 only 8 of America's larger cities mandated TB reporting.[140] By 1906 53 of the 86 cities with populations of 48,000 or more had adopted such requirements. Of the 20 largest cities—comprising a population of almost 11 million—all but 4 had mandatory reporting.[141] By 1921 50 cities had developed visitation plans for TB cases that were modeled on New York's extensive surveillance and monitoring protocol.[142]

In contrast, at the turn of the twentieth century, 32 states and the District of Columbia did not explicitly require any tuberculosis reporting. But by the second decade of the twentieth century, following the recommendations outlined in a "Model State Law for Morbidity Reports" by ASTHO in 1913,[143] a number of states had moved to make physician reporting of TB mandatory, with 38 states requiring reporting by 1919.[144]

Although some officials declared reporting to be a disaster from the perspective of actual public health benefit and physician relations,[145] others were more optimistic, particularly in the early years of the enterprise. Pennsylvania, which instituted morbidity reporting in 1905 for a number of conditions including tuberculosis, found physicians quite compliant with reporting requirements: "It has not yet been found necessary to proceed against any physicians for not reporting."[146] Vermont had some 10,000 physicians who made 75,329 reports for infectious disease the first year the law went into effect. Laboratory reporting played a central role in the extension of TB surveillance, in some instances as a prelude to mandatory notification by doctors, in others as a supplement to physician reporting. But of course, for laboratory-based reporting to be successful, physicians had to know about free lab services. "Our laboratory facilities have been advertised all over the State in the newspapers and by means of circulars," reported Dr. J. N. Hurty of Indianapolis, "yet we occasionally receive letters asking us why we have no laboratory. Evidently some people in Indiana read very little."[147]

As they were extended, tuberculosis reporting requirements were, with a few exceptions, almost universally imposed on physicians alone.[148] The communicable disease law in Vallejo, California—in language reminiscent of nineteenth-century sanitary codes—required both physicians and owners or managers of boarding houses, hotels, lodging houses, and tenements to report all "contagious diseases," including pulmonary tuberculosis.[149] Likewise in Utah, where many with tuberculosis went in search of a healing climate, the law explicitly required the owners and proprietors of hotels and boarding and lodging houses to report tuberculosis.[150] Colorado, too, dealt with "a good deal of imported tuberculosis." Its effort to impose reporting requirements on the laity faced resistance. Dr. Henry Sewall noted, "Public sentiment . . . is not with me in [Denver], and that is true of many other towns that I know anything about."[151]

Even so, health officials would hold fast to the belief that "propositions to register the tuberculous in any community may expect opposition from one source, and only one, namely, the medical profession. If lay opposition arises, one can almost always trace it to a medical source."[152] And indeed it was most often physicians who entered the fray with health officials.[153] Thus as tuberculosis reporting advanced, the concerns of private practitioners echoed those that had first been raised in the Northeast. William Baldwin, chair of the National Association for the Study and Prevention of Tuberculosis, noted that doctors resisted filing these reports "on the ground that they interfered with the confidential relations of patient and physician; that they would be made public, and so cause patients to leave physicians who made such reports and go to those who refused to make them; that such patients would be injured in various ways by allowing others to know they had tuberculosis; and that a stigma would also be placed on the family in which the disease existed."[154] In only three cities that had compulsory notification were the records "open to the public."[155] For Baldwin, such evidence provided conclusive proof that TB could be kept confidential and that objections from physicians about the potential harms that could follow notification were without foundation. To assure that health records remained confidential, Baldwin urged the passage of municipal legislation that would definitively declare that public health morbidity reports should "not be open to inspection by any one outside the department."[156]

ELUDING THE SEARCHING EYES OF THE STATE

During the opening battles over TB surveillance, Herman Biggs proclaimed his certainty that "the belief is never aroused in any class of the population, however ignorant, that the institution or enforcement of any sanitary measure is designed for the restriction of individual freedom."[157] But if some patients welcomed public health attention, there is some evidence, albeit scant, that others tried to elude sanitary supervision.[158] Health officials were well aware, for example, that patient "attempts to influence the statements on the death certificates are therefore common." "Direct bribes are offered, and the remark, 'Well, doctor, if I don't get the insurance I cannot pay your bill,' may well be considered a forcible stimulus to some physicians to seek for other causes of death."[159]

When a name was reported, patients could still fairly readily escape the net of surveillance. In New York City, nearly seven thousand cases could not be found at their reported addresses in 1911. Some gave a false address. Others might provide the correct address but then move immediately upon discharge from a hospital. Even cases identified and visited might suddenly disappear without a trace.[160] Given the extraordinary level of supervision that both the city and charity organizations exercised, it is perhaps not surprising that, while there was no organized public protest surround TB reporting, patients intentionally misreported their addresses as frequently as "the clerk records the address incorrectly."[161]

Working-class immigrants made frequent moves, regardless of whether they wanted to escape health inspectors, and it was these patterns of migration that made surveillance all the more difficult.[162] When a breadwinner suffered from a chronic, debilitating disease, the moves were undoubtedly downward.[163] And tuberculosis was the paradigmatic disease associated with immigrants and economic devastation.[164] For Rose Cohen, who arrived in New York City with her aunt in 1892, the pattern of moving was tied to shifts in economic fortune and contributed to her own illness. They first lived with Rose's father in one room of a three-room tenement with another family of five. Her aunt shortly left to live with another family as a domestic servant. Rose and her father moved to Broome Street in 1893, where they were joined in their two rooms by her mother and four siblings. They paid $7.00 per month in rent. The depression of 1893, however, soon forced the family of seven to move back to Cherry Street when both Rose and her father lost their jobs as fellers, sewing the lining of men's coat sleeves. Three lodgers joined them in a three-room tenement. Rose moved out in 1894 to work as a domestic servant, leaving only nine living on Cherry Street. She lived in the family's kitchen. Before the end of 1894, her father was once again employed and the family moved to Clinton Street.[165] The cycle of change was reflected in Rose's health. Tuberculosis became a "long, drawn-out affair. It had no definite beginning and promised to have no end."[166] It was not visits from health officials or charity workers that Rose dreaded but rather hospitalization.[167]

The TB program was aimed at halting the downward spiral and forestalling or preventing hospitalization. But there can also be no doubt that as the disease progressed, it became more and more difficult to meet the behavioral and sanitary expectations of the health department—which included basic criteria for proper nutrition, personal hygiene, adequate clothing, intimate relations, ventilation, expectorating and disposing of sputum, and sweeping and dusting the home—and the hand of the health department might feel heavy indeed.[168]

It remains clear, however, that no matter how extensive sanitary supervision had become, many escaped the embrace of the state, by accident or intent, exposing the flaws and limitations that would plague case reporting even as it became a central feature of public health practice in the twentieth century.

3

Raising the Veil

Syphilis and Secrecy

In 1920 Dr. William Edler, a PHS officer and director of the Bureau of
Venereal Diseases at the Louisiana State Board of Health, made clear that
he was ready to use the threat of prosecution to compel physicians to report
disease and that public health warranted limits on privacy. He challenged
the "principle of privileged communications between the physician and his
patient" in matters concerning the public welfare: "No system of government could long endure if it were based on any other principle than that of
the right of the individual is always subservient to that of the mass. Any
other creed spells rank individualism, and individualism carried to its logical conclusions means nothing more nor less than anarchy." Thus the individual "has no rights that conflict with society's interests. In other words, an
infected person's rights cease where community protection begins."[1]

But what seemed so straightforward a matter to Edler, as a matter of public health philosophy, touched on the central and contested questions
posed by public health surveillance. The move to extend notification to
venereal disease (VD) would underscore the divisiveness of these questions.
As in the case of tuberculosis control, struggles would emerge between
health officials advocating for venereal disease surveillance and physicians
seeking to protect the privacy of the clinical relationship. Accommodations
would be negotiated, some of which would give a unique character to venereal disease reporting, setting it apart from the notification requirements
that prevailed in the case of TB.

A DISEASE LIKE ANY OTHER

As early as 1905, the Michigan State Medical Society began to debate the
possibility of venereal disease reporting. Dr. Albert E. Carrier's argument

that venereal diseases should be regarded as contagious and reported to state health officials like other conditions was surprisingly well-received by his colleagues, who saw reporting primarily as a means of data collection rather than direct intervention, except with prostitutes. They shared an understanding that "the innocent victims should be protected from the disreputable notoriety attached to the name of syphilis" and supported the idea of anonymous reporting.[2] But despite this early discussion among physicians, a more serious nationwide debate regarding venereal disease reporting would not begin until the next decade.

In 1911 thirty-five states required some form of TB reporting, but only three states mandated either gonorrhea or syphilis reporting,[3] reflecting physicians' opinion that reporting for VD, while desirable, was simply not yet practicable because of the great social stigma attached to these conditions.[4] The health officer in Detroit, for example, observed in 1911 that it was not yet possible to have a reporting law in his city because "in order that a sanitary law may be enforced it must be backed," and not just by medical but also by "public opinion." To build public support, the Detroit Society for Sex Hygiene organized a series of workshops in public schools and churches as a means of arousing popular sentiment and making a reporting law feasible.[5]

But pressure was beginning to build. In commenting on the state of affairs, Dr. Prince Morrow, a New York City physician at the forefront of investigative and educational efforts regarding venereal disease,[6] argued that it was time to treat such conditions like other infectious threats. "Within recent years sanitary science has been markedly aggressive in attacking all other infectious diseases—even tuberculosis," he wrote in 1911, but "the sanitary forces have paused irresolute, baffled, and driven back" in the instance of "the great venereal plague."[7]

In Morrow's analysis, "secrecy" had "been placed above the interests of the public health," and "sanitary control has been represented as invasion of the private rights of the individual."[8] For him, then, secrecy was an obstacle for public health to overcome: a desire for secrecy kept patients from seeking treatment from physicians,[9] and the "professional secret" would keep physicians from reporting cases to health officials.[10] Indeed, cultural notions about keeping venereal information clandestine would make it extremely difficult for health officials even to begin educating the public about the control of venereal diseases.[11] Those concerned with such control argued that prevention and treatment efforts were "but empty strokes in the dark, impotent and exhausting struggles with an invisible Frankenstein, whose return thrusts reach home unrewarded. A blinded health department cannot control venereal diseases, and reporting gives it sight."[12]

The issues first raised in the controversies over TB reporting were replayed as venereal diseases were addressed beginning in the second decade of the twentieth century. Hermann Biggs predicted that "the ten year long opposition to the reporting of tuberculosis will doubtless appear as a mild breeze compared with the storm of protest against the sanitary surveillance of venereal disease."[13] He failed, however, to anticipate the compromises that health officials would be compelled to make.

TWO-TIERED SURVEILLANCE

New York City, once again, led the nation in instituting reporting. In 1911, in what would be his last major initiative before assuming leadership of the state health department, Biggs proposed a system of confidential health reporting.[14] It reflected the department's desire to use surveillance as a wedge for public health intervention rather than a statistical or epidemiological tool.[15] Biggs would reiterate the theme that he had so ardently stressed in his campaign for TB reporting: "The notification and registration of communicable diseases *always* has as its object the supervision of the cases."[16] Health officials and medical organizations alike were liable to criticize any other rationale for collecting data. In 1913 the Medical Association of the Greater City of New York flatly stated, "The mere compilation of statistics in venereal disease has no value."[17] Physicians too were opposed to the prospect of notification for statistical purposes alone. As one local practitioner argued in 1910, "No man is anxious to figure as a gonorrhoeic or a syphilitic in the statistics of the community, even if his be only a number and not a name." What, further, "are we to expect from such reports, excepting from that portion of the population whose imagination is not already cloyed with statistics concerning the enormities of the beef trust, or the wealth and inequities of our millionaires?"[18]

Biggs thus emphasized, "From the first it was definitely planned to postpone the requirement for reporting cases until provision for a special hospital should have been made. It was felt that as soon as any scheme of public surveillance went into effect the Department might be called on to remove and detain certain flagrant and unruly cases as has been the experience in tuberculosis, and therefore it was necessary to preface any plan with the construction of a properly equipped hospital."[19]

Drawing a sharp class distinction, Biggs asserted that while "those in comfortable circumstances who are afflicted with" venereal diseases will certainly "make every possible effort to be cured," this was not the case with the "poorer classes, the dispensary and hospital patients."[20] This class of people would only take treatment until their symptoms were relieved or their treatment was "more or less interrupted by the necessities of their occupation." Therefore, he argued, the city needed a hospital to provide for "their free and continuous treatment." And "when a person . . . is being treated in a public institution, or is being cared for at the public expense, there is really no reason whatsoever for not at once reporting the case to the public health authorities."[21] In 1911 the Board of Estimate and Apportionment allotted $55,000 for the construction for such a hospital. The medical advisory board to the New York City Department of Health quickly resolved to undertake the "sanitary surveillance of the venereal diseases."[22]

As it moved forward, the New York City Department of Health, echoing the words of Prince Morrow, argued that the standard that had emerged since the late nineteenth century should be extended without exception: "These diseases should be treated as other infectious and communicable diseases dangerous to the public health are treated."[23]

As in the case of TB, public health authorities were aware of the opprobrium that surrounded sexually transmitted conditions, the "stigma [placed] upon the moral character of the person involved."[24] Some health officials suggested that, in treating VD as other infections, its stigma would be mitigated: "We should have the courage to make a stand in this matter and strip the subject of the stigma of shame and deal with it simply as we do other contagious diseases."[25] And always, the public health response was to stress the ability and commitment to secure public health records, which were to be "regarded as *absolutely* confidential."[26]

Recognizing that such assurances were unlikely to yield results, health officials modified the "cardinal point" of TB surveillance.[27] Although physicians routinely held back the names of certain TB patients from health officials, at least in principle TB surveillance was egalitarian once notification was fully established—physicians were required to report *all* cases by name. Whereas the "ignorant poor as well as the social outcasts" could not be trusted, the department reasoned that "cases under the care of private physicians may, in general, be assumed to be much less of a public health menace."[28] Accordingly, New York City formalized a two-tiered system of reporting: all institutions (hospitals, clinics, dispensaries) were required to report cases by name and address; private physicians, however, would withhold the names and addresses of their patients.[29] The recommendations were adopted by the Board of Health in 1912, and between May 1 and December 31 of that year more than forty thousand cases were reported.[30]

The anonymity offered to private patients did not prevent the emergence of resistance—sometimes open and fierce, sometimes indirect—to notification. As members of the Medical Association of the Greater City of New York declared in 1913, reporting represented "an undesirable and useless invasion of the most confidential relationship between physician and patient."[31] But while the medical journals were decidedly open to the notion of reporting, provided that confidentiality be safeguarded and the records be accessed "only under pledges of secrecy,"[32] three large hospitals in the city carried protests to the mayor. It was in reference to this encounter with hospitals that Biggs remarked, "The progress of sanitation, like the warfare of science, has been the history of a continuous struggle against opposition, carried on in the name of the law, religion, personal rights, or expediency."[33] Clearly it was the rights not only of individuals but of the medical community that were at stake here.

As with TB, much of the opposition centered on the fear that health officials would encroach upon the domain of private practitioners. To this charge Biggs emphatically responded: "The department does not desire and has never desired to assume any responsibility, nor do any work which is being properly done by other authorities or agencies. . . . The department does not wish to treat the venereal diseases if some other authorities will furnish proper and adequate facilities for this purpose."[34]

In confronting the claims made by both hospitals and private physicians, Biggs was to make arguments that would become standard throughout the course of the twentieth century, as public health officials would compare their commitment to and capacity for the protection of the confidentiality of medical records to that which prevailed in the private health care sector. "The medical history, as well as the diagnosis," wrote Biggs, "is almost invariably accessible to the entire hospital staff, including not only the physicians and nurses in charge of the case but also certain lay employees engaged in clerical work in the office."[35] By contrast, at the health department, "a single official [is] in charge of the work" and the records kept under "strict restrictions."[36] Biggs echoed the words of others before him like Prince Morrow, who wrote, "It is not probable that the notification proposed by the health board would involve any violation of professional secrecy that ought to be respected. Even were the report of all cases required, the information furnished would doubtless be kept secret by the sanitary officials; it would not be proclaimed from the housetops or in any way made public."[37]

Biggs, too, had to address the charge that despite the commitment to securing medical records on the part of health officials, a changed political climate might obliterate confidentiality and "rend the veil of secrecy."[38] For Biggs, such assertions appreciated neither the virtues of those responsible for the public health—who were "all medical men and well versed in medical ethics"—nor the legal foundations of confidentiality.[39] He rested his arguments on a 1912 New York State appeals court case, *Allen v. Department of Health,* in which the court had rejected the effort of a private citizen to examine the health department's typhoid case records.

William H. Allen had petitioned the health department for access to the typhoid registry, which recorded all cases of typhoid and tracked healthy carriers—individuals like Typhoid Mary who were not sick but who harbored the bacteria and could continue to infect others—over time. Allen gave "no reason or explanation why he desires to inspect these records" and made the request solely "upon his presumed right as a taxpayer" under city charter, which stipulated, "All books, accounts and papers in any department or bureau thereof, except the police and law departments, shall at all times be open to the inspection of any taxpayer, subject to any reasonable rules and regulations."[40] The court had, in fact, ruled in a prior case that citizens had the right to inspect records regarding the award of city contracts.[41] But here the court's opinion differed dramatically because of the nature of the records in question.[42]

In rejecting Allen's claim, the court emphasized the critical importance of according confidentiality to public health records and distinguished them from records held by other municipal departments: "In consequence of the nature of its duties [the health department] becomes the repository of the records concerning the most intimate affairs of the individuals resident within the limits of the municipality, and among these records are doubtless to be found many matters of no real public interest, but which might, if disclosed to whomsoever sought to examine them, be used for sinister or unworthy motives." The legislature, the opinion continued, "evidently appreciated the evils which might result from indiscriminate publicity of the records of the department of health, and it left it to the wise discretion of that department to determine what safeguards and regulations should protect the privacy of its records."[43]

As had been true for tuberculosis, it was also necessary to address assertions that mandatory reporting would drive patients away from the most reputable physicians into the hands of those who were less skilled and responsible and would neglect reporting. Thus notification would, from the perspective of public health, be utterly counterproductive.[44] These fears, which were widespread—they were at the foundation of the decision in England not to mandate syphilis reporting—were dismissed by Biggs as having no empirical foundation.[45]

Finally, administrators from some large hospitals complained that "the notification of cases . . . involve[s] so much clerical work that it is impossible for them to comply"[46]—a reprise of arguments made by physicians in the nineteenth century who had said public health reporting imposed uncompensated burdens upon them. Biggs was unmoved by such concerns and viewed reporting as the public responsibility of those the state licensed to provide health care.

Despite his remonstrations, resistance on the part of both private physicians and medical institutions persisted. Indeed, Biggs was compelled to acknowledge that there were no accurate statistics available for venereal disease in 1912.[47] Only fifteen hundred of the city's eight thousand private physicians had reported a single case. The next year the board of health lamented the lack of cooperation, holding out the hope that time rather than coercion would remedy the situation. The department thus chose not to rely on the aggressive measures that it had employed to increase physician reporting in the instance of TB. It counted instead on "the inherent reasonableness of its purpose and upon broadening ideas among the profession and public, rather than upon its great reserve of legal power, to compel compliance with the new regulations, as it believe[d] that the battle [would] be eventually won as surely as it was in the case of tuberculosis."[48]

Seemingly bearing out this faith in persistence and patience, in 1913 the health department estimated that reporting for syphilis increased 156 percent and gonorrhea, 49 percent over the previous year.[49] But further gains were not to follow. As late as 1918 the health department described VD reporting as wholly inadequate.[50]

If physicians could not be compelled to report the names of their patients, they could be compelled to use the state laboratory or other state-certified laboratories for testing specimens. Beginning in 1919, specimens sent to the laboratories were to be accompanied by patient name and address. Laboratories in turn were required to report the results not only back to the physician but also to "the health officer in the district from which the specimen came," the "health officer of the district in which the laboratory is situated and to the bureau of venereal diseases."[51] But while health officials might have gained access to names, they continued to respect prohibitions on initiating follow-up with a patient unless requested to do so by a physician.

In what represented more of a hope than an accurate characterization of the state of affairs, one official at the Bureau of Preventable Diseases claimed that the lab-based system nurtured "the growing tendency toward a cordial and cooperative relationship between private physicians and health officers."[52] By 1923, however, the New York City Department of Health was so exasperated with the low rates of VD notification that it felt compelled to issue a bulletin reminding physicians of the reporting requirements for VD and the sanctions for violations. It concluded: "If we find that physicians . . . continue to disregard the law requiring the reporting of these diseases, we shall have to take the indicated legal measures."[53]

Such threats, even when combined with arguments about bringing syphilis and gonorrhea in line with other reportable conditions, had a limited impact on physician compliance with New York law. Nationally, however, federal funds and patriotic fervor accompanying the outbreak of World War I moved the majority of states to join New York in instituting VD surveillance—on paper at least, if not in practice.[54]

THE FIRST WORLD WAR
AND THE EMERGENCE OF "VEILED" REPORTING

Although the 1913 Model State Law for Morbidity Reports had recommended reporting of gonorrhea and syphilis by name and address,[55] only thirteen states required venereal disease notification by 1917.[56] The typical model was a two-tiered system of name-based reporting. Vermont had been the first to follow New York and adopt universal reporting in 1915.[57] The Vermont legislation stipulated that "all information and reports in connection with persons suffering from such diseases shall be regarded as absolutely confidential, and shall not be accessible by the public nor shall records be deemed public records." The secrecy of the private clinical relationship was preserved. Physicians were only required to report the name, address, sex, age, nationality, and race of every "charitable patient" they encountered in "hospitals, dispensaries, clinics, homes, asylums, [and] charitable and correctional institutions."[58] In Ohio, likewise, the state director of the Division of Communicable Diseases affirmed, "In notifying the existence of venereal diseases the name and address may be omitted."[59] With war, reporting became part of the nation's understanding of what security necessitated: the struggle against venereal disease and the vice that was thought to drive it became an urgent matter of national defense and industrial well-being.[60]

The PHS's Gertrude Seymour wrote in the *Journal of Social Hygiene* that the campaign against venereal disease was necessary "for the sake of protecting not only soldiers and sailors, but the industrial army as well—the men behind the men behind the guns."[61] Another editorial declared that "early notification is a most important factor in the *warfare* against disease. . . . Physicians should *rally to the good cause* and see to it that their districts are furnished with reliable figures concerning the incidence of communicable disease."[62] Promoting industrial efficiency was the resounding theme: "The fighting and industrial needs of the nation demand that sick men be made well quickly and with certainty. Venereal infection among the civilian population must be controlled to maintain the maximum efficiency to work or fight."[63] Health officials also drew analogies to industrial models of scientific management in stressing the importance of surveillance for achieving efficiency.[64] In such a climate, VD reporting amounted to "economic salvation."[65]

Foreshadowing the rush of legislation that would accompany the wartime enthusiasm for controlling VD, the Western Social Hygiene Society in Tacoma, Washington, passed "resolutions of a very radical nature," calling on state legislatures to adopt venereal disease reporting.[66] In July 1918 Congress enacted the Chamberlain-Kahn Act, which authorized the U.S. Public Health Service to provide states with $1,000,000 per year for two years to fund their anti–venereal disease control efforts.[67] To be eligible for such support, state boards had to meet three surveillance-related criteria: venereal diseases had to be made reportable to local health authorities; cases had to be investigated to determine the source of infection; and finally, penalties had to be imposed on those who failed to meet reporting requirements.[68] But exactly how cases were to be reported was not settled. The PHS followed up on this legislation with a campaign to win the cooperation of physicians, urging them to "pledge" to report venereal diseases according to state law.[69] Of great significance, Surgeon General Rupert Blue had suggested that such reporting could be accomplished by using serial numbers in lieu of names.[70]

By 1919 all states required venereal disease notification. A model public health act, which had been proposed by the PHS and had suggested that notification be by name,[71] had, "if not in full, at least in its main point, . . . been passed in forty-two states."[72]

Forty states permitted reports using a serial number or patient initials.[73] Of these, seventeen specified that names were to be reported only when the patient "fails to observe proper precautions."[74] In 1918, for example, Massachusetts adopted what was known as the West Australian method for coded reporting, which required that patients be informed that their case would be reported by code. The method was intended to protect both patient *and* physician identity: "At the first visit or consultation the physician furnishes the patient with a numbered circular of information and advice. At the same time he fills out the numbered report blank attached to the circular of advice and mails it to the state department of health. If the patient has been under the care of another physician previously, the second physician consulted notifies the first one on a special blank provided for that purpose. If the patient fails to return to the attending physician for a period of six weeks, the physician notifies the state department, which, in turn, notifies the local board of the community in which the patient resides." Physicians were required to report names "only when [the patient] will not follow proper medical advice or cease from infecting others." In this manner, the state felt that it was possible, "as far as it is consistent with the best interests of the public health, [to] respect the patient's instinctive desire for secrecy."[75] The vast majority of Massachusetts cases were reported by serial number: in 1918 only 11 percent of VD reports to the state were made by name; in Boston that same year, all but 8 percent of the cases were reported by serial number.[76] Like Massachusetts, California adhered to the West Australian method for reporting. California patients were given a pamphlet upon diagnosis informing them that reporting was anonymous unless they failed to comply with the law: "If you want your name kept secret," the booklet instructed, "follow these instructions carefully."[77]

Illinois adopted a similar system in 1917, allowing reporting by key—a numeric code—if the "diseased person" was under the regular care of a reputable physician, was not a prostitute or "an associate of prostitutes," and was not in active military duty. For their part, physicians had to observe certain standards of care, including keeping a record of the case and placing the key identifier on all prescriptions. In commenting on these requirements, one editorial stated, "Only prostitutes need be reported in full and no sane man"—much less a "patriotic physician"—"will question the wisdom of that."[78] Druggists were also required to keep records of all prescriptions by name and address unless the prescription bore the physician's key number. The law specifically protected druggists' records from all but local and state health officials.[79]

THE MEDICAL RESPONSE

Before the war, while the American Medical Association had acknowledged the role of public health in the control of venereal diseases—calling for "the centralized control of venereal infections through special divisions of the proper public health and medical services"—it withheld any support for VD reporting.[80] But the patriotic imperative generated by the war would linger and help to inform clinical attitudes about reporting.[81]

In 1919 Dr. H. N. Cole, a professor of dermatology and syphilis at Ohio's Western Reserve University Medical School, urged that the venereal campaign persist: "It is the patriotic duty and the moral duty of every physician and parent to report all cases of venereal disease by name and address making a particular attempt to find the source of the infection."[82] Health officials hectored the clinical community that failed to take reporting seriously, suggesting that they undermined the command capacity of public health generals, were un-American, and failed in the duties of citizens to the state. Particularly shameful were physicians who objected to VD reporting on the grounds that it would "injure the doctor's practice." Such calls were increasingly taken up by physicians. The issue of privacy, protected for the sake of the physician, had to be weighed against the social costs of illness: "Shall the medical profession, for the sake of the paltry dollar, treat lightly efforts to learn the prevalence, the method of control, and the cure for the diseases which produce so many sterile men and women, so many chronic invalids who, with their continual suffering, become burdens to their friends and often to the community and the State?"[83]

The African American medical community, like others,[84] supported compulsory reporting and case finding. The nation's only black physician organization, the National Medical Association, took a strong stance against treating VD differently from other infectious conditions. "Is it not evident from the precautionary methods adopted by health authorities in the control and prevention of smallpox, diphtheria and other communicable disease," asked a physician writing for the National Medical Association, "that these same health authorities are negligent and inconsistent, when, solely because of temerity, syphilis and gonorrhea are permitted to live and thrive?"[85] They felt that statistics needed to be full and complete "so that health authorities may . . . throw around the 'Great Society' the strong arm of protection from unnecessary illness and preventable death."[86] "The doctors," said one Nashville practitioner, should "report communicable diseases not primarily because they wish to be 'within the law,' but rather they desire . . . thru love for the commonwealth . . . the conservation of human resources."[87] Echoing the position that Louisiana's William Edler took in 1920, a New York physician who addressed the National Medical Association at its annual meeting said that the doctor regards reporting "as an invasion of the personal rights and liberty of his patient and himself. But individual rights are always subservient to those of the mass."[88] The physician who failed in the duty to report "is guilty of criminal negligence" and little better than "the man who robs a bank, wrecks a train, administers poison, burns a home, bombs Wall Street or takes a life."[89] Indeed, "if such a doctor exists," who "for selfish reasons . . . may remain silent and reap a financial harvest," then "he is a bar to domestic tranquility, a menace to the public health, and a reproach to the 'great profession.' It is needless to say he should be immediately and permanently debarred from the healing art."[90]

This tough stance was matched by an equal determination to prevent questions of race from modulating the public health approach to VD in any way. Black physicians emphasized, "We need not take time to inquire where the greater prevalence lies": "No race, no class, no color is immune." The most active measures should be taken against prostitution, "the great source from which venereal infection is gotten and brought into the family by the male portion of the population."[91] It was a sad paradox that health officials might quarantine a home with a case of smallpox, while "in the adjoining home is a victim of syphilis, with mucous patches in his mouth and leutic ulcerations of his body, the Beau Brummel of the red light district." Why, questioned a Philadelphia physician, did such a man remain "free to invade at will any and every section of the community? He is a regular patron of the public soda fountain across the street; a frequent visitor to the public drinking cup in the park around the corner and his fine clothes and gentlemanly bearing have given him access to some of the exclusive families whose daughters vie for his attentions and affections."[92]

Outside of "the maintenance of clinics for the treatment of infected patients and the enforcement of laws against prostitution," however, the black community wanted sovereignty. The editors of the *Journal of the National Medical Association* thus highlighted the stance of Millard Knowlton, a health officer in North Carolina, who insisted, "Each race can best work out its own salvation from venereal diseases by raising its own leadership."[93]

By the 1930s, systematic neglect compounded by racism made possible the start of a forty-year PHS study of the effects of untreated syphilis. Begun in 1932, the investigation used a group of patients originally identified in Macon County, Alabama, as part of a demonstration project that had recommended mass testing and treatment of syphilis in the South. When money for testing and treatment dried up in the midst of the Depression, PHS officers saw an opportunity to document the damaging effects of the disease and, ostensibly, to pressure southern legislatures to fund new treatment programs.[94] Researchers and physicians involved in the Tuskegee Syphilis Study, however, chose not to inform the study's participants that they were infected with syphilis or educate them regarding its treatment or prevention. The doctors involved deliberately misled the men, telling them that they were receiving treatment for "bad blood"—a generic term that referred to a variety of ailments—rather than syphilis. Nonetheless, during the study's recruitment period, PHS officers deceptively provided inadequate treatment for syphilis as a means of securing the trust of the men and the support of the State Department of Health. Although the PHS's Division of Venereal Diseases—the driving force behind Tuskegee—began using penicillin in several of its clinics across the nation in the early 1940s,[95] it failed to provide the drug to study subjects. Not only did the PHS remain committed to seeing the study through to its end, but it also used the existence of penicillin as a rationale for continuing the study. Never again would the PHS find such a group of untreated individuals.[96] In the closing decades of the twentieth century, as the American AIDS epidemic increasingly affected black communities, Tuskegee would come to crystallize African American mistrust of public health.[97]

THE "USUAL METHOD"

Concerns about the patient's desire for secrecy and the physician's resistance to the provision of names had dictated the course of veiled reporting. It was nonetheless possible to reconcile this departure with the broad mission of public health surveillance. As one medical commentator wrote in 1920, while "the first essential in the control of any infectious disease is to locate the disease," in the instance of venereal infection "the object to be attained in locating a case . . . is not to ascertain the identity of the patient, who is under proper treatment and is respecting the regulations as regards the exposure of others to infection, but to locate, and get under treatment, the sources of infection—the disease spreader."[98] From the outset, then, reporting that shielded the identity of the patient constituted not an exception but rather the "usual method."[99]

Thus while some health officials would have preferred names, few publicly challenged a veiled reporting system as being incompatible with the goals of public health.[100] Indeed in 1926, despite the ubiquity of shielded reporting for VD, the PHS declared that syphilis, gonorrhea, and chancroid had been "made notifiable *in common with* other recognized communicable diseases."[101] An editorial in *Social Hygiene* viewed the veiled reporting schemes in place in most states as giving "health officials the same authority . . . as is accorded them in dealing with other dangerous communicable diseases." The editorial maintained that "this trend is so widely endorsed and laws and ordinances for its affectuation have been so generally enacted as to fairly entitle it to be considered accepted policy."[102] By 1936 ASTHO gave tacit approval to such veiled notification, asserting that "the requirement of reporting by name or other identifying information . . . interferes with [physician] compliance with the rule" and drives patients away.[103]

New York City's veiled reporting system was viewed by its public health officials as entirely consistent with their aggressive campaign to control VD launched in the mid-1930s, which involved providing free laboratory diagnostic testing, distributing free drugs to private physicians, and dispatching teams of epidemiologists to work with clinicians to "bring in for examination possible sources of infection and contact to their patients."[104] Health officials described the program as a service to physicians rather than an obligation borne by them, which was no doubt critical to its success. Physicians forwarded the names of 650 contacts for investigation during 1937, the program's first year. Fifty-two percent of the investigations resulted in a person with previously undiagnosed infection coming in for treatment.

Nurse epidemiologists were also responsible for following up on "delinquent cases," and the health department described them as "agents of the doctors," whose "chief concern is the return of the patient to the referring physician." In 1938 the nurses investigated 360 cases, the majority of which had either given a false address or moved. Of the 167 cases actually located, 50 percent returned to their physicians to resume treatment. The result of the new system was vastly improved case reporting. Prior to 1938 the department had used the count of positive laboratory results to estimate the levels of VD. They ceased this practice in 1938 because physician reporting had increased some 126 percent in just one year. Remarkably, by the second quarter of 1938, the number of cases of syphilis and gonorrhea reported by private physicians exceeded those of public health clinics (whose reporting had also increased 135 percent).[105]

COERCION'S PROPER PLACE

As surveillance was extended, it set the stage for the exercise of the state's coercive authority. But just as citizens with high moral standards need not be subjected to the full requirements of reporting, they also need not be quarantined or isolated; these measures were appropriate primarily for the most "delinquent" cases.[106] Wisconsin, for example, was quite explicit in stating that its quarantine law was "primarily intended for unmanageable persons who are a public menace."[107] Typically, this meant prostitutes and their associates.[108]

While recourse to legal sanctions might be necessary for prostitutes and the occasional "delinquent" or "irresponsible patient,"[109] physicians claimed they bore responsibility for "compel[ling] the indifferent infectious patient to continue under some responsible medical guidance, if not one's own." The "physician is morally obligated to array himself determinedly, if gently, on the compulsory side."[110] Physicians were in the proper position to apply pressure on patients. Thus even if debate about whose authority was superior persisted, public health authorities and doctors were of the same mind when it came to coercion in the instance of VD. It was appropriate. And when the best efforts of those in the field of public health and medicine fell short, it was justifiable to call on law enforcement, not only to detain but also to confine threats to the public health.

Although health officials saw "the need for a place of detention, which is neither a hospital nor a jail," one or the other had to suffice. Jails were primarily used as fertile places to identify the infected rather than isolate them. Officials urged that "the opportunity should be seized to make examinations and institute treatment of all persons confined in these jails."[111] In New York, however, even arrest without conviction made one suspect: "Every person arrested for vagrancy, for violating the tenement house law or for frequenting disorderly houses or houses of prostitution" was required to be held for examination for venereal disease; courts and magistrates were required to report the names of all persons detained for testing.[112]

FROM CASE FINDING TO EPIDEMIOLOGY

In the period between the two world wars, supporters of reporting continued to favor secrecy, for the sake of both physician and patient cooperation (fig. 13). Louis Dublin, the chief actuary and vice president of the Metropolitan Life Insurance Company, and his colleague Mary August Clark— America's leading advocates for the creation of systematic statistical data on morbidity and mortality—stressed, "There is hardly any other problem in public-health education that requires more tact in the creation and management of public opinion than that of venereal-disease notification and control. The idea must be 'sold' skillfully. Any attempt to enforce the provisions of a venereal-disease notification act which ignores the patient's desire to keep knowledge of the case from his friends and neighbor will probably fail to produce results commensurate with the effort." Physicians remained a key constituency to whom it was necessary to cater: "Both physicians and patients," Dublin and Clark underscored, "must be shown by actual examples of confidence maintained that a notice to the local and State board of health will not jeopardize the physician's or patient's social and economic interests."[113]

While the interwar period would see the persistence of privacy concerns, it also saw subtle transformations in the intended uses of surveillance data with the advancement of epidemiology, the basic science of public health. To be sure, notification continued to be seen as a tool for direct intervention

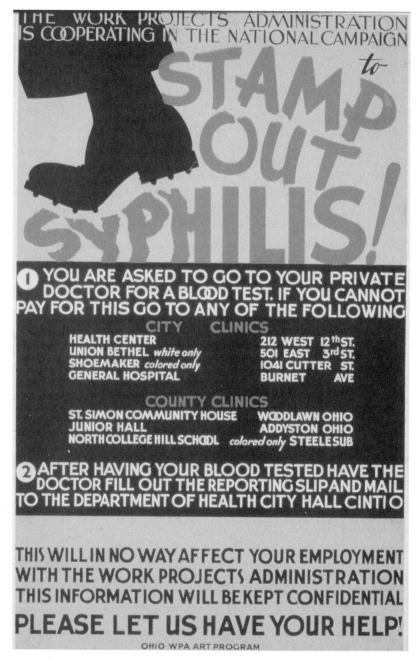

Figure 13. Ohio Work Projects Administration, *Stamp Out Syphilis,* 1940. Both physicians and the public were exhorted to adhere to reporting requirements and were assured of the confidentiality of the records. Work Projects Administration Poster Collection, Library of Congress.

with the contacts of the infected and, in very limited instances, the infected themselves.[114] Indeed, the very concept of surveillance suggested such measures.

Health officials had sometimes acknowledged that surveillance could serve purposes other than intervening with individual patients—that it could provide the basis for research, the allocation of public funds, and the organization and planning of public health programs[115]—but clear expressions of support for the compilation of data for such purposes did not come until the end of World War I.[116] Thus when in 1919 the PHS's Gertrude Seymour wrote, "Whether no other argument on behalf of reporting is given save that of the desperately inadequate information at present concerning the extent of syphilis and gonorrhea—this lack of statistical evidence alone surely should suffice," she entered the vanguard of health officials articulating a new function for surveillance.[117]

In 1928 Tomas Parran, then assistant surgeon general of the PHS, wrote that "statistical research" had to be considered "an integral part of other aspects" of the public health approach to the syphilis problem.[118] That same year, Michigan's health commissioner lobbied for name-based VD reporting because having names made the epidemiological study of venereal disease easier and more efficient, not because they were needed for public health intervention.[119] For the eminent epidemiologist Wade Hampton Frost, a more systematic statistical approach was advisable, even when the health officer believed he knew where interventions were most likely to assist in the control of disease and had concrete measures to apply: "For the defense of many, perhaps most, of the measures" in the public health arsenal, officials quite simply lacked "statistical proof" that what they did worked. Thus while epidemiology might be viewed as "not directly applicable to the health officer's problems," it was time to use epidemiology to demonstrate the effectiveness of public health. This would represent the "strongest asset in winning popular support" for more contentious measures.[120]

Accordingly in 1928, in conjunction with the Social Hygiene Association and state and local health departments and medical societies, the PHS undertook "a census of syphilis cases" in selected communities.[121] These large surveys suggested that the notification system was inadequate for the accurate epidemiological characterization of the prevalence of sexually transmitted diseases. For the PHS, the question was not merely one of being able to identify all cases, but determining the degree to which syphilis shortened life span, reduced productivity, and increased costs of institutional care. Federal health officials were also concerned with assessing the accuracy of physician training in diagnosis and treatment and improving medical school curricula.[122] Ironically, while notification was being justified in the name of epidemiological research, such research was demonstrating the limitations of case reporting. This was a theme that would surface repeatedly as the role and function of notification was debated over the course of the century.

With only a few exceptions, the custom of private physicians reporting by key or serial number or patient initials would continue in most states through the 1930s and into the 1940s.[123] In large measure, health officials considered coded reporting adequate during a period when, given the high cost and long course of therapy, the vast majority of VD patients were treated in public clinics or dispensaries rather than in the offices of private physicians. (Indeed, to this day New York physicians may report "the patients' initials . . . in lieu of the patient's name," while providers must maintain a record of their coded reports with the idea that, at some point, they might be compelled to release the name.)[124]

With the introduction of penicillin as an effective treatment for syphilis and gonorrhea in 1943, health officials renewed interest in reporting for the purposes of contact tracing.[125] Because VD now could be treated rapidly and effectively in private practice—often with a single dose of a slow absorption form of penicillin—"case-holding no longer was the problem. Emphasis was gradually shifted to case finding."[126] On the grounds that "every existing case of syphilis or gonorrhea was caught from someone who had that disease," the PHS, in conjunction with the American Social Hygiene Association, launched its campaign: "Find the Missing Million—and Help Stamp Out VD." Thus the new public health dictum was "It is essential to *find* these infected people—the 'contacts'—who may have transmitted or acquired the disease."[127] This was the context within which the shielded reporting option was subject to reconsideration in some states.[128]

In 1943 Connecticut began requiring reports by full name, age, address, and occupation with the explicit stipulation that "such reports of infected persons shall be confidential and not open to public inspection." Physicians were further required to report individuals who failed to return for observation or treatment. In addition, physicians were required to attempt to determine the source of infection and, if successful, report this name "in strict confidence."[129] In Massachusetts, on the other hand, physicians continued to report the cases that they were treating by serial number. But as of 1946 they were required to report the name, age, sex, race, and marital status of the supposed *source* of infection, unless that source was the husband or wife, as well as all identifying information for any person that the patient may have infected, with one important caveat: reporting need not be by name if the attending physician was satisfied that such contacts "ha[d] been brought under medical observation."[130]

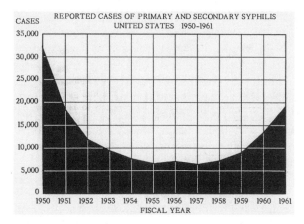

Figure 14. Reported cases of primary and secondary syphilis, United States, 1950–61. U.S. Public Health Service, *The Eradication of Syphilis: A Task Force Report to the Surgeon General Public Health Service on Syphilis Control in the United States.* Washington, DC, 1962.

With the new public health investment in controlling syphilis, the incidence of and death rate from venereal diseases began to drop. According to Leona Baumgartner, commissioner of health in New York City, the rate of syphilis declined from 55.9 per 100,000 in 1948 to 6.2 per 100,000 in 1953. By 1957 the rate was 3.8 per 100,000.[131] In the wake of such successes, public health officials began writing articles asking, "Are Venereal Diseases Disappearing?" and the leading medical journals on venereal disease ceased publication.[132] Congress also cut back federal funding for VD programs in the 1950s.[133] Medical triumph led to complacency: with the new ease of treatment, patients were increasingly treated in the offices of private physicians rather than public clinics, making it more difficult to continue an aggressive contact tracing initiative.[134] Thus while death rates from syphilis steadily declined, the number of cases began to increase in the late 1950s and early 1960s (fig. 14).[135]

In the face of an increasing problem—in 1963 the PHS estimated that private physicians reported only 11.3 percent of their cases and that, even with the efforts of public clinics, only 28 percent of all cases were being reported, drastically limiting potential for health departments to follow up with sexual contacts[136]—there was a growing sense of alarm.[137] As a *Journal of the American Medical Association* article asserted, "Every case should be considered an emergency, be reported, and each patient be interviewed for sex contacts by a trained health department interviewer."[138]

As it became apparent that at least 50 percent of its syphilis cases were not being reported, Philadelphia, which had long offered free laboratory testing and drugs for indigent patients in exchange for a voluntary case report from the physician, adopted the New York lab-based reporting model. Health officials sought to have labs voluntarily report the name and address of all reactive serologies as well as the names of the physicians ordering the tests. After five years, it became clear that a voluntary approach was inadequate, and the city made lab-based reporting mandatory, providing a means for health officials to contact private physicians, solicit more information regarding each case, and inform physicians about the department's contact tracing program.[139]

Reflecting the new sense of urgency, the PHS renewed its interest in VD control. In 1961 Surgeon General Luther Terry created the Task Force on Syphilis Control, which, under the leadership of Leona Baumgartner, was dumbfounded by "the shockingly inadequate reporting of the disease."[140] Speaking for the task force, Baumgartner argued, "The spread of syphilis can be stopped by vigorous efforts to build a bridge, a highway, a transmission line, between the laboratory, the doctor and the public."[141] Thus the primary recommendation of the task force was to aggressively enhance reporting and contact investigation: "The individuals who have syphilis have *got* to be found. . . . It is *not* enough for the physicians to treat those who come to them. They must report their cases to the health officials who are in a position to follow up all contacts." Moreover, "since it is clear that in many instances the physician does not report all his cases of syphilis, health authorities must go to him."[142]

Congress responded to the recommendations of the task force in 1962 with an appropriation of $6.2 million for the nationwide syphilis eradication effort. The goal of the program was to eradicate syphilis by 1972, leaving a structure in place for the subsequent eradication of gonorrhea.[143] Given these aims, and the abysmal levels of VD case reporting by physicians, a major thrust of the program was laboratory-based reporting.[144] At the outset of the eradication initiative, at least fifteen states had laws requiring name-based laboratory reporting of reactive tests for syphilis.[145] Los Angeles, for example, had adopted mandatory lab-based reporting in 1962 after nearly 40 percent of city labs failed to cooperate with a system of voluntary lab reporting "for fear of upsetting doctors and losing business."[146] Indeed, laboratory directors initially resisted compulsory notification, arguing that physicians bore the legal requirement to report. If physicians refused to obey the law, how could laboratories presume to interfere in the doctor-patient relationship? Arguing further that laboratories could not provide the extra clerical staff that would be required to submit reports to the health department, a handful of lab directors, some of whom were physicians, refused to comply. But by 1964 reporting had improved vastly and the health department refrained from taking any legal action.[147]

At least half and possibly two-thirds of the states and some eighty locales had adopted mandatory lab-based reporting for venereal diseases by 1966,[148] accounting for 62 percent of all reported cases.[149] Typical of lab-based systems were strict prohibitions preventing health officials from contacting either patients or their potential contacts directly "until a diagnosis has been reported to the local health officer by the attending physician." In California, this was true not only for VD, but also for tuberculosis, diphtheria, and typhoid, which were considered to be of "particular importance" and had been folded into the mandatory laboratory reporting regulation.[150]

While health department procedures for contacting physicians and patients varied, Norfolk, Virginia, developed a model originally advanced by the CDC.[151] In this locale, after instituting lab-based reporting and requiring all serologic testing for VD to be processed by the city laboratory, epidemiologists would check each reactive serology test to determine whether the individual had previously been reported to the health department. If not, the attending physician would be sent a VD morbidity card with a self-addressed stamped envelope to complete and return to health officials. Lab tests, after all, did not represent a definitive diagnosis of syphilis. For that, the physician had to interpret the lab results in light of the patient's history and a clinical examination.[152] A second card would be sent if necessary, followed by a phone call and then a personal visit. Health officials next requested physician permission to contact and interview cases. "If the physician refuses to permit an interview with the patient, the case is closed without further followup." When the health department persisted in this time-intensive fashion, which ultimately concluded with personal interaction between doctors and officials, physicians characteristically agreed to allow their patients to be contacted; in only one instance did a patient refuse an interview.[153]

Virginia attempted to impress its investigators with the importance of maintaining confidentiality and securing trust: "Never reveal the name of an informant to a contact. . . . never gossip, for loose talk reduces an investigator's effectiveness to zero," leave only unmarked envelopes containing appointment materials for individuals not contacted personally, and "avoid taking medical records into the field (if they must be taken, avoid displaying them and exercise every care to prevent loss)."[154] Virginia investigators sought to be seen "as a helpful friend." To gain trust (and information about the whereabouts of the individuals they sought out), investigators were encouraged to "develop acquaintances in places where people gather to spend their leisure, such as in bars or restaurants." In sharp contrast, "police and sheriff's files should be used only as a last resort, for the investigator must avoid being associated with law enforcement."[155] It was imperative for public health investigators to distinguish themselves from all forms of punitive public authority. Health department investigators were to adopt an undercover posture, to blend into the community, not stick out as health officials as had visiting nurses in the era of TB.[156]

In 1962 federal funding became available to support the recruitment and training of contact investigators to visit private physicians. The program made clear the degree to which access to confidential information did not depend on the physician. The challenge was to win the trust and support of physicians and their consent to contact the patient, not to obtain the patient data itself, for this was already in hand. Physicians who failed to cooperate with health officials, the PHS believed, "most often . . . had . . . a misperception of how we performed our interviews and the lengths to which we would go to protect patient confidentiality" when conducting contact tracing.[157]

Misgivings and misunderstandings would not be limited to physicians. While the vast majority of public health practitioners firmly supported name reporting, a small group remained opposed.[158] In one survey, about 10 percent of state and local health officers surveyed rejected mandatory reporting, typically on the grounds that either voluntary reporting was preferable or that any type of reporting would drive patients away from competent care.[159] In Ohio, for example, while the health officials supported mandatory lab-based reporting in theory, they felt that in Cincinnati physicians would refuse to comply and would send specimens outside the city limits, largely because Ohio law did not recognize health department records as confidential. Health officials in Cincinnati thus proposed an alternative laboratory reporting system based on serial numbers that would work much the same as a name-based system.[160]

In facing the concerns of those who raised questions about reporting and violations of privacy, ASTHO—which had three decades earlier asserted that coded reporting was preferable to the use of names—held, "It should be understood that reporting *by name* implies no loss of confidentiality to the patient. Maintenance of strict confidentiality is a part of the code of public health workers engaged in the epidemiological process."[161] But clearly the secrecy that had been provided by coded reporting no longer existed. The federal field manual for contact investigators stressed that when making contact with physicians the investigator should use information regarding the patient's name, address, marital status, occupation, and medical history "during your conversation with the physician to convey to him that everything you do professionally is done in a personalized confidential manner."[162] Personal visits could accomplish much. But if after such encounters the physician continued to decline either to report the case or consent to have the patient interviewed, the contact investigator still retained the patient's name and other personal information. He or she lacked only the authority to act on that information until that patient was reported as a contact by another individual.[163]

In all, the renewed national effort resulted in a 19 percent increase in reporting in 1963 alone.[164] By 1966 the PHS estimated that "the majority of the physicians in private practice have been visited at least once."[165] Contact tracing was also enhanced: in 1960 only 62 percent of the reported cases of primary and secondary syphilis were interviewed by health officials, whereas by 1966 nearly 90 percent of such cases were interviewed. The PHS estimated that such contact investigation produced thirty-three undiagnosed cases for every report.[166]

DOCTORS DIVIDED

Despite these gains, success once again set the stage for a diminution of attention and effort. The PHS cut back on visits to private physicians in 1967 in the face of continuing personnel shortages created by the failure of funding to keep pace with activities.[167] Although some CDC officials used this as the occasion to advocate for mandatory testing for all hospital admissions,[168] the surgeon general's Task Force on Syphilis Control instead recommended intensified contact tracing efforts in all high incidence areas, dubbing the program Operation Pursuit.[169] The goal was to identify individuals who might be unaware of their exposure, screen them, and provide treatment where appropriate.[170]

Because of the need to provide treatment to the unidentified, major medical associations began to back the war against venereal diseases and, for the first time, forcefully advocate for reporting.[171] The most important of these was the AMA. In 1964 the organization took "official cognizance of the resurgence of syphilis and gonorrhea to the proportions of a national health problem," though only vaguely promised to provide "guidance" to physicians on matters of epidemiology.[172] It studiously avoided the "delicate problem" of "divided loyalty"—the clash between the claims of individual privacy and the needs of the community as a whole.[173] But by 1966 the AMA was forthright and unambiguous: "The physician and the health authorities should understand the importance of reporting *all* cases for epidemiological investigation."[174] In 1971 the AMA would strengthen its resolve to support reporting, urging its members to report cases in a timely fashion. In those states that did not already have lab-based reporting, the AMA called for its adoption.[175]

The endorsement of the AMA notwithstanding, physicians on the ground remained reluctant.[176] A committee of the New York Academy of Medicine advised caution: "Above all in treating a disease relating to sex, exposing a patient to disclosure of his private life seems to the physician to violate one of the cardinal principles in the doctor-patient relationship, confidentiality."[177] The problem was one of trust.[178] Results of a national survey, published in the *Journal of the American Medical Association* in 1967, noted that "doctors do not fully trust the confidential nature of health department records and personnel, and that doctors lack complete understanding of reporting as the basis of contact tracing."[179] Even with the best of intentions and the strictest of security measures, physicians feared "that there is always the *possibility* of a mishap" when they entrusted intimate patient data to health officials.[180]

The "very serious under-reporting" that resulted could undermine the public health war on VD. In 1970 a national study determined that only one in nine private physicians reported cases.[181] William Brown, a VD official at the CDC, thus stressed, "a case of syphilis privately treated and not reported can cause multiple infections to continue to spread geographically."[182] Will J. Dougherty of the New Jersey Department of Health noted, "A doctor may be responsible for respecting his patients' privacy, but he is also responsible for the community when treating a highly contagious disease. We have the medical tools to control venereal diseases . . . if we get cooperation from the doctors in reporting, in allowing their patients to be interviewed about their other contacts and in seeking diagnostic and treatment aid from public health officials on the slightest suspicion."[183] The terms of engagement had thus not changed since Hermann Biggs first challenged the medical profession almost six decades earlier.

PART II

Extending Surveillance

The Politics of Recognition

4

The Right to Know

Detection, Reporting, and Prevention
of Occupational Disease

As efforts were made to expand disease reporting beyond infectious conditions, the interests and institutions engaged in the encounter over surveillance broadened. Tension between clinical medicine and public health, in particular, became less central. In the instance of occupational diseases, debates over reporting turned primarily on questions about the rights of employers to run businesses free of interference on the one hand and the obligations of the state to protect vulnerable workers on the other.

Calls for reporting occupational illness to state governments in the early twentieth century emerged as part of a broad progressive era movement to protect the welfare of workers. Against a backdrop of changes in industrial production, labor unrest, and the growing apprehension that "modern industrial prosperity has been achieved at the expense of the lives and the health of the workers,"[1] a heterogeneous assortment of reformers sought to make capitalist production systems more humane through regulation. The primary advocates for reporting laws were not public health officials associated with municipal or state health departments but rather labor reformers and activists. Reporting of occupational illness was one component of an ambitious social policy agenda that included other innovations in this period such as workmen's compensation systems, minimum wage and maximum work hour laws, and factory inspection requirements.[2]

THE RISE OF OCCUPATIONAL DISEASE REPORTING

On December 29, 1910, Charles Henderson rose to address the factory inspectors, physicians, lawyers, manufacturers, and trade unionists gathered at the fourth annual meeting of the American Association for Labor Legislation (AALL). Arguing that medical practitioners should be required to report industrial diseases to state factory inspectors, Henderson pointed out that mandatory notification to government authorities had been essential in controlling communicable diseases such as scarlet fever and diphtheria. "What is brought to light can be fought in the open," he noted, arguing that employers should be required to keep careful records of all illnesses, to report them by causes and occupation to state authorities, and to allow regular physician examinations to "instruct, warn and fortify" all engaged in potentially dangerous trades. Occupational disease surveillance would give physicians insights into factors aggravating diseases to which workers were exposed and lead to "hygienic devices" to protect them against illness and injury.[3]

F. V. Hamar, president of the Hamar Lead Works in East St. Louis, Illinois, offered a counterpoint. Assured that the AALL "sought to be as just to the employer as the employee," Hamar pointed out that reporting requirements would work only in the unlikely event that all factories used physicians who were equally trained and operating with uniform standards. Absent these utopian conditions, occupational reporting would obscure as much as it clarified. Manufacturers that dismissed sick workers rather than recording their conditions, for example, would appear to be safer than those that reported illness and provided care. Bias could lead physicians to attribute occupational causes to cases with none and thus cause unnecessary deprivation of employment. While assuring those assembled that American improvements in lead manufacturing had eliminated the hazards of the old, dusty workshops of Europe—his own smelter in Kansas, he noted, had not reported a single death or case of "wrist drop," symptomatic of severe lead poisoning—Hamar said his experience in the field raised questions that general calls for reporting failed to address. "What constitutes a case of lead poisoning that justifies a report for your record?" he asked. "Shall we report a case where a single dose of salts has effected a cure? . . . Or shall we report the case of a laborer who we know has a slight attack and is not incapacitated, but who, for family reasons, must continue his employment temporarily until he can find other work?"[4]

The AALL pursued Henderson's vision, launching a lobbying effort that included a four-page leaflet, "Reporting of Occupational Diseases," to press physicians to report cases of occupational disease and the names of the employers to the government. The leaflet—the last page of which contained text for a model law—was sent to lawmakers, editors, and public health officials who might be willing to testify or editorialize on behalf of occupational disease reporting.[5] Part of a broader campaign that included calls for accident reporting and workmen's compensation, disease reporting was seen by the AALL as a step "which may be used in improving . . . work conditions which seriously impair the health, vitality, energy and industrial efficiency of wage earners."[6]

By 1911 six of the eight industrial states in which the AALL had pushed for occupational surveillance—California, Connecticut, Illinois, Michigan, New York, and Wisconsin—had passed laws requiring physicians to report occupational diseases. The laws were similar, with most requiring that physicians complete a form, including employee and employer name and address, whenever a worker was diagnosed with any of six conditions (anthrax, compressed air illness, and poisoning from lead, phosphorus, arsenic, and mercury).[7] All states except Connecticut imposed a penalty, ranging from ten to one hundred dollars, for failure to report, and California and Connecticut offered physicians a fee of fifty cents for each report filed.[8] The Illinois law, in part due to the efforts of industrial hygiene pioneer Alice Hamilton, who in 1910 had directed the state's commission on occupational diseases, required that all employees who came in direct contact with poisonous metals such as lead, arsenic, zinc, or mercury be examined monthly by physicians. Diseased workers were to be reported to the state department of health, which would in turn submit a copy of the report to the department of factory inspection.[9]

In 1912 Maryland and New Jersey joined the states requiring physicians to report occupational illnesses. Maryland's law went beyond diseases linked to metals and poisons, requiring physicians to report "any other ailment or disease contracted as a result of the nature of the patient's employment." This was an amendment that the AALL incorporated into its own lobbying, and one that garnered support from the public health officers, who had become a powerful lobby for infectious disease reporting. At its annual conference in 1913, ASTHO called for a model law that included reporting of twelve specific occupational conditions and "any other disease or disability contracted as a result of the nature of the person's employment."[10]

Even as it enjoyed legislative success, however, the AALL conceded that early warnings about the difficulties of mandatory reporting were being born out. Less than a year after the passage of the first occupational disease reporting laws, the AALL formed a subcommittee to press for standardization, since legislative inconsistencies made it difficult to compare data across states or to make "intelligent use of such statistics rather than merely to compile columns of figures."[11] Some laws required that physicians report diseases to commissions of labor, as the AALL had suggested, while others reported to the boards of health, an approach favored by the state and territorial health authorities. Time requirements varied, with some laws requiring physicians to report the next day, and some permitting a delay of weeks. Most important for the purposes of reform, there were no clear mechanisms for enforcement of reporting requirements, and several states protected employers from legal actions that might lead to a corrective response.[12] The laws in Connecticut, New Hampshire, and Ohio, for example, stipulated explicitly that "no report made pursuant to the provisions of this act shall be evidence of the facts therein stated in any action at law against any employer of such diseased person."[13]

The question of whether a disease was occupational was equally thorny, with critics taking the new legal requirements to task for being both too broad and too narrow. "A man might have been a hard drinker for ten years and acquired arteriosclerosis and Bright's disease therefrom, and he might have worked in lead, which causes the same diseases, for only ten days, yet the present method of compulsory registration would tend to class him under lead occupation," noted W. Gilman Thompson, author of the first comprehensive textbook on occupational disease in America and an opponent of mandatory reporting, shortly after the passage of the New York State law.[14] Cressy Wilbur of the U.S. Census Bureau wondered why efforts ignored diseases found elsewhere that might be aggravated by workplace exposure. Would, for example, tuberculosis exacerbated by workplace conditions be reportable? If so, how would its occupational nature be designated?[15]

STATE AGENCIES AND THE LIMITS OF AUTHORITY

If germ theory made it possible to isolate the organisms that caused diseases such as tuberculosis, typhoid, and cholera, it also provided health officials with authority to track, in the name of the public good, those who harbored such organisms. Diseases of the workplace, by contrast, were often seen as an inevitable by-product of progress, a suffering of the few in the interest of the many. Frederick Hoffman, chief statistician for Prudential Life Insurance, noted at the first AALL conference on industrial disease that "the unfavorable efforts of industry on health have been held to be inseparable from industrial processes required for the needs of the community at large."[16]

But if disease was the necessary price of progress, it was ironic that it proved almost impossible to document that linkage. Alice Hamilton's commission in Illinois, daunted by the complexity of demonstrating causation in most workplaces, had decided to focus only on occupational poisons.[17] The diseases associated with the "dusty trades"—mesothelioma, asbestosis, byssinosis (brown lung), coal workers' pneumoconiosis (black lung), and silicosis—were in the early twentieth century included under the single category of phthisis, believed traceable to infection with the tuberculosis bacillus.[18] Insurance company statisticians had noted the correlation between dust and diseases following the introduction of pneumatic tools: Frederick Hoffman had termed tuberculosis a "trade disease" in 1909, noting that "the degree of frequency in industry is in almost exact proportion to the amount of dust inhalation."[19] In the medical arena, however, the question of cause remained disputed, with many physicians attributing disease among miners, glaziers, and pottery workers to unsanitary conditions at home, to negligence or mental incapacity at the workplace, or to hereditary predisposition.[20]

Deprived of bacteriological backup, public health officials struggled for regulatory authority. Inspectors from state departments of labor were empowered by law to enter the workplace, but no such power was accorded to state public health departments. Commitment to industrial health by the PHS emerged primarily as a preemptive measure after several bills introduced into the 1913 Congress proposed a Bureau of Industrial Safety in the new Department of Labor. Alarmed at the prospect of "another health bureau, in another department of the government," Surgeon General Rupert Blue established the Division of Industrial Hygiene and put Harvard-trained surgeon Joseph Schereschewsky, who had articulated strong opinions about worker fitness when at Ellis Island, at its head.[21] Some companies used state labor agencies to stonewall investigations by the PHS, refused to allow PHS researchers to perform medical examinations on their employees, or agreed only on the condition that researchers share with management the results of medical exams for each employee.[22] By 1917 the PHS had begun withholding the individual results of its examinations from both employee and employer "in view of the confidential character of the information obtained," a policy the PHS would employ in workplace investigations in ensuing decades.[23] While this protected sick employees from dismissal or reprisal, it also denied workers knowledge that they might use to press for the kinds of changes imagined by progressive era reformers.

Legal contests over the limits of corporate regulation were also common. Workers perceived to be particularly vulnerable, such as women, or those in particularly dangerous trades, such as smelter workers, won concessions in court on wages or working hours.[24] The limits of health regulation in the progressive era workplace, however, were most famously captured in *Lochner v. New York,* the 1905 ruling in which the Supreme Court rejected New York State's contention that long shifts in hot, flour-filled rooms put bakers at elevated risk for diseases and should be curtailed. "It might be safely affirmed that almost all occupations more or less affect the health," Justice Peckham wrote for the majority. "There must be more than the mere fact of the possible existence of some small amount of unhealthiness to warrant legislative interference with liberty."[25] Liberty of contract between employer and employed—that is, the "freedom" to work as long as the contract demanded—trumped the regulatory power of the state.[26]

THE INDUSTRIAL PHYSICIAN:
ALLOWING THE MILL TO KEEP ON GRINDING

Company doctors, the linchpin of mandatory occupational disease reporting proposals, were themselves employees subject to rules of contract and the threat of dismissal. The analogies that compared doctor to priest or family member in debates over infectious disease surveillance were hardly appropriate to industrial physicians, whose ranks swelled primarily as a result of employers' interest in protecting themselves against compensation claims and whose salaries were paid by business executives rather than by those for whom they cared. With duties primarily restricted to initial medical screening and treatment of injuries, industrial physicians were also not particularly well-positioned to identify patterns of occupational disease or even to identify individual cases of occupational origin.

"Industrial medicine is, in a measure, a compromise between the ideals of medicine and the necessities of business," Clarence Selby, who was to become the head of the General Motors medical staff and the president of the American Association of Industrial Physicians and Surgeons, wrote in a 1919 PHS bulletin.[27] Selby's report showed how heavily that compromise was weighted in favor of business necessities: of one hundred sixty industrial medical departments surveyed, two-thirds reported to officers responsible for shop floor production or payment of workmen's compensation. Fewer than one in five reported to high-level administrators such as the plant manager or president.[28] While leading figures such as Schereschewsky from the PHS or Sears-Roebuck medical director Harry Mock might portray the shop floor as providing a great human laboratory and an opportunity to study the healthy as well as the sick,[29] most industrial physicians were hired to watch the bottom line of production and cost.

The politics of the medical profession, too, made it less likely that physicians would have the time or inclination to engage in detection and reporting of occupational diseases. Until the formation of its own Council on Industrial Health in 1937, the AMA derided industrial physicians as "finger wrappers," as dispensers of patent medicine, or, most pejoratively, as contract doctors who provided cut-rate services. Condemnations of undereducated hacks spoiling the market for other physicians frequently took the form of backhanded compliments to industrial physicians for having left the practice behind.[30]

When America's entrance into World War I heightened attention to the importance of national production, industrial physicians emphasized how the "scientific" practice of medicine could prevent accidents and help employees work longer. Stressing their intermediate role between engineer and doctor, they routinely referred to workers as human "tools" or "machinery" in need of maintenance or as domesticated animals.[31] "Chickens, race-horses, and circus monkeys are fed, housed, trained, and kept up to the highest physical pitch in order to secure a full return from them," James D. Hackett wrote in his 1925 book *Health Maintenance in Industry*. "The same principle applies to human beings."[32] Harlow Brooks, professor of medicine at New York University, advised the Conference Board of Physicians in Industry that doctors perform their medical inspections with an efficiency that minimized interchange, examining workers "as a horse jockey looks at a horse."[33]

Just as it was along the nation's borders, where immigrant medical exams served to underscore American norms of industrial efficiency as well as to detect disease, the workplace medical examination emphasized intolerance for defective workers and the importance of fitness for duty.[34] As at immigration stations, medical screenings were performed with such speed that they were unlikely to detect any occupational illness beyond a dermatitis, an obvious poisoning, or advanced respiratory disease. This was seen as desirable. The routine physical exam for men proposed by the New England Conference of Industrial Physicians in 1926 included inspection of scalp, eyes and ears, palpitation of neck, chest, liver, kidney and genitals, and examination of spine, feet, legs, and anal canal, all in a suggested completion time of five minutes.[35] Harlow Brooks estimated that one trained physician could inspect "fully one thousand men per day."[36]

Workers themselves regarded these exercises with mistrust, seeing them as a way to weed out "defectives" and union sympathizers.[37] "Have the employers of the United States shown that they are fit to exercise such authority over the lives of their employees?" American Federation of Labor president Samuel Gompers asked in 1914.[38] In 1919 iron and steelworkers included cessation of physical examinations as one of their demands for ending their national strike.[39] Gompers's opposition to medical exams stymied Alice Hamilton's request that they be instituted among munitions workers during World War I.[40]

Thus constrained, occupational disease reporting yielded little reform. Reviewing nearly a decade's progress in 1919, AALL secretary John Andrews noted that the reporting requirements had been useful "mainly as affording occasional clues to individual plants where further precautions should be taken."[41] A representative of the PHS, addressing the National Industrial Conference Board in 1924, told attendees that the agency had great hopes for a standardized form newly created for better record keeping.[42] But Emery Hayhurst, professor of industrial hygiene at Ohio State, suggested that the problems with occupational disease reporting extended well beyond the type of form used. Thirty-one states, he noted, seemed "practically oblivious of the subject of industrial hygiene."[43] Even when the law allowed intervention, he noted, "nothing is done," and officials "simply allow the mill to keep on grinding."[44]

NEW DEAL TO COLD WAR:
LABOR DEPARTMENT ENGAGEMENT AND RETREAT

Workmen's compensation laws, which required companies with high rates of worker injury to pay elevated insurance premiums and barred compensated employees from seeking further redress through the courts, powerfully structured how employers, industrial physicians, and government officials defined the limits of occupational health. Compensation claims would also become a key source of information on occupational disease, for the Bureau of Labor Statistics (BLS), the PHS, and representatives of industrial hygiene trade associations.[45]

Progressive era compensation legislation did seek to resolve the question of what constituted occupational illness—though not in ways that proponents of disease reporting found satisfying. Of the thirty-seven workmen's compensation laws passed by state legislatures in the period between 1911 and 1919, all save Wisconsin's focused on compensation for accidents or injuries while excluding occupational disease.[46] Generally, "occupational disease" was the constellation of conditions *distinct* from those that should be compensated: that is, those conditions whose links to the workplace were either so commonly understood that workers could be expected to know about the risk when they began work or those diseases "ordinary to life" whose links to work were too tenuous to count. Among the latter were tuberculosis and the other long-latency dust diseases. Cancers were also excluded from compensation.

National attention to silicosis in the 1930s—galvanized by a blizzard of worker lawsuits and the Gauley Bridge disaster, in which as many as fifteen hundred workers were killed by acute exposure to silica dust in West Virginia—brought renewed attention to the question of compensation for occupational disease.[47] Rejuvenated by the regulatory ethos of the New Deal and the leadership of Secretary Frances Perkins, the Department of Labor established the Division of Labor Standards in 1934. The division was soon pressing for inspections, inclusion of occupational disease in state compensation policies, and worker participation to make workplaces "as safe as science and law can make them."[48] While conceding the need to contain the skyrocketing claims—more than $300 million in litigation was associated with silicosis by 1934 alone[49]—employers resisted wholesale reform, urging that the definition of occupational disease be limited to those illnesses linked clearly to occupation and that claims made years after exposure be disallowed. Their attack turned on long-standing questions of etiology—how could one know whether a disease was really due to exposure on the current job and not on prior employment or conditions in the home?—as well as on the disjuncture between medical record and actual disability. Was an X-ray indicating the presence of silica in the lungs synonymous with disease? "General and vague language will lend itself to the inclusion of any and every sort of illness and disease to which human flesh is heir," warned Henry Sayer, an insurance company representative.[50]

By 1941 twenty-five states had incorporated occupational disease into their compensation plans. By 1947 thirty eight had done so.[51] Rather than using a uniform procedure, however, each state created its own. Two-thirds compiled lists of compensable diseases and required workers to come before boards or examiners who decided a claim's validity. Many refused to compensate when exposure had occurred years prior to the claim—making it difficult for those with long-latency diseases to collect—and barred rewards for those where the link between occupation and disease could not be proven through X-rays or other "objective" measures.[52]

For all its support for the concept of workplace surveillance, the PHS played a far smaller role than the federal Department of Labor in engaging in debate over compensation criteria, and PHS representatives avoided testifying before state boards to resolve questions of evidence.[53] Instead the PHS focused on laboratory methods—air samples, animal studies, and toxicology profiles of chemicals and poisons—to quantify what levels of exposures would safeguard health.[54]

The PHS approach to occupational disease surveillance was codified by the 1935 Social Security Act, which funded the expansion of public health programs for industrial hygiene and effectively displaced state labor departments from the field.[55] Before 1936 only five state departments of health had industrial hygiene units, but by 1942 thirty-six did. In all but two states labor departments, while critical of what they perceived to be PHS accommodation to industry, shut down their own divisions of industrial hygiene due to lack of funds.[56]

The coming of World War II gave new luster to occupational medicine, reinforcing the notion that its role was to help industry rather than to constrain it.[57] With President Roosevelt and the War Production Board equating industrial mobilization at home with victory abroad, industrial physicians promised to identify sources of lost work time and to incorporate every available worker into manufacturing. As American Association of Industrial Physicians and Surgeons president T. Lyle Hazlett observed approvingly, industrial physicians became the "medical field marshals for the Army of Production."[58] Frank Fulton, medical director of the Eastern Aircraft Division of General Motors, conducted stopwatch studies of ten thousand procedures in plant hospitals to determine how many minutes were required for efficient completion of the medical record, which he termed the "seeing eye" of medicine. Completion of accurate charts, he concluded, added a mere 1.5 minutes to the time required for the delivery of quality industrial health care.[59]

But postwar concerns about communism constrained occupational health interventions. Legislators and corporate lobbyists pressed successfully for further rollbacks to corporate regulation. "I for one shall vote to wean as many [bureaucrats] as possible to keep our government American and from becoming communistic, and we all know that it has been tending that way a long time ago," Oklahoma representative George Schwabe told Congress in a characteristic, post–New Deal attack on the Department of Labor in 1947.[60] Shortly thereafter the department's budget was cut and more than seven hundred employees were dismissed.[61] Congressional efforts to increase job safety in the workplace after the war died in committee, including Senator Hubert Humphrey's 1951 proposal for a bureau to create occupational safety standards and a 1962 effort to provide grants to states for job safety.[62] No postwar job safety bill addressed occupational disease at all.[63]

Organized labor, so energized by the 1935 Wagner Act that had guaranteed the right to collective bargaining, also lost power in the cold war era. The 1947 Taft-Hartley Act limited bargaining rights and required unions to purge officers known to be communists. Calls for such innovations as national health insurance, which Senator Taft would refer to as "the Moscow party line," were soon similarly silenced.[64] This was the era of the so-called Treaty of Detroit, in which labor accepted big industry's offer of wage increases, reduced work hours, and job security but relinquished claims to more radical workplace reform. In the area of occupational health, union emphasis went to securing care for ill workers and their families, now mostly white collar, rather than regulating the conditions that caused disease in the first place.[65]

In such a climate, pursuing mandatory reporting of occupational disease by industrial physicians seemed of dubious value. Victoria Trasko, a junior PHS statistician, piloted a first attempt at a national system of occupational surveillance from 1950 to 1951, combining physician reporting, workmen's compensation data, and occupational information from death certificates in eleven states. Of the more than nine thousand cases of occupational disease she detected, only 20 percent came from physicians' records. "In view of the long experience with required notification of occupational diseases and the continuous inadequacy of resultant reports," she noted, "the need is indicated for a reevaluation of the principle as well as procedures of required medical reporting."[66] For Trasko, greater standardization of workmen's compensation data and greater integration of that data with PHS records represented the direction most likely to provide results.[67]

Trasko's calls for consolidation of medical records anticipated the national movement toward data aggregation that would build in the 1960s. Strikingly, while the idea of centralized medical information would provoke concerns about individual privacy, it would receive a more favorable reception from those at risk for disease in the workplace.

MOBILIZING FOR SURVEILLANCE

The same social movements that began in the 1960s to redefine the politics of privacy also reshaped efforts to track occupational disease. Popular opposition to the Vietnam War, including hostility toward the industrial side of the "military-industrial complex," brought new skepticism about the ability of corporate executives to look after the best interests of either the workers or the public. Rachel Carson's 1962 bestseller *Silent Spring*, with its images of nursing mothers unknowingly passing DDT to helpless infants, as well as Ralph Nader's 1965 *Unsafe at Any Speed* helped replace belief in industrial products as the benign harbingers of progress with a pervasive concern about their devastating effects on humans and nature.

As the environmental movement grew in strength, occupational health would be among the first health issues to be addressed in Washington. A 1968 proposal by Lyndon Johnson to protect "every one of America's 75 million workers while they are on the job" had been defeated by Republicans, conservative Democrats, and business groups, who claimed it would allow the labor secretary to rewrite local fire regulations or cancel football games in the name of safety.[68] Recognition of the need to address questions of industrial safety, however, continued to grow.[69] Studies by Mt. Sinai Hospital's Irving Selikoff documenting elevated rates of asbestosis and cancer among asbestos workers and work by I. A. Buff and Hawley Well establishing the association between coal dust and lung disease among West Virginia miners marked new collaborations between health researchers and labor unions.[70] The deaths of seventy-eight miners in an explosion near Farmington, West Virginia, in 1968 focused federal attention on safety and would bring passage of the Federal Coal Mine Health and Safety Act of 1969.[71]

Labor in other industries was slower to recognize the value of occupational disease surveillance. Of the forty unions surveyed by Ralph Nader's study group in the summers of 1969 and 1970, only four kept records of occupational disease among their members.[72] Nonetheless, a June 1969 conference organized by the Industrial Union Department of the AFL-CIO brought together union representatives and medical specialists to discuss byssinosis, asbestosis, noise, and dust. The textile workers union labeled occupational health "A Must for '70" and condemned the American Textile Manufacturers Institute for failing to sponsor studies of byssinosis.[73] The Oil, Chemical and Atomic Workers Union (OCAW)—among the most aggressive in pursuit of more information on occupational health hazards—held conferences in every district in 1969 and 1970. The format of the meetings reflected contemporary ideas about the importance of a patient-directed approach, with workers addressing panels of scientists and doctors rather than the other way around. Union officials used the meeting transcripts as a guide to data collection about health problems among the membership.[74]

While feminist health advocates emphasized birth control and abortion as choices best reserved for women themselves, the occupational health movement was concerned less with the right to choose than with the workers' right to know about the hazards to which they were being exposed. Toxic chemicals in the work environment were of particular concern.[75]

"We're meeting within the framework of a situation where no one really knows about the problem," OCAW's legislative director Anthony Mazzochi told those gathered at one the first of the OCAW's 1969 health sessions. "Out of the 6,000 or so chemicals in use in industry today, there are only standards for a little more than 400."[76] Echoing environmentalist concern with air pollution, Mazzochi's call for impartial investigation and public discussion of industrial chemicals would in turn be taken up by rubber workers, cotton workers, and others.

Occupational health issues became important enough to warrant strikes. "Our position is that every means should be taken immediately to limit and prevent exposure of the workers to [harmful] chemicals and other materials," Peter Bommarito, president of the United Rubber, Cork, Linoleum and Plastic Workers, explained in 1970.[77] Strikes by rubber and oil workers would wrest commitments from industry to devote as much as five cents per hour worked to occupational research.[78] By 1973 all major oil companies also agreed to establish joint labor-management health and safety committees and to retain independent industrial health consultants at company expense.[79]

Organized labor did not rely on professionals alone. In keeping with the self-help spirit of the time, unions sponsored training sessions to help workers perform occupational health interventions, including air sampling, record keeping, and disease reporting. "Since work-related chronic disease is almost never recognized by medical or labor authorities, a person who goes to a doctor with such an ailment usually cannot expect to have it properly diagnosed as an occupational disorder," advised the chapter entitled "Keeping Health Records" in *Work Is Dangerous to Your Health*, the 1973 guide written "to and for workers" by OCAW chemist Jeanne Stellman and physician Susan Daum (fig. 15). A kind of analog to *Our Bodies, Ourselves*, the volume, which sold more than one hundred thousand copies, included sample medical surveys, instructions on how to preserve medical records and report morbidity and mortality to unions, and descriptions of how to sample air and survey exposure hazards.[80]

The right to know went beyond hazard exposure to encompass workers' access to their medical records. Ivring Selikoff, Howard Buff, and other physicians, aided by journalistic investigations like Paul Brodeur's series on asbestos workers in the *New Yorker*, had documented that employers had tested workers for occupational disease without sharing the results.[81] Coal miners had focused specifically on the "crackerbox breath tests and snapshot X-rays" used by mine operators to deny benefits.[82] They argued successfully that medical examinations should be supplied by independent physicians and that X-rays not be the only gauge of disability. Similarly, a 1974 agreement between U.S. Steel and the United Steelworkers included an explicit agreement giving employees working with coke ovens the right

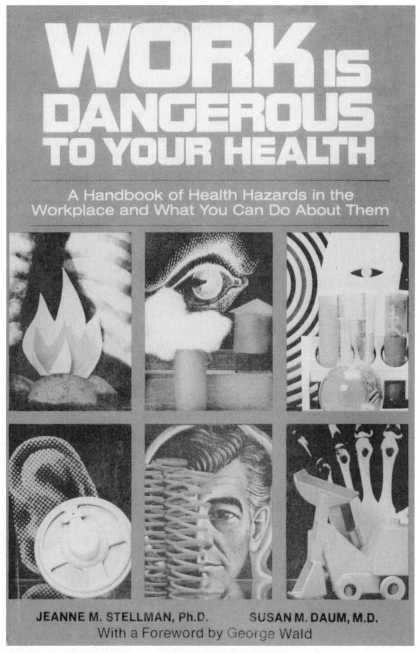

Figure 15. Jeanne Stellman and Susan Daum, *Work Is Dangerous to Your Health.* This 1973 guide on workers' health included a section for employees on the importance of preserving medical records and reporting morbidity and mortality to unions. New York, 1973.

to obtain copies of the examinations and X-rays administered by plant physicians. The agreement was an industry first.[83]

Efforts by government and professional associations to document occupational disease were also clearly in need of overhaul. A 1968 survey found that many states lacked any kind of occupational health entity; where they did exist, the power to advise, adopt, promulgate, and enforce in the arena of occupational health was fragmented among different agencies.[84] Private efforts to document patterns of occupational illness, such as an AMA effort to solicit reports of reactions to toxins from private physicians in 1967, were similarly ill-conceived. "Our hope is that physicians will report these cases to their professional association when they would not report it to the government," AMA representative Henry Howe testified to a Senate subcommittee in 1970. Yet in his own estimation, 98 percent of private physicians had insufficient training to recognize occupational illness.[85] By 1972, after mailing out seventeen thousand report forms and widely publicizing the effort, the AMA had received eight thousand reports from the California government office, to which physicians had long been required to forward all reports of occupational injury or illness, and fewer than five hundred from private physicians. An AMA analyst concluded that voluntary registration was "likely meaningless" and, as they did for venereal diseases at around the same time, recommended compulsory reporting and statistical analysis of data on a national basis.[86]

Registries maintained by manufacturers also offered little of value to public health. Since 1956, for example, DuPont maintained a cancer surveillance program along with a database of hazardous exposures and medical sequelae among employees.[87] The results of this data collection, however, were released only as deemed appropriate to company executives and individuals tested, not to unions or government officials concerned with monitoring larger trends.[88] The Manufacturing Chemists' Association, amid reports that exposure to vinyl chloride caused acreosteolysis, a condition involving destruction of bone and tissue, established a registry in 1969 to track cases of the disease among workers. Less than two years later the association acknowledged that because manufacturers failed to report new cases or financially support the effort, the registry was "dangerously close to collapse." By 1973 it had been abandoned entirely.[89]

THE OCCUPATIONAL SAFETY AND HEALTH ACT:
THE USES AND ABUSES OF PRIVACY

The federal stake in occupational health presaged by the Coal Mine Health and Safety Act of 1969 was fully articulated with the passage of the Occupational Safety and Health (OSH) Act in 1970. A turning point in the legal and rhetorical framing of corporate privacy and occupational disease surveillance, the OSH Act promised the most sweeping regulation of the corporation since the New Deal. The successful passage of an occupational health bill—whose every clause was followed closely by labor and big business alike—has been attributed to the growing awareness of the workplace safety crisis, labor union pressure, the belief by employers that what was conceded in legislation could be constrained by future legal challenge, and the desire by the Nixon administration to capture blue-collar votes.[90]

Whatever its reasons for passage, there was no question that the OSH Act dramatically increased federal investment in the prevention and monitoring of occupational disease. The legislation held out a sweeping promise: "No employee shall suffer material impairment of health or functional capacity."[91] It left intact the long-standing division of responsibility between the Departments of Labor and Health. The Occupational Safety and Health Administration (OSHA), a new agency housed in the Department of Labor, was to set and enforce standards; research to inform those standards would be performed by the newly created National Institute for Occupational Safety and Health (NIOSH), housed in the Department of Health, Education, and Welfare. The first two words in NIOSH's title were significant: unlike previous occupational health efforts located in the Department of Health, Education, and Welfare, this agency was not buried within the bureaucracy but was instead granted the standing and independence of a national institute.

By requiring "accurate statistics on work-related deaths, injuries and illnesses" and requiring employers to "make, keep, and keep available" records on how they were complying, the OSH Act also cut against the growing concern with aggregation of data in corporate and federal government headquarters.[92] NIOSH, as a research institution, would be entitled to perform health hazard evaluations including examination of medical records and testing of employees. Employers selected for participation in the BLS survey of workplace injury and illness would be required to participate. OSHA mandated that employers post an annual summary of all workplace injuries and illnesses for employee inspection. Further, authority to issue and enforce health standards—among the most important and controversial of OSHA's new powers—allowed the agency to prescribe the type and frequency of medical examinations that had to be offered at no cost to employees exposed to hazards.[93]

In theory, these two mandates for disease surveillance—better reports flowing out from the employers on one hand and new government power to come in to inspect records or evaluate health hazards on the other—would form a pincer in which the elusive problem of occupational disease surveillance would at last be grasped. In practice, though, the OSH Act's ambiguities would reprise difficulties that had hampered occupational disease reporting since the progressive era. First, the act offered no precise definition of what was meant by "work-related disease." Second, while OSHA required recording of diseases, it did not mandate their regular reporting to a federal agency and so did not disrupt the ability of employers to shield themselves from the results of disease surveillance. The BLS, for example—afraid to jeopardize employer participation in other, voluntary surveys—chose from the start to make anonymous its annual survey results, declining to require individual companies to reveal their names or locations.[94] While BLS data would give some indication of levels of occupational illness, they would not tell labor advocates which companies were causing the bulk of occupational illness or where to push for change.

Medical screening efforts were similarly constrained by employee fears that physicals would simply be used to screen out the sick, echoing the concerns expressed by labor leader Samuel Gompers a half-century earlier. The 1974 standard that OSHA issued on vinyl chloride, for example, mandated removal of workers at high risk for health problems as a result of exposure but did nothing to guarantee employee salaries or seniority. "It is to me an impossible situation for a worker to be afraid to take a physical examination because he is going to lose the job that he uses to feed his family. It is unbelievable," lamented Dr. Eula Bingham, chair of the advisory committee on coke oven emissions in 1976.[95] A representative of the Oil, Chemical and Atomic Workers Union agreed: "OSHA is fooling itself if it thinks that workers will submit to medical exams when the results may cost them their job, their seniority or their pay rate."[96] OSHA, while noting the "difficult choice" faced by workers, made no provision for wage or seniority guarantees in its 1976 standard on coke oven emissions or on subsequent standards the agency issued on benzene, arsenic, or cotton dust.[97]

In the absence of such protections, the questions of who had access to medical records and who was authorized to interpret them was contested by unions and industry. Regulations mandated that the results of voluntary medical exams be furnished to OSHA, NIOSH, and, "at the request of the employee, to his physician."[98] Workers pressed for the right to hire independent physicians, for long-term retention of records by those employers who performed medical tests, and for union and employee access to those records. Employers urged minimal record retention requirements, that exams be performed by physicians they hired, and that the findings not go automatically to either workers or unions.

OSHA would hover uncomfortably between labor and industry, shifting with the political winds in Washington. For its first five years, a period of Republican presidencies, the agency issued standards that cut against contemporary efforts to grant patients a greater stake in controlling their medical records, allowing company doctors to perform screening exams without any obligation to divulge the results to individual workers. "Since the results are to be made available to the employer, allowing the employer to select the physician has the advantage of both convenience and efficiency," OSHA noted in its first permanent health standard, on asbestos, in 1972. "It seems more reasonable to permit [workers] to utilize present programs and expertise than to permit them to choose a private practitioner."[99] The reasonableness of this argument was not evident to organized labor, which unsuccessfully challenged the decision in court on the grounds that it violated doctor-patient confidentiality.[100]

The election of Jimmy Carter to the presidency in 1976 and the appointment of Eula Bingham as OSHA director increased commitment to providing workers with incentives for taking medical exams as well as with easy access to the results. Debate reached its highest pitch when OSHA proposed a new step to sharply increase employee access to their medical records. "Access to Employee Exposure and Medical Records," a rule OSHA put forward for public comment in 1978, proposed that employers maintain employee exposure records for the more than thirty-nine thousand substances in NIOSH's registry of toxins, that they be required to keep exposure and medical records for a minimum of forty years, and that access to the records be granted to all employees or their designated representatives.[101]

For nearly two years employer representatives and labor unions battled over the OSHA proposal. The fact that both sides deployed the notion of employee protection demonstrated how malleable the concept of patient rights had become and how easily concerns about privacy could be turned to the service of either industry or labor, whose interests were so often antagonistic. Employers argued that the rule would provoke anxiety by exposing workers to confusing medical information and removing control best left with doctors. "The physician," the American Occupational Medical Association noted in characteristic testimony, "should be granted the right to withhold information contained in the records which may be harmful if divulged to the employee." Labor urged OSHA to end the situation where unions had to waste time and resources resorting to grievances, arbitration, or strikes to secure basic medical information.[102] "We're asking the oil industry and chemical industry, tell us what happens to people," Anthony Mazzochi of OCAW told an audience at an OSHA seminar for the news media in January of 1980. "What happens to the facts? Who gets them? Who sees them? . . . Only management is privy."[103]

Leading privacy advocates supported OSHA's move to make medical records more accessible but questioned the government's ability to use the data responsibly. "I believe OSHA deserves the broadest possible praise for its position on worker access," Alan Westin, now at the forefront of critiques of the state of privacy in America, told attendees at a 1978 Occupational Safety and Health Symposium. But, he warned, "there are no safeguards in the regulations to insure that the records, once in Federal hands, will not be shared with any other parties, or will not be used to make any adverse decisions about the individual. It is not enough in my judgment for any Federal agency to say, 'Of course, we will only use it for our purposes.'"[104]

In May of 1980 OSHA ruled in favor of democratizing the medical record. "Unrestricted patient access to medical records has been a major public policy issue during the past decade, and the trend throughout the nation has been to provide direct patient access," the preamble noted. Recommending full access to the record by employees and their designees, OSHA flatly rejected the paternalistic argument that workers would be ill-equipped to make sense of medical uncertainty: "If a worker is incapable of understanding something in a medical or exposure record, OSHA expects that the worker will naturally seek the assistance of someone more knowledgeable whom he or she trusts."[105] A blizzard of legal challenges from industry—including arguments that the rule violated employer rights under the Fourth Amendment, the privacy rights of employees, the Trade Secrets Act, and the jurisdiction of the National Labor Relations Board—were all rejected in a Louisiana federal court in November 1982.[106]

LITIGATING PRIVACY:
CORPORATE CLAIMS AND WORKER INTEREST

In the absence of effective mechanisms to move information from workplace to government, efforts that brought investigators into workplaces to discern health hazards remained critical to disease surveillance. A 1973 NIOSH-funded pilot study conducted by the University of Washington showed the potential of going beyond employer reporting. Offering workers a complete physical exam and interview, the study concluded that as many as 31 percent of medical conditions detected were occupational in origin. Tellingly, only 2 percent of occupational illnesses had been recorded on the employer logs required by OSHA.[107] Department of Labor studies based on employer reports had suggested that dermatitis—of short latency and rarely life-threatening—accounted for the largest share of occupational illness.[108] In the NIOSH study, by contrast, dermatitis accounted for less than one in five cases of illness.

Data from the National Occupational Hazard Survey, in which NIOSH conducted "walk-throughs" in more than forty-six hundred workplaces from 1972 to 1974, also suggested the limits of relying on employers to disclose occupational disease. While unable to document levels of exposure, NIOSH estimated that one in four American workers were exposed on either a full- or part-time basis to toxic substances.[109] In a reprise of debates about medical paternalism, the extent of chemical exposures provoked prolonged conflict about whether the duty to protect workers from disturbing information superseded their need to know. "Cancer is the most fear-provoking word in the English language, and this has been established in academic studies and in tests," a trade association representative told a meeting of the National Advisory Committee on Occupational Safety and Health in 1977. "The end result [of alerting workers to risk] is that you have greater accidents, you have greater absenteeism, and it reduces the employee's morale and is deleterious to the employee's health."[110]

Employers would test NIOSH's own right to know in court. In response to employee requests for health hazard evaluations, NIOSH researchers subpoenaed medical records at plants run by DuPont, General Motors, and Westinghouse in 1977 and 1978. The corporations preferred to sue rather than to comply, claiming that the release of names and confidential information about sensitive medical conditions would violate constitutional protections on privacy even if NIOSH agreed to safeguard the information. In the General Motors case, the Ohio court found that NIOSH had not demonstrated sufficient need for employee names and addresses and ordered in 1977 that the records be released without names.[111] In the 1978 DuPont case, where the NIOSH demand for employee records was part of an effort to investigate the possibility of elevated cancer rates at the plant, the Supreme Court of West Virginia upheld the agency's right to obtain records, including names and addresses. The decision cited the 1977 case of *Whalen v. Roe,* in which the Supreme Court had found a New York State effort to collect the names of patients prescribed controlled substances to be constitutional.[112]

The limits of *Whalen* would be tested in the 1980 case of *United States v. Westinghouse Electric Corporation.* NIOSH employees, acting on a request from a union organizer at a facility in Trafford, Pennsylvania, performed blood and pulmonary function tests on employees in two areas of a Westinghouse plant. Having found evidence of potentially reduced lung capacity and toxic substances in employees' blood, NIOSH requested the medical records of current and former employees to determine the workers' health status before they had worked in the areas where their exposure was suspected to have occurred.

Westinghouse refused, claiming the NIOSH request would violate "the bargain of confidentiality made with its employees" and asserting that it could release records only with names removed and replaced by unique identifiers.[113] Westinghouse cited the Supreme Court decisions on reproductive health, *Griswold v. Connecticut* (1965) and *Roe v. Wade* (1973), as well as the General Motors and DuPont cases, arguing that since medical records might contain sensitive information about impotence, sexual abuse, or other "socially stigmatizing illnesses . . . of extreme sensitivity,"[114] NIOSH had exceeded its mandate. To release the full medical record, the company argued, violated employee privacy and patient-doctor privilege.[115] The danger was particularly acute because of the potential to match records against other databases, NIOSH's reliance on outside contractors, and what Westinghouse termed the agency's "incestuous" relationship with organized labor.[116]

By joining the specter of sexual privacy violations with more general anxieties about confidentiality in the computer age, the company implied that even the strictest security was insufficient: "All the regulations in the world cannot possibly insure against leaks or inadvertence especially where information is stored in computer banks which may be accessed not by a single key, but by the proper keypunch sequence entered at any terminal."[117] More fundamentally, the company rejected the government's right to know. "An unreasonable search and seizure," Westinghouse attorneys argued, "is not redeemed simply because the Government does not tell the public what it has found."[118]

NIOSH rejoined that *Whalen v. Roe,* rather than *Griswold,* was the relevant precedent. Agency lawyers suggested that the case was "virtually identical" to *Whalen,* except that here—contradicting Westinghouse's claim of concern for employee interests—it was "the employees' *own representatives* whose request initiat[ed] the investigation." NIOSH attorneys reminded the court that disclosure of information on the part of NIOSH, its physicians, or its contractors was prohibited by law, and that it needed names to link company records with those of the agency itself in order to "warn those employees whose health might be endangered by further exposure."[119] As NIOSH pointed out, workplace conditions, rather than simply the chemicals used, were under study: to allow Westinghouse to decide what information NIOSH could use for the study was clearly inappropriate.[120] NIOSH also noted that both the Privacy Act and the proposed rules and legislation on informed consent and the use of medical records explicitly exempted data gathered for epidemiological research and public health investigations.[121]

The District Court for the Western District of Pennsylvania agreed with NIOSH. State law, Judge Rosenberg noted, privileged medical information only when it might "blacken" the patient's reputation.[122] Further, citing the DuPont case, the court found that NIOSH safety precautions for maintaining and disclosing records were "sufficiently adequate." As to Westinghouse's claim that it was responsible for protecting its employees' privacy interests, the court noted that NIOSH's responsibility for protecting worker interests took precedence: the government, Judge Rosenberg wrote, "stands thus as the chief guardian for the protection and promotion of health." Accordingly, the ruling granted NIOSH access to "the entire medical records in personally identifiable form."[123] On appeal, Westinghouse would retort that in giving NIOSH and OSHA a duty to protect, Congress did not "give those Agencies the power to trample upon individual privacy in one's medical affairs."[124] *Whalen,* the company scolded, "did not offer carte blanche to every Government agency to rummage at will through the medical files of any citizen who comes under the Federal Government's baleful gaze."[125]

The Third Circuit Court of Appeals upheld the lower court's decision in October 1980, though it seemed responsive to what Westinghouse lawyers had described as an "arrogant wholesale demand for total medical files without even informing the employees involved."[126] Specifically, the court required that NIOSH set a time period in which employees could request that portions of their individual records be withheld. More generally, the court offered a five-point calculus for "the delicate task of weighing competing interests" when societal interests appeared to justify intrusion into private records. It recommended consideration of (1) the type of record requested and the nature of the information it contained; (2) the potential for harm in subsequent disclosures unauthorized by the individual; (3) the degree to which release of the private information might injure relationships, such as between doctor and patient or employer and employee; (4) the adequacy of safeguards to prevent unauthorized disclosure; and (5) the degree to which recognizable public interests established a need for access to the information.[127]

As in *Whalen,* the court warned NIOSH that individual claims to privacy might not always be outweighed. Rather, NIOSH had a duty to notify individuals when it sought to examine their medical records and to offer them an opportunity to object. "The touchstone," the court stated, "should be provision for reasonable notice to as many affected individuals as can reasonably be reached; an opportunity for them to raise their objections, if any, expeditiously and inexpensively; preservation of confidentiality as to the objections and the material itself from unwarranted disclosure; and prompt disposition" so as not to hamper the research.[128] The ruling added a new dimension to the right to know, requiring NIOSH to inform workers when medical records containing their names were to be used in research and offering them a chance to object.

Even as it forced companies to disclose their medical records, NIOSH found itself on the horns of its own disclosure controversies. As early as 1977 Ralph Nader and Sydney Wolfe, from the consumer advocacy group Public Citizen, sparked debate and Senate hearings by charging that the agency had the names of as many as seventy-five thousand workers exposed to harmful toxins in the workplace who had never been warned that they might be at increased risk of disease. This time, it was NIOSH that raised the question of whether disclosure might do more harm than good. "I do not mean to imply that it would not be possible to write letters telling people they had been at risk," NIOSH director John Finklea told a Senate subcommittee in May of 1977. "But I think if we are to assure that they have adequate medical counseling and adequate medical follow-up, that is where we run into the problem."[129]

At the request of the subcommittee, NIOSH issued an internal document, *The Right to Know,* that emphasized the complexity of notification.[130] Measurements of exposures were imprecise, so some workers might be notified who in fact were not at risk. Exposed workers were not guaranteed salaries if they were shown to be medically impaired, and worker compensation systems were not equipped to deal adequately with occupational health problems. Health insurance did not cover tests or follow-up examinations made necessary by toxic exposures. "Notification without counseling services can have a number of undesirable results," the report authors concluded, "and lead to an undermining of confidence in government and perhaps also in private industry or even labor unions."[131]

Was surveillance meant to expand scientific understanding of disease determinants or to allow workers the means to intervene? Listening to Finklea at a 1977 meeting of the National Advisory Committee on Occupational Safety and Health, OSHA director Eula Bingham suggested that reluctance to notify represented a "rather poor attitude" that ignored the government's obligations and stood in marked contrast to the lessons of infectious disease surveillance: "I don't know whether it's NIOSH's jurisdiction or whether OSHA can do it or not, but even if immediate remedies are not available, [I feel] that workers have a right to know that they have been exposed to benzidine for five years and this is a carcinogen. . . . I would like to point out that if a person came through who had some very contagious disease, let's say smallpox, the PHS would do everything within its means to track down the people who had contacted that individual. If we can do it for smallpox, why can't we do it for benzidine?"[132]

At regular intervals in the period between 1978 and 1984, workers' rights groups, medical ethicists, and NIOSH staff members themselves would challenge the agency's reluctance to notify. As at OSHA, NIOSH response depended in part on leadership in the White House. During the Carter administration, NIOSH director Anthony Robbins recalled, notification was taken for granted among NIOSH staff, part of a larger ethos that made it clear that the agency's first priority was protection of the health of the worker.[133]

The election of President Reagan and the replacement of Robbins with Centers for Disease Control career employee J. Donald Millar in July 1981 reignited debate. Pro-labor forces within NIOSH referred to the CDC as "the Plantation," seeing the agency as a cost-conscious, conservative entity that siphoned funds from NIOSH while providing little in return. The decision to move NIOSH headquarters to Atlanta, made while Millar was NIOSH head, further fueled concern that the agency lacked commitment to workers' best interest.[134]

"There has to be exposure notification," said Joe Velazquez of the Worker's Institute in a 1981 front-page *Washington Post* story titled "Millions Not Told of Job Health Perils." "Society has the responsibility to take care of these people."[135] Philip Landrigan, director of NIOSH's Division of Surveillance, Hazard Evaluations, and Field Studies, followed the article with a memo to Millar urging notification. "Sooner or later our responsibility to notify members of NIOSH epidemiologic studies of their participation and our results will be tested in court," Landrigan wrote. Against claims of potential damage, Landrigan invoked the language of self-determination. "Beyond the law, we believe participants do have a right to know information that involves them . . . even though we realize that in some instances . . . no possible good and sure harm (anxiety, depression, or worse) may stem from notification."[136] Ethicists addressing a CDC committee in 1983 emphasized that NIOSH had no alternative but to proceed with notification. As the only entity that knew the names of those exposed, NIOSH carried a particular obligation to share that knowledge.[137]

Millar, however, urged CDC ethics committee members to consider the economic and political backlash that might proceed from notification. A 1981 pilot program to alert workers in Augusta, Georgia, about increased risk of bladder cancer following exposure to beta-naphthylamine had already resulted in $300 million in lawsuits against the corporations involved.[138] When the ethics committee voted for notification, Millar sent the recommendation to Assistant Secretary of Health Edward Brandt accompanied by a memo emphasizing potential costs.[139] Although Brandt reminded the NIOSH director that his agency's first commitment should be to public health, the Department of Health and Human Services (DHHS) would deny a NIOSH request for funding to begin notification.[140] Congressional representatives regularly took up the call for notification. Supported by organized labor and opposed by trade associations, the legislation was never enacted.[141]

THE CRISIS IN CONFIDENCE: OSHA CALLED TO ACCOUNT

Created by the same piece of legislation, NIOSH and OSHA had interlocking political fates, with concerns about one agency shaping popular perceptions of the other. If Don Millar became the subject of scrutiny at NIOSH, the 1981 appointment of Thorne Auchter as OSHA director did far more to awaken anxieties about the Reagan administration's commitment to occupational health. A construction executive and self-proclaimed supporter of deregulation, Auchter cut the OSHA budget within a day of his appointment. The "Reagan revolution" he heralded also brought repeal of requirements that workers be paid while accompanying OSHA inspectors on "walk-arounds," suspension or reconsideration of standards issued under Eula Bingham, and sharp reductions in the number of workplaces inspected.[142] When OSHA followed the reduced inspections with announcements of record lows in workplace injuries and proposed restrictions to the access to medical records rule, the AFL-CIO, the United Auto Workers, and the Public Citizen's Health Research Group charged the OSHA director with launching "assaults on worker safety," "dismantling enforcement," and "making a shambles" of the agency.[143]

Debates over infectious disease surveillance in the 1980s, such as those that erupted around HIV reporting, pitted individuals affected by disease against the specter of a prying, stigmatizing government. In occupational disease, by contrast, it was those at risk who urged greater record keeping at the federal level and increased intervention by government investigators.[144] OSHA's retreat from an already limited disease surveillance effort provoked open conflict with labor and a series of congressional hearings. In 1984, following hearings on OSHA inspection practices, a subcommittee of the House Committee on Government Operations convened to examine whether the government was meeting its responsibility to monitor and prevent occupational disease.[145] The subcommittee's report—*Occupational Illness Data Collection: Fragmented, Unreliable, and Seventy Years Behind Communicable Disease Surveillance*—painted a dismal picture of what it called "a bipartisan failure over four administrations." Irregular reporting of occupational illness had resulted in a "gross underestimate."[146]

Testimony from government witnesses made clear that responsibility for occupational disease surveillance, divided among multiple government agencies, rested with none. Asked why the BLS relied on logs and surveys of questionable veracity, the BLS commissioner responded that its job was data analysis: OSHA was in charge of enforcement. OSHA's deputy director, when asked about the inadequacy of the statistics, replied that his agency's mandate did not include data collection. The subcommittee offered NIOSH more praise than condemnation; the phrase "70 years behind the field of communicable disease control" was taken from Don Millar's testimony. NIOSH's cooperative disease surveillance agreement with six states was singled out as a promising model. But the subcommittee also noted that the agency had no plans for expansion of surveillance and that it had shied away from using its regulatory authority or from producing a single national estimate on illness or death from occupational disease.[147] It contended that $2 million and nine staff positions could help NIOSH bring surveillance of key occupational diseases to thirty states.[148]

In 1986, however, in follow-up hearings, the Committee on Government Operations would learn that while the CDC's budget had increased by 28 percent since 1980, NIOSH's budget and staff had fallen by approximately 20 percent in the same period.[149] The report from these hearings—this time entitled *72 Years Behind and Counting*—would again urge NIOSH to step up surveillance efforts, noting that the United States remained "the only large developed country without a national system for reporting occupational disease" and was spending approximately two cents per worker on surveillance.[150]

Fueled by the congressional hearings and reports by government and not-for-profit research organizations such as the National Academy of Sciences,[151] a significant number of key policy makers had begun to look to NIOSH as the best source for accurate data on occupational disease. In 1983, seventy years after the national organization of state health officials had endorsed a model act for the reporting of work-related illnesses, the Council of State and Territorial Epidemiologists recommended a national, mandatory reporting system for occupational disease.[152] Now Congress and some of the most prestigious research policy institutions in America were lending their support for NIOSH to take the lead in realizing that recommendation.

THE FEDERAL-STATE COMPACT:
SENSOR AND COOPERATIVE DISEASE SURVEILLANCE

Emerging as much from the suggestions of its own staff as from the recommendations of outside auditors, the call for a national disease surveillance system did not find NIOSH unprepared. In 1983 the agency had worked with Harvard Medical School to compile a list of fifty diseases of the workplace, ranging from dermatitis to cancers to tuberculosis, whose diagnosis would signal a breakdown in disease prevention. Termed SHE(O)s—Sentinel Health Events (Occupational)—each was coded according to the *International Classification of Diseases.*[153] NIOSH had funded pilot surveillance projects in a handful of states as well as a study to gauge state disease surveillance capacity more broadly: surveying fifty-two health departments in 1985 (from all states, New York City, and Washington, DC), researchers found that 60 percent included occupational information on death certificates, 52 percent had such information on worker's compensation claims, and around a third included occupational data in cancer registries and on birth certificates. Further, when asked about reporting laws for six deadly, primarily long-latency occupational illnesses that DHHS had identified as preventable—byssinosis, asbestos, silicosis, mesothelioma, pneumoconiosis, and lead poisoning—researchers found that more than half of states already required reporting of one or more of the conditions. Only sixteen, however, had mandatory reporting of all six diseases.[154]

Edward Baker, a former officer of the CDC's Epidemic Intelligence Service who was appointed NIOSH deputy director in 1986, would be charged with turning this potential into a formal system of coordinated data surveillance. Baker altered surveillance at NIOSH physically, putting staff in Atlanta to supplement office operations in Cincinnati, as well as metaphorically, shifting emphasis to the more active, case follow-up model familiar from infectious disease control. In 1987 NIOSH alerted all states that they could apply to participate in the new Sentinel Event Notification System for Occupational Risks, or SENSOR.

Funded through cooperative agreements with state governments, SENSOR linked a network of providers, including individual practitioners, laboratories, and clinics, to a state surveillance center. Once notified of a case of occupational disease, the centers were responsible for confirming diagnosis using a standardized case definition, providing quarterly reports to NIOSH, and evaluating appropriate follow-up. While states were free to add other conditions, SENSOR specified six from which states had to choose: occupational asthma, pesticide poisoning, lead poisoning, carpal tunnel syndrome, noise-induced hearing loss, and silicosis.[155] Ten states received funding in the first year.

In deciding what conditions would be reportable and where the surveillance centers should be located, Baker made clear that he believed what had worked for infectious disease reporting would work for occupational illness. In nine of the ten states where SENSOR began, state departments of health received funding and were responsible for disease reports.[156] While SENSOR would draw on data from other sources—NIOSH, for example, made some funds available to add occupational health questions to the 1988 National Health and Nutrition Examination Survey conducted by the National Center for Health Statistics—the physician remained the pivotal point for reporting.[157]

Equally strikingly, SENSOR's architects addressed what dean of infectious disease surveillance Alexander Langmuir had called the baffling "little problem of definition" in occupational disease by sidestepping it entirely.[158] The original SHE(O) list included diseases with complex and contested etiologies such as occupational cancers; the SENSOR list did not. With the exception of silicosis, the long-latency diseases around which labor, business, and OSHA had battled—byssinosis, asbestosis, mesothelioma, and pneumoconiosis—were also excluded. A focus on short- and medium-latency diseases, NIOSH argued, made it more likely that the conditions that caused disease would still be in place and that intervention could protect others from succumbing.[159] While SENSOR would expand to include accidental amputation, work-related dermatitis, and injuries to miners, and while some states chose to add long-latency or fatal conditions, the program's emphasis on short- and medium-term latency diseases would remain undisturbed.

A number of states enacted legislative changes to make reporting of occupational diseases mandatory or to improve data collection.[160] The efforts resulted in substantial increases—albeit from very small starting points—in the numbers of occupational conditions reported.[161]

In sharp contrast to contemporary debates around HIV surveillance, measures for named reporting of occupational diseases provoked grumbling from a few physicians but virtually no public outcry.[162] Employers also raised little opposition to SENSOR surveillance, a silence that may have spoken as eloquently to the limits of SENSOR's utility as to the boldness of its proponents. With the vast majority of SENSOR programs administered by health departments, efforts to move beyond data collection to workplace reform meant seeking support from labor departments or federal or state OSHA programs. Commitment to that process varied greatly from state to state and depended on local political context.

The case of Massachusetts captures some of the difficulties inherent in collaboration between departments of health and labor even in well-coordinated circumstances. A 1913 law requiring physician reporting to the labor department had long gone unenforced. Hoping to improve physician reporting, the state's SENSOR program sought in 1991 to institute mandatory reporting of occupational diseases to the Department of Health. Since even sympathetic physicians feared loss of business or lawsuits if they brought occupational diseases to light, the Department of Health reasoned that a mandatory reporting law would provide cover to those physicians who wished to report but feared the consequences.[163]

What the Department of Health proposed as a step toward improved occupational health, however, was seen by the Department of Labor and Industries as an invasion of its turf. The labor department questioned the legality of passing a new regulation and countered with the suggestion that it be the arm of the state to reinvigorate occupational disease legislation. In the end, the departments worked together to promulgate an acceptable compromise—reports would be made to the Department of Health but all information save patient name, confidential by law, would be shared with the Department of Labor.[164] In states with less of a history of collaboration between departments, such obstacles have proved impassable. In Maine, for example, the departments of health and labor filed separate and competing applications for SENSOR funding in 2004.[165]

The problem of physician motivation remained even more of an obstacle for SENSOR's success. The new NIOSH approach to occupational disease surveillance left open the old question of why physicians would want to report. Ethicists and professional associations throughout the 1970s had stressed that the occupational physician's first loyalty should be to workers rather than employers. But this did little to remove the obstacles to reporting on the ground. A 1976 study in Massachusetts, done when reporting was voluntary, had sought to develop "sentinel physicians," a cadre of occupational doctors who, sensitized to the need for reporting and trained by the Department of Health, would be most motivated to bring work-related diseases to light. From a pool of eighty physicians, eighteen were selected as sentinels: of these, only a third completed their reports. If mandatory reporting laws were envisioned, as a 1991 Massachusetts health department memo put it, as a "carrot" intended to encourage communication between physicians and the health department,[166] no state approached occupational disease reporting with anything resembling a stick.[167] A 1992 evaluation of SENSOR noted that despite numerous attempts at recruiting, the few physicians who participated frequently reported only a single case. In language familiar from earlier studies, the evaluators concluded that a model that relied heavily on physician reporting of occupational disorders was "not realistic."[168]

The most serious constraint on SENSOR, however, was lack of funds. NIOSH conceived of SENSOR as a way to provide seed grants: at meetings of surveillance staff, a recurring theme at the agency was how to get states to commit funding of their own or to press Washington for increased allocations.[169] States, for their part, found NIOSH funding difficult to obtain and inadequate to their needs.[170] Resources for SENSOR remained so limited that no more than twenty states, tracking a subset of the already limited number of SENSOR conditions, participated in the program at any point between 1987 and 2004.[171] Although Edward Baker would travel to Washington meetings armed with the National Academy of Science's call for a national, NIOSH-led occupational surveillance system, neither he nor his successors found the financing to make the rhetoric real. The Department of Labor, for its part, was careful to ensure that financial commitments to NIOSH did not come at its own expense and lobbied successfully to launch its own Census of Fatal Occupational Injuries in 1992.[172]

In the end, the NIOSH surveillance efforts that have been most effective in providing a national picture are those few that require little money and no physician involvement. NIOSH tracking of adult lead poisoning, for example, has been achieved through the Adult Blood Lead Epidemiological Survey (ABLES), a program based on mandatory laboratory reporting of elevated blood lead levels that also began in 1987. Including thirty-seven states in 2004 and engaging both OSHA and NIOSH, the ABLES program offers a valuable counterpoint to stories of lack of progress in occupational disease surveillance. Neither costly nor cumbersome, the program—albeit incomplete—provides a partial vision of what national surveillance could be.

ABLES: SURVEILLANCE WITHOUT THE DOCTOR

In the broadest sense, public concern about lead poisoning throughout the twentieth century set the stage for surveillance of elevated blood lead levels. From debates over the dangers of leaded gasoline in the 1920s to door-to-door blood testing by Bronx residents in the 1960s, lead poisoning prevention has engaged both government and community groups.[173] Concern about hazardous exposures in the wake of the Love Canal scandal—the upstate New York neighborhood built over a toxic waste dump—had proved a particularly powerful lever, moving New York State to implement mandatory laboratory reporting of elevated blood levels of lead and other heavy metals in 1982.[174] By 1987 several other states required laboratories to report elevated blood lead levels to a registry, usually maintained by the state department of health.[175]

NIOSH's ABLES program benefited from this political legacy. ABLES began in 1987, the same year as SENSOR, in four states with lead registries: California, New York, New Jersey, and Texas.[176] Like SENSOR, ABLES sought to build on existing state activities, offering grants to states to establish a program capable of tracking, consolidating, and analyzing reports. As with SENSOR, the ABLES program in each state was made responsible for sending NIOSH data to help build a national picture of the problem of lead exposure.[177]

Unlike SENSOR—though similar to some sexually transmitted disease surveillance efforts—ABLES put primary responsibility for reporting on laboratories rather than on physicians. For each of the four states where ABLES started, and for all those that subsequently received funding, laboratory reporting of elevated blood lead levels was mandatory. The relatively small number of laboratories performing blood lead level analysis and that laboratory licensing gave states a way to enforce participation resulted in compliance that far surpassed any achievements in physician reporting. Audits after the passage of mandatory laboratory reporting requirements in New York, for example, found that more than 90 percent relayed results.[178] In virtually all states, less than a full-time commitment from a single staff person was sufficient to enable the transfer of reports from laboratories into a database at the health or labor department and from there to NIOSH.[179]

As with SENSOR, state ABLES programs varied widely in their commitment to workplace interventions. Some state health departments maintained their own industrial hygienists, while others were reluctant to do more than send a letter of notification. Virtually all established a level at which employers who failed to respond to department of health inquires were referred to OSHA.[180] Aggressive education and surveillance efforts brought action to reduce lead hazards for workers in industries that had been previously unmonitored, including bridge cleaners in Connecticut and painters in California.[181] In Alabama, ABLES data triggered a 1991 health hazard evaluation by NIOSH and an OSHA inspection that resulted in one of the largest penalties for an occupational health violation: a fine of $1.2 million levied against Birmingham tire and battery distributor G. T. Jones.[182] California supplemented NIOSH funding for ABLES by requiring industries with a documented history of lead poisoning to pay the state an annual fee.[183]

Political attention to lead poisoning and the reliability of reporting have in turn drawn support from entities whose interests are normally restricted to infectious diseases. The National Health and Nutrition Examination Survey, which conducts medical examinations and blood tests on randomly selected Americans, has included tests for blood lead levels since 1976.[184] In

1992, using ABLES data, the CDC made elevated blood lead levels the first occupational disease to be reported quarterly in its *Morbidity and Mortality Weekly Report.*[185]

By 2001, twenty-one states had made laboratory reporting mandatory and were participating in ABLES.[186] Some states, including New York and Michigan, had broadened requirements to ensure that any laboratory, including those out of state, report blood levels for residents of their state to the ABLES registry. Unlike SENSOR, which included virtually no southern states, all parts of the country were represented in ABLES. Perhaps most important, while SENSOR remained based on a competitive grant system, NIOSH changed ABLES to a contract-funded approach in 2002, essentially guaranteeing funding to all states who met program requirements. The change provided incentive for states unwilling to spend resources on a small grant of uncertain longevity: the year after ABLES changed to contract funding, the number of states participating in the program increased from twenty-one to thirty-five. By 2004, thirty-seven states participated.[187]

FROM WORKER RISK TO PUBLIC RISK:
THE LIMITS OF OCCUPATIONAL HEALTH

A 2003 Institute of Medicine report on the future of American public health made brief mention of occupational disease, and that only after discussing employer provision of health insurance and ways that workplace programs can help individuals reduce obesity, smoking, and other health risks.[188] National acceptance of the employer as a source of health benefits and the workplace as a site for personal health promotion stands in contrast to the ways in which the government has held industries accountable—or, more accurately, failed to hold them accountable—for worker health. Technological advances such as genetic screening are likely to raise new controversies about the degree to which employers are entitled to screen employees and restrict them based on toxic exposures or predisposition to disease.[189] If history is any guide, these new measures will do little to increase government authority to remove causes of disease in the workplace.

The next chapters, describing more successful efforts to rally resources for tracking environmental causes of cancer and birth defects, raise questions central to occupational disease surveillance. Even with conditions that disproportionately strike vulnerable minorities, environmental advocates have managed to mobilize resources by stressing the threat posed to all. Strikingly, albeit exposed to particularly concentrated levels of the same environmental toxins that threaten the general public, workers historically have been seen as separate from that public. The limits of occupational disease surveillance in the twentieth century are a testament to the relative weakness of the labor movement and the degree to which that plea has yet to be heard.

5

The Right to Be Counted

Confronting the "Menace of Cancer"

After an initial period of enthusiasm for routine surveillance of cancer incidence in the 1910s and 1920s, the idea of universal reporting along the lines of infectious disease notification dropped off the radar screen for several decades.[1] By midcentury only about half the states had established population-based registries to collect data on cancer incidence. Surveillance more commonly took the form of hospital-based registries, which did not measure incidence or prevalence but rather provided detailed information on selected groups of patients.

The piecemeal and relatively tardy development of population-based registries is the result of what one analysis called a "triangular accommodation."[2] First, the biomedical research establishment dominated the cancer agenda and focused on bench science at the expense of prevention. Second, the medical profession resisted the establishment of public-sector detection and screening centers that might have been sites for surveillance. The third leg of the triangle was private industry, which, as we saw in the previous chapter, resisted all attempts to conduct epidemiological research that might indict occupational carcinogens or malignancies associated with consumer products such as cigarettes. Within this triangle, efforts at public health surveillance remained marginal. Whereas constituencies such as the labor movement had aggressively pushed for reporting of occupational illnesses from early in the century, the politics of surveillance and privacy surrounding cancer did not become fully democratic until the 1970s, when broad social changes galvanized the public to demand that cancer cases be counted more completely.

Against the backdrop of the burgeoning environmental movement, communities who feared exposures to cancer-causing toxins demanded that states create population-based registries to provide data that could support or refute hypotheses about suspected hazards. Building on these developments, breast cancer activists who believed the government was paying insufficient attention to their condition demanded that information on every person with the disease be collected in order to gain precise figures on incidence and better understanding of etiology. In contrast to demands to be left alone from the searching eyes of government, it was the opposite claim—citizens' right to be counted—that brought cancer registration more fully into the realm of public health practice. The distinctive feature of contemporary cancer surveillance has been the extent to which patients themselves, along with people who believed they might be at risk of cancer, have led the calls for expanded reporting.

EARLY WARNINGS ON A NEW MENACE

Early investigations into the etiology of cancer were prototypical epidemiological studies, such as Percival Potts's classic 1775 analysis showing high rates of scrotal cancer among chimney sweeps.[3] But the emergent public health profession paid scant attention to cancer during the sanitary and bacteriological revolutions; as a source of morbidity and mortality, it was dwarfed by contagious menaces. There were exceptions, however. The Massachusetts health department, the country's first such statewide authority, took an early interest in the prevalence of cancer in the commonwealth and published groundbreaking reports on the subject in 1896 and 1899.[4]

The only medical intervention available at this time was surgical removal of the tumor, and it was common interest in the problem of cancer that led to the founding in 1913 of the American College of Surgeons (ACoS). The ACoS quickly became a leading advocate for increased public awareness and research that might lead to new treatments.[5] That year, several prominent surgeons struck an alliance with representatives of the insurance industry, who were greatly interested in health issues and, because of the mortality information they held on policy holders, were far better positioned to study patterns of illness than government agencies.[6] Along with some leading philanthropists, the surgeons and insurance professionals formed the American Society for the Control of Cancer (ASCC). They followed the example of other charitable organizations devoted to health problems, such as the National Tuberculosis and Health Association and the Association for the Aid of Crippled Children, that proliferated during the progressive era.[7] The ASCC would lead a chorus of calls for cancer surveillance.

The ASCC's most ardent proponent of surveillance was Frederick Hoffman, the chief statistician for the Prudential Life Insurance Company. Hoffman detected intriguing and ominous patterns in Prudential's actuarial tables—policyholders who smoked cigars and cigarettes had greatly elevated rates of cancer, for example—and he proselytized about the urgency of the problem with his talk "The Menace of Cancer," which he gave before a wide variety of civic and professional organizations around the country.[8] Hoffman wrote, "The need of trustworthy statistical data regarding local cancer frequency was clearly recognized and it soon became apparent that the work of the Society would be materially facilitated by a thoroughly trustworthy compilation of the essential statistical facts of the cancer problem, medically and sociologically considered."[9]

Hoffman did not question whether cancer surveillance was a legitimate concern of public health practitioners. "I am decidedly of the opinion that Cancer should be made a reportable disease," he declared. "It is the proper function of the Health Department to take cognizance of the conditions frequently met with in Cancer cases previous to qualified treatment."[10] He was further convinced that such reporting should be mandatory. "I am satisfied that voluntary registration is a hopeless effort," he wrote. "The matter must be made a statutory requirement and derelict physicians must be held accountable. . . . Compulsion alone will ensure success."[11] Hoffman believed that resistance from private doctors could be overcome through diligent enforcement, just as it had been surmounted with opposition to reporting of tuberculosis and other communicable diseases.

In a similar spirit, the 1913 "Model State Law for Morbidity Reports," prepared by the Surgeon General's office of the U.S. Public Health Service, called for cancer reporting, describing it as a disease of unknown origin.[12] The office's interest in tracking cancer reflected an expanding notion of the responsibilities of public health and the function of reporting. In 1913, for example, Assistant Surgeon General John Trask observed that "originally the duties of the health officer were very simple, and related only to the control of certain diseases associated with popular dread. As knowledge, however, of the causes of diseases and their means of spread has been acquired, the responsibilities of the health department have rapidly increased, so that at present time the health department is properly the guardian of the community's health."[13]

But public health action in the area of cancer fell far short of the expansive visions of Hoffman and Trask. Like occupational diseases, cancer presented a conundrum to the public health profession, which at the time was highly oriented toward laboratory techniques aimed at identifying specific disease-causing germs.[14] The American Public Health Association (APHA) was resigned to the fact that the condition could not be prevented or controlled with the same techniques that had been applied to contagious threats. While surveillance of tuberculosis had presented numerous logistical difficulties, at least its value for intervention was clear: once reported, a case of the illness could be traced, treated, and, if necessary, confined. But what could be done with a cancer patient? The traditional role of surveillance in stopping the spread of illness seemed not to apply. There was little possibility of intervening at the population level because the cause, or causes, of the condition remained baffling and were thus hotly disputed. Chronic irritation or inflammation were considered precipitating causes.[15] There had long been evidence of high rates of cancer in certain occupations, and substances common in industry such as tar, pitch, and analine were considered likely culprits.[16] But these theories hardly explained, for example, breast tumors in women. Scientific consensus remained elusive.

As a result, the public health profession's response largely remained limited to public education urging early detection and treatment. The APHA did call upon health departments to undertake surveys of physicians, nursing organizations, and hospitals about the number of cancer cases and deaths within their jurisdictions and to compare their data with those of adjacent areas. But in contrast to the PHS, the APHA stopped short of recommending that cancer become reportable. Routine surveillance of cancer, in the APHA's view, simply did not promise enough benefit to justify the time, expense, and labor that it would require. "Cancer has generally been regarded by departments of health as a degenerative disease and one against which there is no definitive and effective procedure such as is available for the control of infectious diseases," explained the APHA's Committee on Cancer. "They have felt that cancer should best be combated through the joint action of patients and physicians and that departments of health, which are charged especially with the prevention rather than the cure of the disease, could co-operate best in this crusade by helping to instruct the public in the part which it should play."[17] The APHA's claim that it was impossible to intervene against cancer was an ironic echo of the arguments physicians had put forth in resisting the notification of tuberculosis cases. Thus dissent within the public health ranks, exemplified by the opposing positions of the surgeon general's office and the APHA leadership, kept the profession from bringing cancer cases within the ambit of surveillance.

Even if there had been unanimous public health support for making cancer reportable, it would no doubt have faced resistance from the physician rank and file, as with tuberculosis and venereal disease. Cancer was a highly feared illness, which decreased the likelihood that health departments could rely on the cooperation of physicians to report it even if called upon to do so. Indeed, doctors at the time frequently recorded the cause of a cancer death as heart disease or pneumonia out of deference to the family, to spare them the "taint" associated with the illness.[18]

Finally, many medical professionals argued that expanded surveillance was unnecessary because the disease was not really on the rise. Cancer had not ranked in the ten leading causes of death at the turn of the century, but it climbed to second place by the 1920s, surpassing all of the contagious threats of a previous era to rank just behind heart disease. While no one disputed that infectious diseases were declining, there was considerable disagreement about whether the concomitant increase observed for cancer cases was real or simply artifactual, the result of better diagnosis or the increased longevity of the population.[19] Some doctors attributed the rise in cases to more people living in large cities, where the availability of laboratory and microscopic facilities increased the likelihood of diagnosing cases that would previously have gone undetected.[20] Typical were the comments of Wendell Strong, a gynecologist at Columbia University, who wrote in the *Journal of Cancer Research,* "We cannot now determine whether the cancer mortality is slightly increasing, practically stationary, or slightly decreasing, but we can be sure that it is not greatly increasing."[21]

In 1925, in response to these debates, the PHS undertook a retrospective study of cancer mortality in ten states since the turn of the century. The study found that about one-third of the apparent increase in mortality could be attributed to increasing diagnostic precision. The remaining two-thirds of the increase, however, was determined to be real.[22] By the end of the 1920s the debate about rising cancer incidence was largely settled. The notable holdout on this point was Louis Dublin, the prominent health statistician and chief actuary at the Metropolitan Life Insurance Company, who maintained as late as 1937 that the rise in the cancer death rate was "spurious" and that "the cancer situation in the United States is far from alarming although much can be done to improve it."[23]

THE ROOTS OF THE MEDICAL MODEL

Just as the public health community was divided over the value of reporting, so too did clinicians disagree about the potential benefits that more systematic documentation of cancer cases might offer. A few prominent physicians saw surveillance as an avenue to enhancing the profession's ability to treat the disease and improving the outcomes for individual patients. Francis Carter Wood, director of the Institute of Cancer Research at Columbia University, decried the inadequacy of death records, the profession's primary source of information about the course of disease: they "are of but little value in the practical evaluation of the results of treatment, or lack of treatment, for any given individual with cancer."[24] Noting the wide range of possible outcomes for cancers of different types and sites, Wood claimed that reporting would provide information to help doctors diagnose and treat the condition in their patients. "The first step that must be made is to have the disease notifiable," Wood wrote in a 1930 issue of the *American Journal of Public Health.* "We will then be able to get at the present crying need, which is not of mortality records, but of the number of people who have cancer in a community and the length of time which they live after such a cancer is discovered."[25]

The desire to find more effective treatment provided the impetus for a few physicians who recognized that data on a larger number of patients than they saw in their own practice might enhance their ability to diagnose and treat the condition. One such advocate was Ernest Codman, a Boston surgeon and founding member of the American College of Surgeons, whose efforts at increasing his clinical skills led him to create one of the earliest cancer registries, albeit one with a purpose fundamentally different from public health surveillance.

In 1920 Codman sent a form letter to every member of the ACoS:

> Dear Doctor: Have you any living cases of bone sarcoma? . . . I have a patient with a sarcoma of the ilium, who is having treatment with radium, and I am most anxious to get in touch with other surgeons who have similar cases. . . . Dr. Bloodgood and Dr. Ewing are joining me in this investigation and it is our intention to keep a file of all living cases in which the diagnosis is reasonably certain, and to send to each surgeon who contributes a case, a duplicate file of all the other. In this way each case will have the benefit of the experience of the rest.[26]

Codman and his two colleagues went on to develop an elaborate system of record keeping. They gathered detailed information on individual patients into folders, each containing a standardized personal information form, a typewritten abstract of the case, prints of the X-rays, photographs of the patient and the bone specimen, and any additional correspondence or files that might be relevant. The folders were placed in cardboard boxes, which the three surgeons sent to laboratories, hospitals, and doctors' offices all over the country so that other medical professionals could examine the contents of each folder (figs. 16 and 17). Responding to those who were concerned about the materials circulating so widely, Codman opined, "It is far better to run the risk of losing some of the material than to lose the opportunity of having other minds study the data."[27]

It is significant that the concerns raised by Codman's colleagues had to do with the materials being lost or mislaid—not with the patients' right to privacy being compromised. Within the era of paternalistic privacy, physicians viewed such sharing as posing no risk to patients. Codman asked doctors to submit the patient's name, address, sex, age, and race, along with the name and address of a close friend who could be contacted for follow-up questions. That the data would be circulated only within the medical fraternity obviated any concerns about privacy. The procedures Codman developed for submitting cases to the registry said nothing about informing the patient whose personal information would be viewed by doctors all over the country; Codman believed that patients could only benefit from having their cases reviewed by others, and this expert judgment about what was in the patient's best interest was unquestioned. "In cases where the patient is

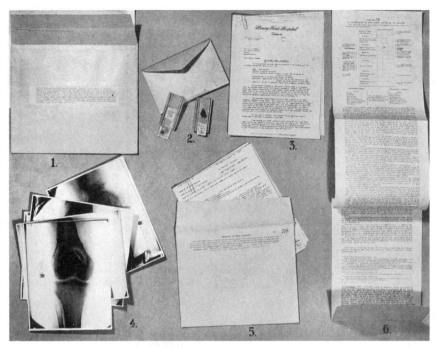

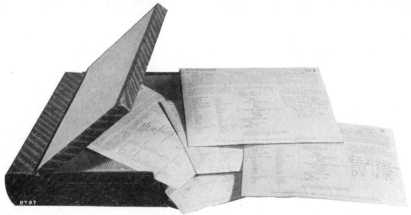

Figures 16 and 17. The Bone Sarcoma Registry established by Ernest Codman and his colleagues consisted of folders on each patient; each folder contained a standardized personal information form, an abstract of the case, prints of the X-rays, photographs of the patient and the bone specimen, and any additional correspondence or files that might be relevant (*above*). The folders were placed in cardboard boxes, which the three surgeons sent to laboratories, hospitals, and doctors' offices all over the country so that other medical professionals could examine the contents of each folder (*below*). Reprinted from E. A. Codman, "The Cases of Bone Sarcoma," *Surgery, Gynecology, and Obstetrics* 34 (1922), with permission from the American College of Surgeons.

of sufficient intelligence," the doctor might explain the purpose and benefits of the registry, but there was no requirement to do so.[28]

Within two years of his invitation, more than four hundred fifty of his colleagues had contacted Codman about cases they suspected might be bone cancer. They contributed detailed records, photographs, and X-rays to the traveling registry. Because of the favorable response, the ACoS agreed to provide financial support and give the registry a permanent home at its Chicago headquarters.[29] While Codman believed that the registry might shed some light on the epidemiology of bone sarcoma, it was primarily a tool for building the diagnostic and therapeutic skills of physicians. The majority of submitted cases, it turned out, were judged by Codman and his colleagues to be not true cases of the condition.[30] This model of case reporting—selective rather than universal, focused on individual patient outcomes rather than population-level patterns and preventive interventions—would become the dominant form of cancer surveillance in the coming decades.

Inspired by the model of Codman's registry, the ACoS also began to advocate that hospital managers set up registries of all tumors seen at their facilities in order to track clinical outcomes and assess what types of therapy were most effective. Most institutions lacked systems for making the information available, however. Writing in a 1922 issue of *Modern Hospital* magazine, Dr. Nathaniel Faxon of Massachusetts General Hospital urged that all statistics be routinely transferred from patient charts onto perforated index cards that could be run though automatic sorting machines—a technology originally developed for use with financial records in accounting firms—in order to easily and quickly sort cases by demographic information and illness. Such tabulations, Faxon argued, would greatly "increase medical and surgical knowledge, aid public health administration and, through comparison, assist in hospital management."[31] In 1932 the ACoS began accrediting hospital cancer programs and used the process to encourage facilities to set up registries.

As the ACoS and a few hospitals were taking the first steps toward systematic collection of data on cancer patients, two state health departments moved to bring the cancer problem under their purview. The Massachusetts health department, an early leader in cancer studies, created a multifaceted clinical and research program, starting with a small "tumor diagnostic service" in 1919 and expanding steadily over the following decade to include twelve permanent cancer clinics in the largest cities and a dedicated cancer hospital.[32] Henry Chadwick, the Massachusetts commissioner of public health, saw a more expansive role for his profession than many of his colleagues. He was untroubled by the expansion of his department into what some saw as the terrain of the physician. In Chadwick's view this was "a logical development of health service. The great reduction in the morbidity and mortality from gastrointestinal diseases of infancy and childhood and the acute communicable diseases, and the aging of the population, have placed chronic disease in the forefront. . . . A department of public health must keep in step with these fundamental changes and readjust its activities to meet the problems incidental to an older population."[33] Chadwick's vision reflected the thinking of the more progressive wing of the public health profession that saw the hospital not so much as a center for treatment but as a site for health maintenance and prevention.[34]

Although Chadwick steered the department of health toward a more activist role in applying public health approaches to medical problems, he stopped short of mandating that all cases of cancer be reported to a central registry.[35] The department had attempted a trial of routine reporting in the late 1920s in the town of Newton as a prelude to a possible statewide requirement, only to find that a scant one-third of physicians complied.[36] Nevertheless, the program had a very strong component devoted to statistical studies, which were carried out using death records, hospital admission records, physician questionnaires, and sometimes interviews in house-to-house surveys. In 1926 the state began collecting data on cases seen in the largest hospitals (fig. 18).[37]

In neighboring Connecticut, meanwhile, physicians at New Haven Hospital, affiliated with the Yale University School of Medicine, began laying the groundwork for an innovative program. The effort was led by C.-E. A. Winslow, a professor of public health at the medical school who had written the admiring biography of Hermann Biggs, the pioneer of TB and venereal disease notification in New York. Like Chadwick, Winslow sought to move public health beyond its long-standing focus on contagion and apply a preventive approach to a wide range of illnesses. In 1926 Chadwick directed a study of the health facilities and needs of New Haven. Noting a striking rise in local cancer frequency consistent with the increase being seen nationwide, Winslow and his colleagues mounted a comprehensive program in New Haven, including public education campaigns and new cancer clinics.[38] In 1933 the Connecticut State Medical Board established a statewide Tumor Study Committee to recommend possible ways to build upon the New Haven model. At the committee's urging, the governor signed a bill in 1935 authorizing the department of health "to make investigations concerning cancer, the prevention and treatment thereof and the mortality therefrom and to take such action as it may deem will assist in bringing about a reduction in the mortality thereto."[39] With this vaguely worded mandate, the state created a Division of Cancer Research within the health department. The staff included a statistician and a tabulating machine operator who would keep track of cases using a newly developed standard record form on which physicians noted the name, age, sex, race, place of residence, and pertinent lifestyle information of all cancer patients.[40]

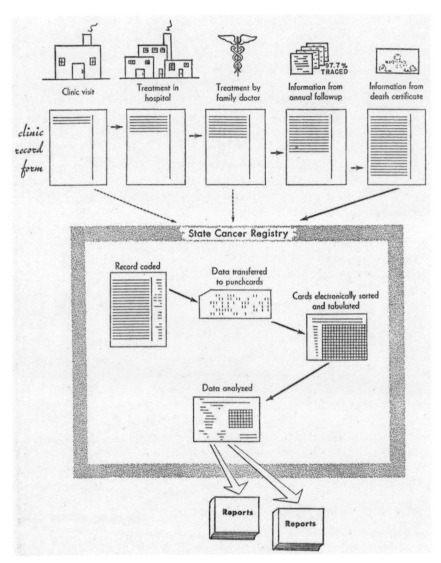

Figure 18. "Evolution of the Cancer Clinic Record." Massachusetts was an early leader in cancer surveillance. In 1926 the state began collecting data on cases of the disease diagnosed in large hospitals and later expanded to include other sources of information. This schematic, reproduced in *Public Health Reports* in 1953, illustrates the flow of data to the cancer registry from hospitals, clinics, and private physicians.

While the operation was housed administratively in the health department, the state medical society had ultimate authority over the Division of Cancer Research. The buy-in from the state's physicians and the ongoing involvement of the medical society enabled Connecticut during the mid-1930s to achieve universal reporting of cancer to local authorities on a voluntary basis, without legal or statutory requirements.[41]

In 1941, when the legislature allocated additional funding, Connecticut's program was ready to go one step further than the one that had been created in Massachusetts: it would establish a complete registry of every hospitalized cancer case in the state. Eleanor MacDonald, a research statistician who had worked as a registrar with the Massachusetts program for ten years, took a new position in New Haven to supervise the program. Since mostly complete records were available from all over the state going back to 1935, the year the Division of Cancer Research had standardized reporting procedures, MacDonald and her staff decided to make the registry retroactive to that year and set to the daunting task of collecting and abstracting some ten thousand annual records for each of the state's thirty-seven general hospitals along its clinics, laboratories, and outpatient facilities. The task took almost two years.[42] The Connecticut Tumor Registry was the nation's first statewide cancer registry.

In the interwar years, Connecticut and Massachusetts remained outliers among the states in their strong approach to cancer control and the extent of their surveillance for the disease. It was not until the 1940s that a substantial number of state health departments, inspired by the example of the Connecticut Tumor Registry and a new interest in the disease on the part of the federal government, began to take action on cancer. Even as surveillance expanded, however, it would become even more firmly entrenched within a biomedical approach, with an emphasis on providing better treatment rather than on understanding cancer's causes and preventing its occurrence.

THE COMING OF THE NATIONAL CANCER INSTITUTE

During the 1930s, cancer garnered heightened attention from politicians and the lay public. The new head of the American Society for the Control of Cancer undertook an aggressive publicity campaign to draw attention to the disease, which resulted in a flurry of articles in newspapers and leading magazines such as *Time* and *Life*. This push dovetailed with increasing interest among members of Congress and, more generally, in the idea that the federal government should devote money to fighting disease. Since the 1920s legislators had sought to create a National Institute of Health; as the Depression worsened, there was a rising expectation that it was appropriate for the federal government to intervene in urgent matters of domestic policy. These threads coalesced with the founding in 1937 of the National Cancer Institute (NCI) within the PHS.[43]

One of the NCI's priorities was to be the first nationwide survey of cancer prevalence. "It is not easy to obtain accurate information concerning the number of persons with cancer," wrote an NCI official. "Experience has demonstrated that inquiries made by a house-to-house canvass do not obtain reliable data since many people do not know that they have cancer, while others will not admit the fact even if they know it to be true."[44] Furthermore, the scope of the undertaking seemed much more daunting than previous local or statewide efforts, encompassing as it did not only urban areas but also sparsely populated rural regions with few medical facilities. Ultimately, the need for accurate data trumped the desire for an exact count in all areas of the country: the survey would be conducted "only in areas with superior medical and hospital facilities which were reasonably accessible to all groups of the population. This necessarily restricted the communities studied to urban areas."[45]

Officials selected ten metropolitan areas from which they would extrapolate nationwide prevalence. Atlanta, Pittsburgh, Detroit, Chicago, and New Orleans were surveyed in 1937; Dallas/Fort Worth, San Francisco/Alameda County, Birmingham, and Philadelphia in the following year; and Denver in 1939. The combined population of the surveyed areas totaled just over thirteen million, or about 10 percent of the U.S. population. The agency sent detailed questionnaires to every physician and hospital in the ten areas asking for reports of any person under care for a malignant growth. Since many patients received care at more than one facility, names and addresses were recorded for each case in order to avoid duplicate records. Survey workers paid in-person visits to any hospital or physician who failed to respond.[46] The AMA offered measured support for the effort. Responding to the survey "may entail considerable labor and some inconvenience, but it is desirable and in the public interest," the *Journal of the American Medical Association* editorialized. "The first step toward conquest of any disease is a complete knowledge of its prevalence."[47] Getting doctors to respond to a one-time survey was, of course, a far simpler matter than gaining their cooperation with ongoing cancer reporting.

The formation of the NCI, the attention garnered by the ten-city survey, and the successful model of the Connecticut Tumor Registry all prompted activity among states related to cancer surveillance. More than twenty states made cancer a reportable condition in the 1940s. Most modeled the reporting after that for communicable diseases: the health department collected a single report on the diagnosis of a case of cancer but tracked no information about the subsequent clinical course of the case.[48] Even in "incidence-only" registries that did not follow cases over time, named reporting was the norm.

New York, for example, made cancer a reportable condition in 1940 following a study by a legislative committee. All cases except those from New York City were reported by physicians, hospitals, and laboratories to a central register in the state capital in Albany. In making its recommendation, the commission noted that the burden of reporting would fall primarily on a few large hospitals and laboratories where the majority of cases were diagnosed. "The average physician," the committee noted, "sees fewer than 10 cases a year, probably less; the average hospital admits less than 20 patients with cancer each month."[49] Because of the cooperation of the state's physicians, reporting for cancer was relatively complete.

Some states undertook surveillance activities but declined to mandate universal reporting. In California, a selective but still extensive system of reporting was instituted under the guidance of the pioneering epidemiologist Lester Breslow, who headed the state health department's bureau of chronic diseases. The seeds of the system were planted when Los Angeles County General Hospital established a tumor registry under the aegis of the state medical association in the early 1940s. Within several years almost sixty other large hospitals in the state had set up such registries. When Breslow joined the state health department, he became interested in the problem of cancer and the ways that the information being gathered in hospitals around the state might be put to use. Breslow visited the cancer control programs in Massachusetts, Connecticut, and New York, and in 1947 established the California Tumor Registry. Like the one in Massachusetts, it drew reports from large hospitals, which accounted for about one-third of the state's cancer patients.[50] Breslow decided against compulsory reporting of cancer, believing that active surveillance targeting hospitals with the most cases would provide better-quality data and would be more effective and efficient than universal notification.[51]

The California registry proved to be a valuable tool in increasing the skills of clinicians, providing the participating institutions with reports based on the data that gave doctors a better idea of what they were doing right and what could be improved with respect to their patient care. The state health department reported that "putting these statistical registries in the various private hospitals has been one of the best educational influences in these hospitals for better cancer control, better than anything they have done before."[52]

By 1948 cancer was reportable in twenty-four states.[53] But only in a few states, such as New York, Massachusetts, and Connecticut, was there anything close to complete reporting. Most state health departments were perpetually underfunded and lacked the needed resources and technical assistance to take action on cancer. Some turned to the NCI for help in setting up registries, but they did not find a receptive audience in Bethesda. On the contrary, the NCI's grant making focused almost exclusively on basic science research. This priority was set by the National Advisory Cancer Council, a six-member body that was charged with setting the organization's research agenda and making decisions on extramural funding. The council included several of the nation's most eminent researchers, all of whom favored laboratory work. Council members looked askance at public education and prevention, which they considered the domain of the medical profession and voluntary associations such as the American Society for the Control of Cancer.[54] This is not to say that the NCI was not interested in uncovering the causes of cancer; at one of its first meetings the council endorsed the idea of—but did not provide money for—studies of cancer incidence in various occupations.[55] But they saw basic molecular and biological research as the most promising path to the conquest of cancer and had little use for traditional public health approaches. As we shall see in the next chapter, an emphasis on bench science also prevailed among the voluntary organizations that were concerned with the problem of birth defects.

The advisory council even looked with skepticism on programs such as Ernest Codman's bone sarcoma registry. Within a few years of its formation, the council had received numerous applications from medical specialty societies seeking support for similar registries of particular cancers. But the council's policy was "to support research, *real* research."[56] Said one council member, "The history of these registries is very interesting. When they start there is a great deal of interest, and then they sag. It seems to me the very fact that they sag indicates that they are not very necessary."[57] Another concurred, claiming that since "the work in question is taken up more and more in institutions and hospitals of various kinds . . . the time for this sort of thing is passing."[58]

Further, there was general skepticism on the advisory council about the quality of the data that reporting would yield. It was widely acknowledged that common sources of information on cancer were fraught with problems of reliability and validity.[59] "You are going to end up," predicted one council member, "with a couple of filing cabinets full of stuff of no use to man or beast."[60]

THE LIMITS OF DATA

There were numerous sources of information on patients with cancer, including death certificates, records of clinics, hospitals, and private physicians, and targeted surveys, but all had major limitations and often contradicted each other. The number of cases diagnosed in a given area was subject to bias according to the number and quality of diagnostic facilities, the training and capability of physicians, and the willingness of people to present for medical care following the appearance of suspicious symptoms. Hospital statistics were skewed because many institutions did not collect data on patients who applied for care but were rejected because their disease was too advanced for treatment.[61] Death certificates were notoriously unreliable and, of course, provided no information about people who did not die from their condition or whose cause of death was masked. Studies found wide discrepancies between what physicians recorded upon diagnosis and what was noted on the patient's death certificate.[62] Well into the 1940s, deaths from cancer were often reported as from some other cause in order to spare survivors the "shame" of the disease.[63]

Finally cancers, like occupational diseases, were far more complex than infectious illnesses that had been targets of surveillance. Although colloquially referred to as a single disease, cancer in fact represented a wide range of malignancies. While many infectious diseases could be confirmed by identifying the causative agent under a microscope, cancer diagnosis was often a matter of pathologist's judgment in deciding whether a growth was benign or malignant. Once the tumor had metastasized, determining the original site of the cancer could be difficult. Worst of all was the data on the cancer's life span. Many tumors were occult or slow-growing, and if the patient came under the care of a physician only in the later stages of illness, the recorded duration was only the tip of the iceberg.[64]

Given the many sources of error and bias in the available cancer data, even as ardent a proponent of surveillance as Surgeon General Thomas Parran doubted the value of applying to cancer the methods that had been successfully used for infectious disease. In 1938 Columbia University's Francis Carter Wood asked Parran if the PHS might undertake more forceful efforts to establish state laws covering notification of cancer. But Parran—who had made case reporting by physicians one of the central pillars of his campaign against syphilis—demurred. "I would not feel warranted now in recommending to every state that they establish notification," he explained. "We need a background of experience and different methods of ascertaining the presence of types of cancer."[65] The etiology of cancer was so poorly understood and the potential factors that might contribute to its development were so diverse that surveillance—even assuming a high level of completeness in reporting—would shed little light.

The focus of the federal cancer program remained on laboratory science rather than prevention throughout the post–World War II years, a time of explosive growth in the budget and resources of the NCI and the other components of what had now become the National Institutes of Health.[66] But the success of Lester Breslow's reporting system in California did lead some members of the NCI's advisory council to question whether supporting surveillance might in fact be an appropriate role of the institute. Council member Robert Stone, noting the concrete benefit that surveillance could have on patient care, made a "strenuous objection" to the decision not to support statistical registries.[67] A special NCI committee investigating gastric cancer recommended that the council assist in the establishment of uniform statewide cancer registries in all states.[68] But these remained minority opinions.

The NCI did not completely ignore research into the potential causes of cancer. An epidemiology section was established in the NCI's Cancer Control Branch in 1948. Chronic disease epidemiology was a still-young discipline at this point, two years before the landmark studies of Richard Doll and A. Bradford Hill in England and Ernst Wynder and Evarts Graham in the United States used statistical methods to link smoking with lung cancer.[69] The NCI's epidemiology section conducted analyses of data that came from the few states that could provide good-quality records; it also undertook its own studies in collaboration with hospitals and medical societies. Among the investigations were studies of environmental exposure and cancer among retired railroad workers, of leukemia in Boston patients, and of the potential effect of radioactive waters in Hot Springs, Arkansas, on masseurs and attendants.[70] In addition, the NCI sought to measure the population distribution of cancer by repeating the ten-city survey in 1948 and 1949; it would do so again in 1968 and 1969.

NCI statistician Harold Dorn endorsed the universal reporting of cancer, seeing it as a tool for measuring the effects of education programs on getting people to seek early detection and treatment and learning where the disease was distributed geographically. But Dorn did not envision that statistics derived from reporting would, by themselves, shed much light on the causes of cancer. "A routine reporting system," Dorn wrote in 1949, "is not the proper means for the collection of detailed data for the epidemiological study of human cancer although it can provide the basis for the selection of a representative sample of cases for intensive investigation of specific problems."[71] As Alexander Gilliam, the NCI's head of epidemiology, explained, "A cancer register for epidemiologic purposes is an expensive undertaking and requires a great deal of statistical competence in its design and inauguration, and considerable technical skill in its operation and evaluation. Other less expensive means, such as well designed sampling studies, may successfully serve at least some of the epidemiologic needs met by good case reporting systems." ASTHO endorsed the idea of statewide cancer registries "only where the dual purpose of serving as a basis of local cancer service programs and supplying epidemiological data can be utilized."[72]

At midcentury the causes of cancer remained as much in dispute as they had been decades earlier. "Lifestyle" factors such as diet and smoking, occupational exposures, unknown viruses, economic status, climate, membership in racial, ethnic, or religious groups—all were potential but unproven risk factors.[73] Routine collection of all possible variables of interest would require impossibly long and detailed forms. "Experience has demonstrated," Dorn pointed out, "that extensive or complicated forms will not be accurately completed, and that resistance to reporting increases rapidly as forms become increasingly complicated."[74] The head of statistical surveys for the Massachusetts cancer control program advised limiting the number of data items collected "to avoid disturbing the patients unduly."[75] Thus the primary means of investigating the causes of cancer were targeted studies of specific risk hypotheses—for example, the pathbreaking research comparing lung cancer rates in smokers and nonsmokers in the late 1940s and early 1950s in Britain and the United States.[76] Significantly, such research rarely extended to workplace populations. The NCI's Gilliam lamented in 1953 that "studies are sorely needed" of industries where workers were routinely exposed to chemicals known to be carcinogenic in animals, and that detailed evidence from different industries is "conspicuous by its infrequent appearance in the industrial cancer literature."[77]

Meanwhile, hospital tumor registries became more common and served as tools for enhancing the institutions' patient care. When the ACoS issued its revised standards for hospital cancer programs in 1956, the document included a requirement that every cancer program include a registry with information on the diagnosis, treatment, and end results of all patients admitted to the institution.[78] The NCI began to support hospital-based surveillance when it established the End Results Group in 1956. The program was a collaboration among hospitals around the country affiliated with medical schools that pooled their data on the survival experience of patients diagnosed or treated in their facility. Records from the participating hospitals were submitted, including information on primary site, disease stage, treatment, length of survival, and cause of death. The purpose of the program was to conduct studies on subjects such as the survival of patients who did not receive treatment and the results of different types of chemotherapy.[79]

Although by the 1970s the number of hospital-based tumor registries had grown to almost eight hundred, there was some question about just how useful they were. "Most clinicians learned long ago not to rely upon data in Tumor Registries," noted a highly critical analysis in the mid-1970s, "because the lists of patients were usually incomplete and the abstracted data unverified, making it necessary to do an independent search for charts in the medical record library."[80] The problem, the authors argued, was not specific to cancer records but reflected a more far-reaching problem: the sorry state of hospital data management. "Elementary recordkeeping practices of business have never been introduced into most of our hospitals," the article lamented. Another analysis argued that the staff in tumor registries "have been untrained and poorly paid [and] overwhelmed with the massive number of cases to be abstracted."[81]

THE WAR ON CANCER AND SEER

Reviewing the approach to cancer that prevailed during the middle decades of the century, Raymond Kaiser, director of the NCI's Cancer Control Branch, later recalled that cancer researchers "were never convinced that [cancer] ought to have been in the realm of public health activities. . . . It's okay for [health departments] to keep statistical records and maintain their tumor clinic records and that sort of thing, deaths and so forth, and maybe do some epidemiological studies, but that was usually thrown in as an after-thought."[82] The NCI's biometry program did give technical assistance to some states on setting up uniform reporting procedures for their reg-istries.[83] But population-level studies of cancer remained a marginal piece of the NCI's program; few states established robust cancer control programs, and the landmark studies on smoking and lung cancer simply underscored how meager the evidence remained on other potential etiological agents. "Compared with the vast accumulation of literature based upon the clinical observation of individual cases and the experimental study of cancer in ani-mals other than man, the amount of reliable, verified epidemiological knowledge concerning cancer in humans is relatively insignificant" was the candid assessment of a 1959 report from the PHS. Echoing the views of those who had, since the turn of the century, lamented the failure to extend surveillance, the PHS concluded that the failure was "all the more surpris-ing since the value and necessity of epidemiological investigations have long been recognized in the study of infectious and communicable diseases."[84]

The 1960s were a time of increasing societal attention to cancer, as the rising burden of lung cancer captured public attention. The 1964 surgeon general's report on cigarette smoking sent shock waves through the country with its claim that one of the nation's most deeply engrained habits was deadly. But public attention to the disease did not translate into an expan-sion of reporting or alter the NCI's long-standing emphasis on basic science and, to a lesser extent, treatment research over prevention. The decade was a time of administrative travail for the federal cancer control program. Major reorganizations within the PHS resulted in the NCI's cancer control program and its epidemiological studies being shunted to the PHS's Bureau of State Services, which funded traditional state public health activities. There the program languished. States, for their part, were slow to take up more aggressive cancer control activities because the condition fell outside their traditional purview of infectious diseases. State health officers, many of whom were battling to improve the reporting of venereal diseases, were reluctant to make a major new incursion on the turf of the medical profes-sion.[85] The PHS's approach to the emergent concern about smoking remained largely one of accommodation to the powerful tobacco industry, which was focusing on efforts to develop a "safer" cigarette.[86]

The sense that the nation's struggle against cancer had stalled—in 1967 federal support for research leveled off for the first time in years as escalat-ing expenses for the Vietnam War siphoned money away from domestic pro-grams—raised alarms among some influential policy makers. The push to restore federal leadership was led by the health philanthropist Mary Lasker and Senator Ralph Yarborough of Texas, Congress's leading advocate for biomedical funding. A specially convened congressional committee, the National Panel of Consultants on the Conquest of Cancer, issued a report at the end of 1970 calling for a renewed commitment and a massive influx of funds. The development of the atomic bomb, the Salk polio vaccine trials, and the 1969 moon landing provided powerful models for what might be accomplished with an all-out push under government leadership: a cure for cancer would be medicine's "giant leap for mankind." In the legislation that was drafted, the emphasis remained on finding effective treatments and research leading to a cure; prevention and population-level control measures remained marginalized, as they had been since the creation of the NCI three decades earlier. After more than a year of congressional wrangling, much of it over whether the NCI should become an independent agency like NASA that reported directly to the president, Richard Nixon signed the bill into law two days before Christmas, 1971.[87]

Buried amid the emphasis on "conquest" and "cure" in the National Cancer Act of 1971 was a directive, added almost as an afterthought, for the NCI to "collect, analyze, and disseminate all data useful in the prevention, diagnosis, and treatment of cancer."[88] An expert panel convened by the NCI recommended an expanded surveillance effort to aid the war on cancer. The panel further recommended that the NCI's two surveillance activities—the periodic ten-city surveys, which had gauged national prevalence in 1937, 1949, and 1969, and the End Results Group, which had studied clinical outcomes through hospital tumor registries—be folded into one. This recommendation led to the creation of SEER: the Surveillance, Epidemiology, and End Results Program. The purpose of SEER was to determine cancer incidence and prevalence nationwide and in selected regions, to gain information on cancer survival trends in various types of cancer, and to identify etiologic factors that might warrant further study. SEER registries would collect data on patient demographics, primary site of cancer, extent of disease, therapy, and underlying cause of death.[89]

SEER's creators wanted to include registries that had a demonstrated track record in conducting cancer surveillance and doing studies—a small pool of candidates from which to choose. Although in 1970 about half the states had cancer incidence registries, a far smaller number—only about six, according to one expert—had reliable and complete data and the capability of tracking patients over time.[90] The NCI began with five statewide registries: Connecticut, Iowa, New Mexico, Utah, and Hawaii. Only in Connecticut was the registry run by the state health department; in the other four it was operated by a major university under contract to the state. The original SEER family also included registries in the metropolitan areas of Detroit and San Francisco–Oakland. Although these registries covered only about 14 percent of the U.S. population, NCI statisticians were able to extrapolate from the data to estimate cancer incidence and prevalence for the nation as a whole. For the first time, the nation had a permanent system, albeit an indirect one, for measuring the extent of its cancer burden. William Haenszel, the head of biometry at the NCI and a primary architect of SEER, later reflected that the epidemiology of the disease at the time remained "a big unknown" and noted that SEER was "the first attempt to get a handle on the extent of cancer."[91]

In the three decades following its creation, SEER would expand incrementally, as the NCI added state and regional registries that were sufficiently advanced to provide reliable and complete data. In 1974 two more metropolitan areas, Atlanta and the thirteen-county Seattle–Puget Sound area, were added. Subsequent additions were chosen to include as much data as possible on "underserved" populations: racial and ethnic minorities and low-income groups. In 1978 ten predominantly African American counties of rural Georgia and Native Americans within Arizona were added. In 1992 five California counties—Los Angeles and four counties south of San Francisco—were added to increase coverage of Hispanics. In 2001, Kentucky, Louisiana, New Jersey, and all of California joined the program. Over the years a few states also joined the program but were subsequently dropped because they stopped meeting SEER's standards for data quality and completeness. By 2005 SEER would grow to include fourteen areas representing about 26 percent of the U.S. population.[92]

Concerns about patient privacy were notably absent from the establishment of SEER. This was partially because the individual state registries that made up the program sent their information to the NCI without patient names. More broadly, the public awareness of and engagement with cancer reporting was limited. But radical social changes would soon alter that landscape.

CANCERS AND COMMUNITIES

The creation of SEER marked a turning point in the ability to ascertain the extent of cancer nationwide. But for all the quality of its data, it presented only a broad picture of the nation's cancer situation, one that was largely insensitive to regional or local variation. It was this inherent limitation in SEER that led to another series of events—grassroots rather than governmental—that would transform cancer reporting.

In the 1970s and 1980s concern about the effect of contaminants in the environment, first galvanized by Rachel Carson's landmark 1962 book *Silent Spring*, increasingly gripped the popular imagination. As the idea that lurking carcinogens were a by-product of modern industrial society seeped into the nation's consciousness, citizens around the country engaged in what one analysis called "popular epidemiology," detecting potential hazards in their communities and taking political action to hold corporate polluters responsible.[93] The media became preoccupied with reports of suspected "cancer clusters," such as the cases of childhood leukemia in Woburn, Massachusetts, that led to civil suits against R. W. Grace and Beatrice Foods and were subsequently dramatized in the book and movie *A Civil Action*. In 1978 and 1979 the back-to-back dramas of Love Canal and the accident at the Three Mile Island nuclear power plant in Pennsylvania captured national headlines.[94] In 1980 Congress created the "Superfund" program, administered by the Environmental Protection Agency, which devoted billions of dollars to cleaning up toxic waste sites around the country and drew further public attention to the hazards in the environment.[95]

Around the country, communities in the 1980s clamored for better information on their cancer incidence. The American Cancer Society, which conducted no surveillance of its own, felt "a constant press for local data."[96] Such concerns about cancer in the environment led to a spate of political activity as lawmakers around the country moved to make cancer a reportable condition, and more than a dozen states created registries to track cancer incidence.[97] In some states it was a particular episode involving a suspected carcinogen that led to action; in others it was more generalized concern about the unknown effects that living or working near environmental toxins might have. For most of the registries, a case report of cancer with demographic information on the patient and medical data on the cancer was included. No follow-up information on treatment or survival was tracked other than the date of death.

In the late 1970s New Jersey legislators became alarmed at their state's apparently high rates of cancer—it had the highest death rate from the disease in the nation—and feared that environmental toxins and pollutants might be responsible. The state had a high concentration of chemical industry plants, which many residents believed were a source of cancer-causing agents. Salem County, where a quarter of the men worked in the chemical industry, had rates of bladder cancer more than twice the national average, while investigations found carcinogens in the water supply in communities in the Passaic Valley and at Toms River. Disparate data such as these led the state health commissioner in 1977 to declare that the connection between cancer and the environment, especially the workplace, was "a plausible hypothesis— although as yet an unproven one."[98]

In response to these concerns, the state legislature convened a commission on cancer incidence in 1976 and created a cancer registry the following year to track all cases of the disease.[99] The state senator who chaired the panel noted the apparent inconsistency in public health requirements: infectious diseases must be reported but cancer need not be. "We have no idea," he declared, "how many cases are being diagnosed and treated or what types of cancer are currently prevalent. Such a lack of statistical knowledge is an obvious hindrance to any cancer control program."[100]

In Pennsylvania, even before the drama of Three Mile Island, concern about dangers of excess radiation among residents living near a nuclear power plant led the governor to appoint an expert panel to investigate the possible increased risk. In 1974 the panel determined that it was unable to reach any conclusions because there was inadequate data about cancer incidence in the state. This outcome led to the appointment of another expert panel, which recommended that a statewide cancer registry with mandated reporting be established. The legislation creating the registry was signed into law in 1980—one year too late to provide data relevant to the accident at Three Mile Island.[101]

Over the next decade such statewide registries were used in analyses of several high-profile cases of suspected clusters. Many of these investigations refuted or failed to confirm links between a given environmental contamination and cancer. For example, during the 1980s four members of the New York Giants were diagnosed with cancer after the football team relocated to a newly constructed sports complex in East Rutherford, New Jersey. Subsequent analysis using the cancer registry data indicated that the cluster most likely was the result of chance and not due to environmental toxins at the sports complex.[102] When residents in a small town in Idaho suspected that cases of brain cancer were due to contamination from a nearby landfill, one study using registry data found no elevated rates of the disease, while a second study found higher rates of brain cancer but lower rates of four other types of cancer.[103] And an analysis of the most infamous environmental disaster of the era, Love Canal, found no elevated rates of cancer in the neighborhood compared to the rest of the state.[104] In spite of these negative findings, environmentalists and cancer activists remained strong supporters of registries.

Such investigations implicitly gave priority to the public's right to know about the hazards to which they were exposed. More broadly, the activity around cancer reporting beginning in the mid-1970s threw into sharp relief the extent to which state public health departments lagged in dealing with cancer and chronic diseases more generally. Although by 1985 some thirty-one states had established registries, only five had robust cancer control programs.[105]

"THE CANCER WEAPON AMERICA NEEDS MOST"

The activism of citizen groups around cancer clusters exemplified the effects that the environmental, feminist, and civil rights movements had on the relationship between communities and the public health establishment. A parallel and closely related social movement during this period was the rise of patient advocacy groups who mobilized around particular diseases. Most prominent were AIDS activists, who lobbied for changing the way clinical trials were designed and experimental drugs were approved.[106] It was this type of activism that ultimately led the CDC to fund the development of a cancer registry in every state.

During the 1980s the breast cancer patient activist movement gained prominence, exemplified by the work of pioneering activist Rose Kushner, whose 1979 memoir *Why Me?* was a watershed in the movement for greater patient empowerment. Activists were inspired by the examples of Kushner and public figures who "came out" as breast cancer survivors, such as First Lady Betty Ford; Happy Rockefeller, wife of New York governor Nelson Rockefeller; and the journalist Betty Rollin, who wrote of her experiences with the disease in her memoir *First You Cry*. By writing and speaking publicly about their experiences, women with cancer sought to remove the stigma and silence they saw as surrounding the disease; they challenged existing treatment paradigms and demanded a greater role in medical decision making. Transforming "the personal into the political," they also demanded to be counted.[107] This demand, in addition to its symbolic resonance, had a concrete political purpose: a key claim of activists was that the government was devoting paltry financial resources to a problem of unrecognized magnitude. Surveillance thus became a lever in a struggle for greater government funding that would drive research agendas.

In 1990 the National Breast Cancer Coalition was formed under the leadership of the well-known surgeon Dr. Susan Love. The following year the group launched a grassroots letter-writing campaign in which people across the country flooded the White House with letters urging the federal government to devote more funding to breast cancer research.[108] As this campaign was underway, a group of breast cancer activists in Vermont—one of the states that had no cancer registry—pushed forward the issue of greater surveillance. Two breast cancer survivors in the state organized a letter-writing campaign parallel to the national "do the write thing" effort but focused specifically on establishing universal cancer reporting. Although most states had some type of central cancer registry by this point, most had only partial coverage of total cancer incidence in the state. Ten states had no registry at all.[109]

Early in 1992 activist Pat Barr and several other breast cancer survivors visited their senator, Patrick Leahy, and their representative, Bernie Sanders, and urged them to introduce legislation that would establish a national program to collect data on cancer incidence. Legislation was introduced in the Senate and House in February 1992. Speaking in support of his bill on the floor of the House of Representatives, Bernie Sanders—a socialist, one of Congress's most liberal members, and its only registered Independent—repeatedly invoked claims of a public "need to know."

"Clearly, if we are going to be effective in fighting cancer in general, and breast cancer specifically, we need more information—we need better than estimates," Sanders declared. "Our researchers need information that they do not have today. . . . We need to know the age of people who are coming down with cancer. We need to know where they live. We need to know the kind of work they do. We need to know their racial and ethnic backgrounds. We need to know the relationship between early detection and the success of treatment. In other words, we need as much information as we can gather."[110]

Throughout 1992, as the bills to establish the national program of cancer registries wended their way through Congress, a highly charged debate about statistics raged in activist circles and the popular media. In March an article by the *New York Times* health reporter Sandra Blakeslee titled "Faulty Math Heightens Fear of Breast Cancer" challenged the widely cited—but, some argued, spurious—figure that a woman had a one in nine chance of contracting breast cancer during her lifetime. Activists seeking to convince the public of the urgency of their cause were frustrated at their inability to prove, through reliable statistics, that the problem was grave enough to warrant greater political attention and commitment of funds. "A little investigation reveals that our statistical gathering apparatus leaves much to be desired," declared activist Nancy Bruning in the June 1992 issue of the newsletter of Breast Cancer Action, a national advocacy group. The *Times* article, Bruning claimed, "forced many thinking people to ask: Just how are these statistics derived? Can we trust them? How do we know the incidence isn't *higher* rather than lower? . . . There's no question that we need numbers in which we can have confidence. There are many who believe founding a national tumor registry is a crucial step on the road to establishing statistics that are less open to debate."[111]

The push was galvanized when *Reader's Digest* published in May 1992 the article "The Cancer Weapon America Needs Most" by John Healey, the head of orthopedic surgery at Sloane-Kettering Cancer Center in New York. "Why does the United States lag behind many other Western nations in gathering cancer data that could save thousands of lives and billions of dollars?" Healey asked in the article. "Perhaps policy makers have always assumed that money is best spent on research and patient care. Record-keeping pays off only well into the future, after data have been collected long enough to reveal trends. Thus we tend to gamble it won't be necessary."[112]

The political debate over cancer registries represented a stark reversal of positions in the fights that were erupting at that very moment over named reporting of HIV cases, the topic to which we turn in chapter 7. While people with cancer demanded the right to be the *subjects of* surveillance, people with HIV sought *protection from* surveillance. Basic characteristics of the diseases and those who suffered from them as well as the potential for public health intervention help explain this apparent paradox. A central rationale of increased cancer surveillance was to enhance understanding of its etiology; HIV's causative agent and modes of transmission were, by the mid-1980s, well known. Because HIV was infectious and fatal, surveillance carried the threat of triggering coercive, even draconian, control measures. Further, people with HIV—primarily gay and bisexual men and drug users and their sexual partners—were highly stigmatized; they feared they would be the targets of discrimination, even violence, should their condition become known. The middle- and upper-class women leading the charge for breast cancer reporting had no such concerns. In the context of HIV, privacy was a civil liberty that was critical to defend; in the context of breast cancer, it would have to yield in the name of health.

The proposal received strong support from the Congressional Caucus for Women's Issues and from representatives of states in the Northeast and mid-Atlantic, where the issue had special urgency because of data suggesting that these regions had breast cancer mortality rates in excess of other areas of the country. The measure (attached to a foreign appropriations bill) passed the House by a large majority, and the Senate version passed on a unanimous voice vote. President George H. W. Bush signed the Cancer Registries Amendment Act into law in mid-October 1992. The act authorized the CDC to set up a program to provide financial and technical support for population-based cancer registries in every state.[113]

Before states could receive federal funding, they had to have laws in place that provided for the confidentiality of the registry data.[114] Indeed, a major hurdle for states in establishing their registries once Congress passed the act was ensuring that a panoply of legal regulations were in place: laws that mandated case reporting by hospitals, laboratories, and health care providers; laws that provided the registry with access to medical records; and laws that allowed studies to be conducted using the data. In 1993 only nine states had all the statutes in place that the CDC deemed essential.[115] By 2000 all states had established statewide population-based registries, most of which tracked cancer incidence only. The CDC's National Program of Cancer Registries provided financial support for forty-five states, including some states that also received funding through the NCI's SEER program.

It is significant that in the decade following its enactment in 1992, the only time the Cancer Registries Amendment Act was amended was in response to demands from activists with a particular type of cancer that they, too, be counted. Less than half of state registries collected data on benign brain tumors, which accounted for about half of all brain tumors. In spite of their classification as "benign," they could be as life threatening as malignant brain tumors. Advocacy groups such as the National Brain Tumor Foundation, which increasingly tapped into the organizing power of the internet to mobilize supporters, sought mandatory reporting of the condition nationwide and urged people with the disease and their loved ones to lobby their members of Congress.[116] Congressional testimony on the bill featured poignant personal testimony from a survivor of a benign brain tumor who invoked the public "need to know" that had been a leitmotif running through the calls for surveillance in the 1992 hearings: "In Norway, where data is kept on benign brain tumors, the incidence rate for men has increased by 250 percent. . . . Is this happening in the United States? We cannot know without data."[117] The bill's Senate sponsor, Jack Reed of Rhode Island, made explicit the link between surveillance and funding: the "lack of consistent data on the incidence of benign brain tumors has hindered the ability of the scientific community to invest appropriate resources into brain tumor research."[118] The Benign Brain Tumor Cancer Registries Act was signed into law in October 2002.

THE RIGHT TO KNOW AND THE RIGHT TO BE LEFT ALONE

Patients, doctors, concerned citizens, and researchers all had a stake in the data that was held in cancer registries—and in the policies governing when and how the data could be released. Community members who feared carcinogens in the environment wanted access so that they could judge potential risks to themselves and their neighbors; researchers wanted access so that they could enlist cancer patients in clinical trials and epidemiological studies. Patients themselves wanted privacy, of course, but many also believed that too strict a commitment to privacy could hobble the usefulness of registries, while others felt they had a right to choose whether to be included in a registry. The shifting and sometimes unpredictable stances toward appropriate procedures for confidentiality of data illustrated the complex politics of privacy. As universal reporting of cancer became a reality in the United States in the 1990s against a backdrop of heightened public concern about the sharing of medical information, conflicts over access to registry data played out in public meetings, legislatures, and courtrooms.

The same force that catalyzed the creation of many state registries—popular concern about incidence of cancer in communities—would eventually bring citizens in conflict with public health officials, who sought to balance their duties to the public with their responsibility to protect individuals listed in registries. The most contentious and protracted controversy unfolded in Illinois, which in 1986 had created a health and hazardous substances registry—a set of linked databases collecting information on birth defects, occupational diseases, and cancer—to track conditions potentially related to environmental hazards. Within two years of its founding, a tug-of-war over the data began between the health department and community members. After four cases of neuroblastoma, a rare cancer, were diagnosed in children in Taylorville, in southern Illinois, the children's parents suspected the illnesses were caused by exposure to coal tar, a known carcino-gen that was released into the environment during the cleanup of an energy plant in the community. The parents sued the utility company responsible for the plant; in addition, one of the mothers filed a Freedom of Informa-tion Act request asking the state cancer registry to release data on leukemia and childhood cancer in the county. The request did not ask for patient names but did ask for data broken down by zip code, year of diagnosis, and type of cancer.[119] The state health department refused, arguing that even in the absence of names, the identities of individual patients could be inferred from those three pieces of information. The health department offered instead to release the data but with the county of residence substituted for the zip code—a compromise unacceptable to the parents. The case ulti-mately ended up in a state appellate court.

In determining whether the data should be released, the judges sought guidance from the legislative language of the act that created the registry—language that bore the clear imprint of public concerns over cancer. The purpose of the registry was to "inform and protect the citizens of Illinois"; further, the act explicitly stipulated that "all information contained in the Registry shall be made available to the public upon request."[120] At the legal heart of the matter was the interpretation of a section of the act regarding privacy. "The identity, or any group of facts *which tends to lead to the identity,* of any person whose condition or treatment is submitted to the Illinois Health and Hazardous Substances Registry is confidential and shall not be open to public inspection or dissemination."[121] Would the pieces of infor-mation requested by the Taylorville mothers "tend to lead" to the disclosure of identities in the registry? The judges in the case determined that they would not, and after the department failed to comply with a subpoena demanding the data, a judge held state health commissioner John Lumpkin in contempt of court. Lumpkin eventually negotiated a compromise under which the expert who would analyze the data would protect patient confidentiality.[122]

That agreement did not end the story, however. The controversy was re-opened—with essentially the same issues at stake—in 1997, when the news-paper *Southern Illinoisan* asked the registry to provide data on the incidence of neuroblastoma from 1985, again without names but with zip code and date of diagnosis. As it made its case for access, the paper stated, "If there are clusters of neuroblastoma in Southern Illinois . . . we want to know that."[123] The health department's refusal to turn over the data, on the same grounds as before, reignited the debate over whether fragments of infor-mation from the registry were sufficient to identify individual patients.

The centerpiece of this new trial was the testimony of a Carnegie Mellon University professor who served as an expert witness for the health depart-ment. LaTanya Sweeney, who held a doctorate in computer science from the Massachusetts Institute of Technology, testified at trial that, through a six-step matching process using a standard laptop computer and commercially available software, she had been able to identify a single correct individual for eighteen of the twenty cases provided to her. While the Department of Public Health defended their continued shielding of the registry data by pointing to Sweeney's success—and arguing that "one does not need to be a professor from MIT" to determine the identities in the data sets—a three-judge panel on the appellate court rejected the state's "alarmist conjecture."[124] "We find it difficult to believe," they wrote, "that an individual with less knowledge, education, and experience than Dr. Sweeney would have been able to navigate the six-step process as adeptly as she did."[125] "Are there two people in the entire state of Illinois who could replicate [these] results with the same limited data or are there two thousand? Are there zero or are there a million? These questions are significant because without some sense of the magnitude of the alleged threat . . . it is very difficult for this court to determine whether the data in question reasonably tends to lead to the identity of specific persons."[126] In 2004 the three appellate judges affirmed a lower court ruling ordering the release of the data, and in early 2006 the Supreme Court of Illinois unanimously upheld the verdict.[127] The publisher of the *Southern Illinoisan* declared the ruling a victory for "the public's right to know."[128]

In New York, however, a similar request by a citizens' group produced an outcome that stood in sharp contrast to the extended battles in Illinois. In 1999 the grassroots group St. Lawrence Environmental Action filed a Freedom of Information Law request with the state health department asking for the release of cancer diagnoses and deaths for St. Lawrence County for the previous twenty years. New York state law contained the following provision: "The reports of cancer cases . . . shall not be divulged or made public so as to disclose the identity of any person to whom they relate" and prohibited the release of information "that identifies, or could lead to the identification of, an individual cancer patient." Registry staff argued that the requested records fell under these exemptions. They also argued that, in combination with the Social Security death index available via the internet, the information could be used to identify individuals in the registry. A panel of judges in the appellate division of the state supreme court agreed, and the records were denied.[129]

Nationwide, no clear pattern of dealing with such cases emerged. A survey in 2003 found that it was the policy in at least twenty-one states not to make neighborhood-specific data from cancer registries available to citizens who requested it.[130]

Equally contentious were questions about access to the data by academic researchers. In 1981 the Department of Health and Human Services had ruled that researchers could conduct epidemiologic studies using previously collected data, such as cancer registry records, without obtaining the informed consent of subjects, provided certain conditions were met.[131] But cancer registries also played an essential role in studies on patient care and outcomes by providing a pool from which participants could be drawn. In cases where researchers wanted the ongoing participation of a person with cancer, a critical question arose: What procedures for the recruitment of cancer patients into studies would be most ethical, effective, and respectful of privacy? Patients could be solicited directly by researchers but might feel their privacy had been violated if contacted by someone they had never met. The patient's physician could serve as a gatekeeper, deciding whether a given patient should be solicited and making the initial contact, but some people might feel pressured to participate in the study because the request came from their doctor: "I feel I have to because my doctor wants me to."[132] A 2004 study found considerable variation around the country in the way state cancer registries dealt with the issue. Between 2000 and 2004 several registries made policy changes that displaced physicians as gatekeepers, reflecting a general sense that they should not have the right to decide whether a patient should be given the option of participating in a trial.[133]

The question of how to enroll patients in research reignited the broader question of whether people diagnosed with cancer should have the right to be informed that their personal information was included in the registry in the first place. "One of the complaints that was heard from consumers was that people don't know that the cancer registry exists," recalled Janice Platner, a breast cancer survivor in Massachusetts who served on the state registry's advisory committee. "It's not even an issue of consent so much as knowledge that their information goes to the cancer registry. . . . People get a call out of the blue saying we're doing this research on blah blah blah. Some people get quite upset. How did they get my name? Where did that come from?"[134] Registry directors often received angry phone calls and letters from individuals who learned to their dismay that a state-run database had large amounts of information about them and their condition. In most cases, these patients were mollified once the purpose of the registry and the extensive confidentiality procedures were explained to them.[135] But some cancer patients sought changes in law and policy.

Of registries that were established after the Cancer Registries Amendment Act, only Oregon had included in its authorizing legislation a requirement that all patients be notified that their case was being added to the registry. But other states moved to implement a notification requirement at the urging of patients who were disturbed to learn about the registry after being contacted by a researcher. In Massachusetts such complaints led a state legislator to introduce a bill in 1996 that would have required patients to give written informed consent before their information was sent to the cancer registry. The measure "was a pen stroke away from being enacted" when alarmed registry staff intervened, Platner recalled.[136] As a member of the advisory committee, Platner opposed the measure, believing that it would hinder needed research. But her view on the matter was complicated: in addition to being a breast cancer survivor, Platner was also a lawyer and self-described "committed privacy advocate" who served on the privacy committee of the Massachusetts American Civil Liberties Union. To the extent that these roles were in tension, Platner's views on the necessity of surveillance trumped her concerns about privacy. The registry's staff and their allies was able to scuttle the legislation; instead a protocol was developed for research recruitment whereby patients would be notified by letter when they were added to the registry and given the option of declining to be contacted by researchers in the future.

Other states confronted similar threats. "It is not possible to collect data for population-based statistics and public health purposes if informed consent is required" was the blunt response of a manager at the Virginia cancer registry when a bill similar to the one in Massachusetts was introduced in 2000.[137] Drawing on long-standing arguments about the necessity of mandatory reporting for other notifiable diseases, Virginia health officials claimed that the addition of a consent requirement would inevitably lead to an unknown number of cancer patients opting out of the registry, thereby undermining the quality of the data. Registry staffs across the country further feared that an informed consent requirement would place an unmanageable burden on registries that were already stretched thin in terms of financial resources and staffing. Echoing the Virginia officials, an editorial in the *New England Journal of Medicine* declared: "Public health is threatened by incomplete data more than individual privacy is threatened by disease registries."[138]

Some patients argued that even if they were not able to give *consent* before being included in the registry, then at least they should be *informed*. When Seattle-area resident Darla Eastman was contacted by a researcher who had gotten her name from the Washington cancer registry, she was shocked at how much knowledge about her the investigator already had gotten from the database. "My Social Security number was even out there," Eastman said. "It upset me, to say the least." Eastman contacted her representative, who introduced a bill in the state legislature that would require the registry to send a letter to anyone whose information was added explaining the registry and its purpose. "The cancer registry is an important program that we want to preserve," said the state representative who sponsored the measure. "But we don't want people to be surprised that data about them is in the database. They deserve to be adequately informed." As of mid-2007 the bill had not passed the legislature.[139]

CANCER SURVEILLANCE IN THE TWENTY-FIRST CENTURY

Together, the federal government's two major cancer surveillance efforts provide depth and breadth. The fourteen state and regional SEER registries are widely seen as the "gold standard" for data, with high standards of accuracy and completeness.[140] While most experts agree that the knowledge supplied through the CDC's National Program of Cancer Registries is a valuable component of the nation's cancer control armamentarium, there are dissenting voices. In a 2002 commentary in the *American Journal of Public Health*, David Thomas, a physician with the Fred Hutchinson Cancer Center in Seattle and a former SEER grantee, argued that routinely collecting data on all cases of cancer in the population through state-level registries was an ineffective and inefficient tool for cancer control. Trends in incidence and mortality could be estimated from the SEER program, Thomas contended, while information on treatment and survival patterns could be more effectively and cheaply gained from the information in hospital-based tumor registries or through clinical trials. "There are good enough alternatives to registry data," Thomas argued, "that funding for a statewide registry is difficult to justify based only on its value for cancer control purposes."[141] Thomas's blunt assessment—which, not surprisingly, ruffled more than a few feathers among those who ran state cancer registries—embodied the long-standing disagreement about how best to apply the techniques of surveillance and would be replayed in the debates over HIV.

6

Who Shall Count the Little Children?

From *"Crippled Kiddies" to Birth Defects*

Although birth certificates had tracked congenital defects since the early twentieth century,[1] the surveillance of "crippled kiddies" was spearheaded in the 1920s by white, middle-class men and women concerned with restoring a generation of children to their full economic potential.[2] Building on the efforts of their progressive era predecessors, fraternal clubs, business groups, and cause-based volunteers would create the foundation for a surveillance effort that would broaden in scope until it ultimately included congenital birth defects. In the years after World War I, as business and fraternal groups emerged as the leaders of the movement to assist "crippled children," certainty of the value of private-public partnerships informed their efforts. Eventually such efforts would become institutionalized in state public health and child welfare departments with the rise of the New Deal state. All these initiatives represented an effort to provide direct services.

In the 1960s, with the thalidomide disaster, and in the 1970s, as the environmental movement came into full swing, the preeminence of service provision would be eclipsed by a new imperative to use surveillance to support a research enterprise. This would create new tensions, and conflict would emerge over the goals of surveillance. The public urgently wanted to understand who and what was responsible for alarming clusters (or presumed clusters) of birth defects. But birth defects surveillance expanded in a context where a clear legal right to reproductive privacy had been upheld by the Supreme Court. Thus while birth defects surveillance would proceed by popular demand, a competing set of public demands would also subject it to limits in the name of privacy.

ORIGINS: FROM POLIOMYELITIS TO CRIPPLED CHILDREN

Although tuberculosis inspired some of the earliest efforts to create surveillance systems for crippled children, it was the epidemics of poliomyelitis, which began sweeping the nation after the turn of the century, that became central to successful initiatives to identify, track, and guide crippled children to services.[3] Polio first appeared in the United States in 1893. During the first major epidemic of 1916, the number of severe cases totaled 29,000.[4] From the mid-1890s to the 1950s, on average, 16,000 paralytic cases were reported each year, with a peak incidence of 13.6 cases per 100,000 in 1952.[5] In general between 2 and 10 percent of paralytic cases resulted in death. Polio—an infectious, epidemic threat—was rapidly made a notifiable condition.[6] The New York City Department of Health declared polio a communicable disease and mandated physician reporting beginning in 1910. California imposed reporting by physicians and authorized compulsory isolation and quarantine for cases and contacts beginning in 1912.[7] Thirty-eight states required reporting by 1919.[8]

The first systematic efforts to register all crippled children, as opposed to individuals with infectious polio, were motivated by recognition of the devastation caused by the epidemic of 1916. In New Jersey, for example, polio was responsible for over a third of the crippled children; the same was true for the nation as a whole.[9] Whereas in the progressive era tuberculosis accounted for the greater portion of crippled children, by the 1920s those paralyzed by polio represented "a larger portion of the present cripples." Children crippled by polio were followed in numbers by cases due to congenital deformities.[10] When Illinois created a registry of crippled children in 1932, the state identified some 2,308 children who suffered some loss of function or mobility due to polio—representing 20 percent of all children identified.[11] In general, half of those who survived paralytic polio regained normal muscle functioning. Another quarter were left with mild paralysis, the remainder with severe, permanent paralysis involving limbs, respiration and swallowing, or both.[12] Conservative estimates tell us that polio left some 3,000 children and young adults with "crippling deformities" each year.[13] But despite the tradition of surveillance for acute poliomyelitis, by and large it was not the state that drove efforts to register crippled children.

In the mid-nineteenth century, a variety of voluntary charity, fraternal, religious, and business associations had begun to address the needs of crippled children in urban settings.[14] Orphanages, hospitals, and other institutions were opened to care for the children of a society's "brothers." The Masons, Odd Fellows, Knights of Pythias, and members of the Loyal Order of the Moose had opened as many as a hundred institutions serving thousands of children by the early decades of the twentieth century.[15] By the 1920s some of these organizations were no longer focused exclusively on assisting the families of the fold and began to serve a broader community; as they did so, they began to move away from institutionally based services.[16]

America's businessmen in the 1920s, like their counterparts in the charity movement who had spearheaded the tuberculosis effort, were also vitally concerned with child education and welfare and the kinds of future citizens (and, critically, employees) those children would become.[17] Merchants, bankers, lawyers, and other businessmen were central to the financing of charity endeavors throughout the progressive era and held prominent positions in charity organizations.[18] Yet they were involved in their capacity as citizens, not specifically businessmen, in an era in which the people sought to participate in civic life. In the period after WWI, however, the politics of reform would shift.[19] A variety of civic, fraternal, business, and women's clubs—including the Elks, Masons, Rotarians, Lions, Kiwanians, and Junior League—were drawn into the identification of crippled children and delivery of services. These efforts, which intensified in the 1920s, were based in the idea of business "associationalism,"[20] voluntary cooperation between business and government.[21] Economic stability and commercial and industrial productivity were the primary goals of associational government.[22] But these public-private collaborations were also aimed at meeting public needs.[23] They were active, working collaborations: "This . . . ever enlarging group of people in each state who are intelligent in regard to the peculiar nature of the social problem of the cripple . . . register . . . that intelligence" by participating in social welfare administration.[24]

CRIPPLED KIDDIES: SURVEILLANCE FROM THE BOTTOM UP

The collaboration of business, citizens, and the state in initiating surveillance is illuminated by the history of crippled children's registration in New Jersey—credited as the first state to have developed a birth defects registry.[25] The original focus of this initiative, however, was not on birth defects. Beginning in 1922 the Benevolent and Protective Order of Elks, a white men's mutual aid and fraternal society dating from the mid-nineteenth century, formed the Crippled Kiddies Committee and began to identify children in need and link them with social, educational, and medical service providers.[26] In 1926 the Elks led a coalition of fraternal and business groups—inspired by the national concerns with child welfare that would blossom alongside the women's suffrage movement from the progressive era through the Depression years[27]—to persuade the state to create a temporary commission to establish the scope of the problem and respond to it.[28] The *New Jersey State Temporary Commission for Inquiry Relating to the Distribution and Condition of Crippled Children* included not only representatives of fraternal and business organizations but also, beginning in 1930, a representative of the "public-at-large."[29]

The first major undertaking of the New Jersey commission was a statewide census in 1927 to determine the number of crippled children and assess how their health care, educational, and vocational needs were being met.[30] Although it also called on physicians and health care organizations to report the names, addresses, and case details for crippled children, it emphasized the role of teachers, principals, insurance workers, fraternal organization members, clergy, motion picture theater managers, and the police in ensuring that all crippled children were identified.[31] While there was an organization of black Elks, it was not involved in the crippled kiddies initiative.[32] There is no evidence that the New Jersey Elks *failed* to register and assist blacks, but the history of neglect for minority populations in the instance of tuberculosis, at least, suggests that any concerted effort to seek out and assist minority racial groups was improbable, particularly given the strong popular associations between polio and white, middle-class children.[33]

The commission distributed some thirty-five thousand census cards that asked recipients to collect detailed information on the name, address, economic situation, and physical ability of each child named and the means of the parents to meet his or her needs. There was no question about whether the benevolent citizens who spearheaded this effort should have access to information and be empowered to share it. Indeed, the commission encouraged home visits to ensure that the fullest possible information be obtained. The census cards did not address the possibility that participation might be refused and noted only, in advice that indicated the centrality of the schools to their surveillance effort, that "special care should be taken to avoid attracting attention to the defects of children in the classroom or of making crippled children self-conscious."[34]

Reflecting the service goals of the surveillance efforts, in 1929 the records of some 11,671 crippled children were distributed to one of the fifty-five local Elks lodges, which in turn hired nurses or welfare workers "to definitively check each case and secure the names of additional cripples in each community."[35] By 1930 the Elks had visited the homes and interviewed the parents of 80 percent of the cases they were charged with managing.[36] These visits included an initial assessment and referral to services and extensive follow-up. When medical treatment was warranted, noted the commission, "the case must be continually followed up by frequent periodic visits until correction of the deformity has been brought about or no further care is indicated."[37] The Elk leaders were not only managing but actively engaged in the social work enterprise. Contemporaries involved in the delivery of crippled children's services from both the public and private sectors referred to such efforts as "fraternal social work."[38] The crippled children's commission thus explained that "various lodges have sought out the crippled children, taking them to clinics, provided regular transportation, follow-up nursing care in the home, and have purchased braces, appliances and other equipment, when required."[39] That the fraternal order carried out "real quantities of work" would have been considered a robust measure of citizenship in the postwar period.[40]

In 1931 New Jersey broadened its vital statistics law requiring the reporting of congenital defects at birth to ensure that private organizations could receive and follow up on the "confidential" information.[41] The only hints that some parents may have objected to the intrusion of well-meaning citizens into their homes were occasional oblique references to the need to educate "reluctant parents and children to accept the necessary care."[42] On the surface it appears that resistant parents objected primarily to efforts to undermine their authority and decision-making capacity, not the registration of their child as "crippled" or the local community access to confidential information.[43] The response of the commission to the hesitant parent was paternalistic persistence: the offers for treatment, education, and training "are being repeated, and shall be continued until the last reluctant parent in the State has been brought to understand the best interests of the child."[44]

When the temporary commission was made permanent in 1931, the continuing legal participation of representatives of the Elks, Rotarians, Shriners, Kiwanians, and Lions together with a health department officer, a representative from the state medical society, and a government appointee indicated the degree to which this undertaking remained associational even as the Great Depression ushered in a new era of state-initiated social reform. Because the job of case management was considered "too great a burden to be placed on the taxpayers of the State," the Elks assumed an "important and permanent part of the process."[45]

The Elks invested considerable time and financial resources on the problem of crippled children in New Jersey—$152,000 in 1929 alone for investigators' salaries and direct care for children.[46] By 1935 they had invested over one million dollars in the problem of crippled children in the state.[47] Beginning in 1931 and 1932, the Kiwanis and Rotary clubs took on the responsibility for assuring that crippled children received vocational training; the Lions, for ensuring eye care for all registered children.[48] The Shriners likewise invested $20,000.[49] Thus, the state department of health was able to continue reporting cases to the commission so that it might continue its work of registering and then managing the care of crippled children.[50]

For these fraternal organizations, this was an investment in local communities.[51] The community, after all, might someday be required to support children without adequate educational or vocational training.[52] Promoting self-sufficiency was, therefore, the leitmotif, not only of this effort but of many initiatives—both public and private—involving handicapped children beginning in the 1920s.[53] In 1932 one of the local Elks' lodges described their efforts to restore to independence more than one hundred children who otherwise would have become "helpless cripples for life."[54] Indeed, the definition of the crippled child did not attempt to describe physical traits but rather focused on "reduce[ed] normal capacity for education for self-support."[55] The commission used success stories to champion "early reporting" of cases so that children might be treated and "permanently removed from the ranks of crippled children."[56]

In 1931 the New Jersey Crippled Children's Commission acknowledged that surveillance might serve ends other than direct medical or educational intervention with the child. But it concluded that "the important problem of the prevention of crippling" must remain a somewhat distant goal, "a matter for discussion in future reports."[57] The polio epidemics of that same year would help advance realization of that goal, providing the occasion to expand the rationale for case finding and registration to include research. Following the outbreak, in cooperation with the state department of health, the state medical society, and the Elks, the commission conducted a special survey of the 828 surviving cases of infantile paralysis to determine whether serum treatment was efficacious in preventing the crippling effects of the disease. Although the study proved inconclusive, it was of a piece with the overriding motivation for cancer reporting—improving medical care.[58]

THE RISE OF THE WELFARE STATE

New Jersey's surveillance efforts had begun on the eve of the Great Depression. During the early years of economic crisis, New Jersey clung tenaciously to its decentralized, collaborative approach to case finding and management in which community organizations played such a vital role.[59] So strongly did the commission feel that this should remain primarily a community-based and community-funded effort that it opposed appropriations in the Social Security Act for the state-based care of crippled children.[60] Only if communities remained vitally involved in the funding and implementation of efforts to identify and care for crippled children would they "have a voice locally in the making of county appropriations" and remain "fully informed in regard to the expenditure of the funds. Therefore, no particular part of the State feels that it is assuming a burden which ought to be borne by another section."[61]

But as the decade wore on and the polio and economic scourges worsened—indeed, economic want was framed as a "handicap" that demanded the state play the leading role in "rehabilitation"[62]—societal views of the role of government and the responsibilities of the private sphere for self-support would shift. The promise of President Franklin Roosevelt's New

Deal was the promise of economic security in which the state took a more prominent role in assuring the social welfare of communities.[63]

Despite her extensive affiliations with voluntary charity organizations, Katharine Lenroot, chief of the U.S. Children's Bureau, sought to expand conceptions of the obligations of the state to all of the nation's children, with a particular focus on its handicapped children.[64] While acknowledging the lead that private agencies and community groups had taken in addressing the needs of such children, by 1940 federal officials were convinced that further progress could not be made except through state-driven, "nationwide measures."[65] Lenroot observed that "much devoted service, life-long commitments, and a variety of sacrifices ungrudgingly brought to the service of children by the supporters and workers of private agencies have earned them the gratitude of the community."[66] But, she continued, both the Depression, which depleted the resources of individual organizations, and the changing nature of government contributed to the growing inability of communities to continue playing a leading role in the provision of services. As important as the labors of well-meaning citizens had been, the New Deal state defined as a "menace" to democracy the idea that "every man is as capable as any other of holding and performing the duties of any public office." Public and private leaders in the maternal and child health field argued that "the business of government" now required a kind of technical and professional competence that was well beyond the reach of the ordinary citizen.[67] Social workers, increasingly cognizant of their authority as professionals, also sought to minimize the role that communities might play in the future. While "approving" the continued participation of communities in efforts to assist physically needy children, attendants of the 1940 White House Conference on Children in a Democracy, chaired by Lenroot, "recognize[d] the ultimate *public* responsibility" for crippled children.[68] In this new political context, public responsibility clearly meant state responsibility.

The Social Security Act's grant-in-aid program for Crippled Children Services was a significant force in shifting the balance from community to state. Voluntary agencies would continue their efforts to provide services, but in the next decades the practices would change.[69] The Social Security Act resulted in the registration of some two hundred ninety thousand "physically handicapped" children.[70]

As federal funds supporting the New Jersey crippled children's program became available under the provisions of the Social Security Act, private funding dwindled. The Elks and their partners began to take a backseat to hospitals and state agencies in evaluating and referring crippled children to services.[71] The New Jersey Crippled Children's Commission grew into a full-fledged social service agency with separate divisions devoted to medical social work, statistics, rheumatic cardiac care, nursing, administration, and psychology.[72] It spawned other programs, such as the New Jersey State

Cerebral Palsy Program, which was supported almost entirely by federal funds and in which private, voluntary clubs and organizations played little role.[73] Thus the early efforts at finding and registering the crippled children of New Jersey became part of the institutional structure of the welfare state.

SURVEILLANCE FROM THE BOTTOM UP
MEETS SURVEILLANCE FROM THE TOP DOWN:
THE POLITICS OF ENUMERATION IN THE NEW DEAL STATE

As the surveillance of crippled children was institutionalized and the idea of governmental associationalism became a relic of the pre-Depression era, a popular desire to contribute to the social welfare—particularly when it involved the welfare of children—did not simply fade. By the 1940s cooperation between the state and groups such as the Elks, Rotary, Lions, Shriners, Salvation Army, Red Cross, Kiwanis Club, Junior League, American Legion, and other local charity and religious societies and private foundations continued to characterize registration efforts in most states and counties.[74] The challenge, in the new era of an emerging welfare state, would be how to negotiate public participation in surveillance.

Organized on behalf of Franklin Roosevelt in 1938, the National Foundation for Infantile Paralysis was devoted to raising funds for polio prevention and research and popularized the fight against polio by carrying its fund-raising efforts directly to the public, enlisting Hollywood personalities to appeal for donations. In so doing the National Foundation—whose fund-raising campaign was dubbed the March of Dimes by radio personality Eddie Cantor during its first national drive, in which it raised $1.8 million—rallied the public behind the cause of polio and its courageous victims.[75] By the 1940s National Foundation local chapters were developed enough for the national office to recommend that they create local registries of polio cases in order to deliver services to children left paralyzed by polio.[76] In 1940, without intending to suggest that they cease notification to health departments, the National Foundation appealed to doctors to report cases *directly* to the organization, sending out letters along with blank reports and return envelopes.[77]

The National Foundation organization also felt that state health officials should report cases directly to local chapters "rather than depend, as we are now doing, on the public health officer's weekly statement, as the information is two weeks old when we receive it."[78] To achieve this goal the organization wrote to all state crippled children's agencies asking for cooperation and data on all cases of poliomyelitis. While the foundation indicated that "nearly all expressed a willingness to assist us," it was also clear that the data-gathering initiative, in sharp contrast to the prior political era of associational government, now raised key questions in the mind of state agencies.[79]

Why did the foundation need the data? What did it plan to do with it? Indicative of state officials' concern with confidentiality, they further pressed the organization on how the registries would be compiled and maintained. The response sparked a national discussion not only with officials at crippled children's agencies but among public health officials as well.

The National Foundation—echoing the arguments that health officials consistently put forward in support of surveillance—insisted that it required the data because "no organization can function properly unless it knows the magnitude and extent of its problem. . . . Without records showing who is in need of care it is impossible to be sure our obligation" to care for all crippled children "has been fulfilled. An additional reason for compiling and keeping current such records is that this very act will publicize the fact that services are available for all poliomyelitis victims, regardless of race, age, creed, color, or place of residence." The foundation stressed that it would draw on "every available source of information" to complete its database. It stressed, "All suitable and ethical methods of learning of all cases will be used. The press, radio, parents groups, hospitals, etc., will be appealed to for their help in compiling as complete a record as possible."[80] The National Foundation intended to use the records to ensure that each patient "*is* under treatment," to help those without care into treatment, and to provide any other needed assistance to patients. It would further use the records "for the first time to provide a picture of the scope of the problem." Hence, it would "analyze the records *and furnish to interested agencies a breakdown in respect to sex, age, color, geographical distribution, and such other information as may be pertinent to evaluating the problem*" (fig. 19).[81]

As the scope of the National Foundation's agenda became evident, the response of public health professionals was to assert their authority. ASTHO praised the "noteworthy services given in behalf of handicapped children by the large number of voluntary organizations unique to America which constitute a contribution to the common welfare." But it also sought to circumscribe the contributions of volunteers. ASTHO was particularly concerned about coordination between the state and volunteers and was alarmed by the prospect of multiple registries of cases within each state that would necessarily result in a duplication of records and, hence, services. ASTHO tried to impress upon the National Foundation that "official agencies have primary responsibility for assuring that poliomyelitis patients (as well as patients with other physical handicapping conditions) receive adequate care. In carrying out this responsibility the official agency administers the function of case finding, case follow up, diagnostic and consultation services, and referral to care or the provision of care under safe-guards as to standards or quality. In relation to this responsibility the National Foundation for Infantile Paralysis should act in a *supporting* capacity" only.[82]

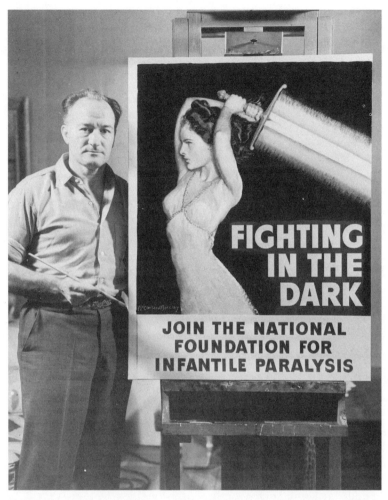

Figure 19. McClelland Barclay, *Fighting in the Dark*, c. 1941. Although this March of Dimes poster was intended to underscore the challenge of fighting polio in the midst of World War II in the context of a campaign for greater access to information, it also resonated with the century-long theme of giving "sight," through data, to those seeking to confront the challenge of infectious diseases. Reproduced with permission of the March of Dimes Birth Defects Foundation.

The National Foundation was quick to concede that "there is no question that the average Chapter, made up of volunteer lay people, is not in a position to determine proper hospital facilities, proper charges therefore or to obtain the best follow-up care for polio patients."[83] But because the organization viewed itself as "a force in the community for the improvement of facilities for the care of infantile paralysis patients," it continued to maintain a vital presence.[84]

For its part, ASTHO was prepared to support the foundation's recommendation that each state create a polio planning committee, which would include not only the state health officer and director of the State Crippled Children's Program but also members of the National Foundation for Infantile Paralysis, the Red Cross, and other key state professional associations, like medical societies.[85] It offered no objections to the National Foundation's recommendation to its local chapters that they report the names of children to the Crippled Children's Services program in the county and that the Crippled Children's Services program keep a statewide register of all children in need of rehabilitative services.[86] Thus the national office of the National Foundation was prepared to recognize that health officials had a certain primacy.[87] But the tensions over surveillance would not fade until the mid-1950s, when the foundation became fully focused on the effort to evaluate and distribute the Salk vaccine.[88]

THALIDOMIDE BABIES

Beginning in the late 1950s, a different set of anxieties would begin to motivate the call for birth defects surveillance. Worries about nuclear fallout combined with very early suspicion about the "river of chemicals that all of us use and breathe" sparked an interest in the root causes of birth defects.[89] As the infant mortality rate declined and the seeds of the environmental movement were sown, "whether birth defects are on the increase" came to represent "one simple question that surely ought to be answered."[90]

But if there was growing uncertainty about the hazards posed by exposure to new chemicals in the environment and the home, it was balanced by what the National Foundation for Infantile Paralysis called the "folklore" of congenital malformations. Still needing to be overcome was "the prevalent belief that most birth defects are due to hereditary factors and therefore, by implication, to deficiencies in the parents."[91] Thus, in 1958, after it determined that "the Salk vaccine had made it possible to eliminate polio as a serious threat to public health," the National Foundation looked to birth defects as it sought a new direction.[92]

Birth defects held a great deal of appeal for a foundation that wanted to focus its efforts on a new area of "*major* unmet needs" and "sufficient statistical importance" that was broader than polio but that would still lend "itself to the strategy of the small giver and the broad base." Public participation and "community level decisions by volunteers" continued to be viewed as essential for this organization that described itself as the "greatest non-governmental force for public health in the United States."[93]

But while the National Foundation would rally the public by citing the tremendous increase in birth defects—noting that "while 12,413 children died as the result of congenital malformations in 1939, the number had risen to 20,012 in 1953"—it would not initially focus on surveillance as a critical feature of its efforts. In a document that the foundation dubbed "the Bible," the organization's leaders set forth the parameters of their new mission: "to determine the cause and methods of prevention, to assist the medical and allied professions in improving methods for diagnosis and treatment and to fill present broad gaps in services to the congenitally malformed." Mirroring the focus of the NCI, the National Foundation explained that research activities—virology, embryology, genetics, endocrinology—were to be "at the heart" of its expanded program. Epidemiology remained conspicuously absent even as organizers lamented the weakness of vital statistics and the absence of a "central way of collecting information."[94]

The medical disaster of thalidomide—a drug to induce sleep and relaxation that, when taken during pregnancy, produced major limb deformities in newborns—would grimly reveal the limits of existing birth defects surveillance systems. In 1959 Richardson-Merrell, Inc., a company based in New York, began sending the new drug thalidomide to U.S. doctors for testing. It had already begun marketing the drug in Germany.[95] A year later the company filed for test marketing permission with the Food and Drug Administration (FDA). The application was famously reviewed by Frances O. Kelsey, a new medical officer whose predecessor had resigned over lax FDA review standards. She elected to subject the drug to more exacting scrutiny, and by November 1961 the reports about birth defects began coming out of Germany. John F. Kennedy awarded her the President's Award for Distinguished Service for having averted "a human tragedy."[96] The next year, U.S. hospitals began to report the birth of "thalidomide babies."

Despite the efforts that had been made to register crippled children in order to direct them to services, there was little by way of systematic surveillance of all newborns at *birth* in order to monitor congenital defects. Few states made any effort to use the limited data that was recorded as part of the birth certificate. Determining the impact of thalidomide in the United States, then, was pure guesswork.[97] Further underscoring that public health was "in the dark," the thalidomide disaster was followed by another. A 1964 outbreak of rubella—German measles—produced an epidemic of birth defects in 1965. In the period after 1965, then, the issue of "congenital defects as a national health problem was more clearly defined than ever before."[98]

But while the hope had been to institutionalize birth defects surveillance in order to prevent "other 'thalidomides,'"[99] few efforts came to fruition in the wake of that disaster.[100] The Metropolitan Atlanta Congenital Defects Program—created in 1967 and managed by the triumvirate of the CDC, the Georgia health department, and Emory University—was the signal achievement.[101] Although initiated just two years after *Griswold v Connecticut*, in which the Supreme Court had declared a constitutional right to privacy, the Atlanta program did not encounter any challenges on those grounds. Coming as it did upon the heels of the thalidomide disaster, which had illustrated the need for detecting the first warning signs of an outbreak of birth defects, the professional epidemiologists who had advocated for and developed the registry viewed it exclusively as a research venture. Reflecting the ethos of paternalistic privacy, physicians served as the gatekeepers to patients and only rarely denied the requests of health officials to contact a woman for follow-up investigations.[102]

Next to follow was New York. Although it had utilized the confidential information available regarding congenital defects on birth certificates since at least 1948, it attempted to recreate this system in the wake of thalidomide.[103] But the Birth Defects Institute, housed in the state department of health, bore the hallmark of the long tradition of crippled children's surveillance. Although formally charged with locating the causes and treatment of birth defects, it heavily emphasized service provision.[104] This was not the research enterprise that professionals at the forefront of birth defects surveillance believed would provide the necessary answers to the new questions posed in the context of detecting and preventing birth defects.

GRAND VISIONS, LITTLE PROGRESS IN AN ERA OF TECHNOLOGICAL AND SOCIAL CHANGE

The twin tragedies of thalidomide and congenital rubella syndrome unfolded in the midst of technological advances that were rapidly changing the medical approach to pregnancy, delivery, and birth. Ultrasound technology had been introduced in the late 1950s followed by amniocentesis a decade later.[105] These developments would usher in an era of feverish interest in identifying and categorizing congenital anomalies.[106] As one sociologist has argued, the new focus on congenital anomalies and "the advent of prenatal genetic testing precipitated a profound shift in how doctors, women, and society at large viewed babies with birth defects. What had previously been regrettable now became, in the context of legalized abortion, 'preventable.'"[107] Viewed within the context of postwar hereditarianism, with a focus on the genetic counseling of white, middle-class American couples, birth defects surveillance would not so much encounter the specter of malevolent eugenics but would, rather, stand it its late-afternoon shadow.[108]

Virginia Apgar, the renowned pediatrician who had pioneered a metric of newborn vitality, was part of the vanguard of physicians who were increasingly attentive to the condition of the infant at birth. Her awareness was not limited to the realm of the delivery room. Apgar, who immediately grasped the import of the data vacuum relating to birth defects, was also at the forefront of efforts to have the National Foundation—which had already dropped "Infantile Paralysis" from its title and would soon formally adopt March of Dimes (MOD) as its official name—take the lead in the "new venture" of birth defects registration (fig. 20).[109] She was quick to note the dismal quality of the data produced by inadequate vital statistics and was not optimistic that PHS efforts to improve the quality and amount of data captured on the birth certificate would represent a sufficient fix. Life insurance companies, she complained, had done a better job of documenting the incidence and prevalence of birth defects.[110] Surveillance was simply "a 'must.'" Apgar envisioned not just state systems but a national registry with consistent standards for reporting.[111] She was not alone in underscoring the importance of surveillance data. Charles Gardipee, chief of the Bureau of Crippled Children's Services in California, which was housed within the state department of health, was committed to delivering services to children. But, viewing the need for services as a measure of the *failure* on the part of public health to determine the causes of birth defects, he expressed a willingness to shift priorities: "If a choice had to be made between funding research and funding services, funding research would be the better decision."[112]

But no such tradeoff was necessary. Apgar's proposal for state and national birth defects surveillance would provide the basis for both research and intervention. "A crucial first step toward an expanded attack on the problem of birth defects," she wrote, "would be improvement in the quantity and quality of the underlying mortality and morbidity data for these conditions. Detailed and up-to-data state and national registration of children with handicapping conditions. . . . would assist materially in defining the scope of the problem for the purpose of planning adequate programs of medical care and research." Apgar appeared to have few reservations about the effort. Underscoring the extent to which confidentiality concerns were not foremost in her mind, a key argument for registration was its broad public utility: "Aside from the importance of genetic studies which can be derived from such a registry, many persons concerned with services to the handicapped would make frequent use of it. Teachers of mentally retarded children and young adults, of the blind and deaf, employers of the handicapped, architects, transportation officials and prosthetic engineers are among those to whom a registry would be useful."[113] Her vision, like that of others taken with the promise computerization held out for both public health and medicine, ran counter to the intensifying national concern about the erosion of privacy in a computer-driven dossier society.[114]

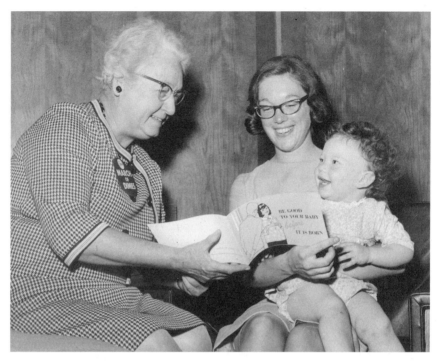

Figure 20. Virginia Apgar with a mother and child in 1968. As director of the March of Dimes' Division of Congenital Malformations and later its vice president for medical affairs, Apgar was a figure emblematic of the new national focus on both fetal and neonate health. The MOD pamphlet "Be Good to Your Baby Before It Is Born" underscored the new emphasis on preventing birth defects, which would both stimulate the extension of surveillance and provide grounds for resisting those efforts. Reproduced with permission of the March of Dimes Birth Defects Foundation.

But as growing anxiety about how computers posed a threat to confidentiality came to national attention, questions regarding large electronic databases could not fail to capture the attention of the bioethics committee of the March of Dimes, provoking discussions about "how to guarantee a patient's privacy and protect his identity." As it addressed this matter, it did not challenge the legitimacy of surveillance and, indeed, rejected the generalized fears of the "tyranny of the computer." Thus, the committee saw no ethical distinction between computerization and "simply monitoring birth certificates very carefully."[115]

What the committee did underline was the applicability of the Code of Fair Information Practices, which had been promulgated by the federal government in 1973. In so doing it threw into bold relief a fundamental challenge to the practice of public health surveillance. The committee left unanswered questions about how to proceed in the event that parents objected to having the diagnoses of their children computerized.[116] Such, questions, however, would be almost immediately resolved by the Supreme Court's 1977 decision in *Whalen v Roe*, which upheld the constitutionality of public health surveillance. Despite this nod toward privacy concerns and surveillance in the late 1970s, the MOD ethics committee remained focused on traditional questions of biomedicine throughout the 1980s and 1990s. Patient autonomy within the clinical relationship, not privacy versus the public health, remained the committee's central concern.

ENVIRONMENTAL CAUSALITIES
AND THE IMPERATIVE FOR DATA

As neonatal intensive care units developed and helped to further lower an already declining infant mortality rate in the United States, birth defects assumed greater salience and became an increasing cause for alarm. By the early 1980s birth defects came to represent the leading cause of infant deaths; they were identified as the cause of half of infant hospital admissions.[117]

In part, birth defects surveillance developed at a slow pace because of the challenges of diagnosis, which rivaled those presented by cancer.[118] Many conditions—like spina bifida and cleft palate—were readily apparent and unmistakable. Others, however, were far more subtle. Fetal alcohol syndrome, for example, was difficult to diagnose and often not recognizable at birth, when the most basic source of surveillance data—the birth certificate—is completed. There was no universally accepted definition, and diagnosis relied heavily on the subjective judgment of the physician to classify its range of often subtle craniofacial features, which varied with age and race.[119]

Furthermore, the issue of birth defects surveillance lacked urgency. The United States, thanks to the vigilance of Kelsey, had largely been spared the thalidomide disaster. In the wake of these events, health officials uniformly saw the need for surveillance as self-evident, but their conviction was not shared by the public. The United States lacked a critical mass of thalidomide parents who might collectively demand a system for ensuring that children were directed to services or sound a call for surveillance in order to spare other families from a similar burden. Thus while the MOD put forward a synoptic vision of national birth defects surveillance in the years after thalidomide, and research into the etiology of birth defects remained high on its agenda, little headway was made. By 1973 only four states had any kind of birth defects surveillance in place.[120]

The emerging environmental movement would reenergize the call for birth defects surveillance. Beginning in the early 1970s, there were signs of

growing concern about the effect of environmental pollution on birth outcomes.[121] Ordinary men and especially women were developing grave concerns about the role of the environmental toxins and pollution in the creation of birth defects clusters and felt increasingly compelled to speak out.
Their activism stood in contrast to the situation in occupational health,
where advocates felt straightjacketed by the politics of regulation during the
Ford administration. Concerns about the health risks of polyvinyl chloride,
for example, were originally focused on the plastics workers exposed to this
chemical.[122] By 1974, however, this chemical crossed over from representing
purely a hazard to workers to being a threat to consumers who used products like plastic wrap and hair spray.[123] It was not long before communities
surrounding petrochemical plants began to be concerned that they might
be affected by the release of the chemical into the air.[124] Clusters of birth
defects in communities with vinyl chloride polymerization plants would
come to national attention by 1976. Jet fuel, toxic waste dumps, pesticides,
and herbicides would all be linked to elevated rates of birth defects.[125] This
would set the stage for the major advances in birth defects surveillance in
the 1980s and 1990s.[126]

No agency claimed responsibility for monitoring birth defects surveillance.[127] The Environmental Protection Agency, for example, had little
interest in studying the biological manifestations of environmental toxins
and pollution. This agency was focused on finding more accurate technologies for measuring levels of substances in the environment.[128] For the
CDC, the problem of birth defects, while significant, was subordinate to the
broader issue of public health and the environment.[129]

But if convincing the state to track and protect the health of workers
would prove all but impossible for much of the twentieth century, bereaved
parents—mothers in particular—who could also warn of a more generalized threat to *all* of the unborn found they held the power to move elected
officials to action.

"SERVING THE PUBLIC THROUGH DATA"

In the late 1970s California experienced an outbreak of Mediterranean
fruit flies. The response was massive spraying of pesticides in the agricultural regions of the Central Valley—where the water supply for the San
Francisco Bay Area was located. While the spraying itself had provoked environmental concerns,[130] alarm about the "Med fly" episode was heightened
by a cluster of birth defects in San Francisco that the community felt was
linked to contaminated drinking water.[131] In 1983 the California Department of Health established "the largest birth defects registry in the world"—
the California Birth Defects Monitoring Program. In contrast to the Atlanta-
based registry, which had been spearheaded entirely by professionals, a

broad coalition that included environmental safety and child and maternal advocates worked to secure passage of the California legislation.[132]

The California system represented an important landmark. Its monitoring program built on the legacy of the regional Atlanta program and stressed research to the exclusion of services. Indeed, the mottos of the California system were "Preventing Birth Defects through Research"[133] and "Serving the Public through Data." Epidemiology, rather than medical, rehabilitative, or educational services directed to the individual child, was the hallmark of this effort.[134]

The MOD played a central role in the passage of the California legislation. The program that was developed was administered by the MOD. It served as a model for the voluntary organization as it sought to spearhead similar efforts across the nation. The MOD noted that California and Atlanta were the only "complete monitoring-research programs."[135] Expansion along the research front "in every state" was viewed as essential if investigation into the causes of birth defects was to advance and vigilance was to be maintained.[136] What the MOD did not anticipate, however, was the extent to which a focus on research to the exclusion of concrete benefits to children or consideration of questions of privacy and stigma could thwart legislative efforts to advance surveillance in a realm touching on sensitive issues of reproductive rights.

As state-based birth defects surveillance systems developed—sixteen states would authorize new systems between 1980 and 1995, the years before CDC funding became available to support such efforts—clusters of disease would continue to play a central role in sparking legislative efforts. As they unfolded, the politics of surveillance were anything but straightforward.

Success in creating birth defects surveillance systems depended not only on bipartisan but also cross-class and cross-racial or -ethnic alliances. For example, health officials, physicians, and the MOD had been advocating for a birth defects registry in Texas for at least ten years when, in 1991, a cluster of children born with anencephaly was reported in Cameron County.[137] Within this Gulf Coast area along the Mexican border, Brownsville and Harlingen became the sites of an intensive investigation conducted jointly by the CDC and the Texas Department of Health. The concern was with the hazard posed by more than nine hundred "twin plants" situated along the U.S.-Mexican border engaged in "production sharing."[138] Parts manufactured in the United States would be sent to this region along the border to be assembled at lower cost before being shipped back to the States. The twin plant, or *maquiladora*, industry had produced a "200-mile-wide-by-1,900-mile-long industrial zone" with factories stretching from Matamoros, just across the border from Brownville, to Tijuana and its U.S. border city, San Diego.[139]

After a year-long investigation, which resulted in the identification of another nineteen cases of anencephaly, health officials determined that the cases did not represent a cluster. But what they found was more alarming. While the rate of anencephaly among whites did not differ from the national average, the rate among Hispanics was significantly higher than that among whites. "We spent a lot of time and money answering the wrong question," said Dr. Dennis Perrotta, chief of epidemiology at the Texas Department of Health.[140]

That time and money would be spent again after a similar cluster appeared in east Texas.[141] The conclusions were similar, but this time the locale was the Woodlands, an affluent suburb of Houston. Whereas the cases in Brownsville lacked a particular face and name to rally behind, an affected Woodlands parent came forward to fight for surveillance legislation and a powerful coalition emerged. Ann Andis, a Houston-area mother and educator at a breastfeeding center whose anencephalic baby died five days after birth, continued to believe that her child had been part of a cluster of environmentally induced birth defects despite the conclusions of local and federal investigators: "The state is dependent on [a petrochemical] industry that is toxic," Andis insisted.[142] Along with another mother, she aired her convictions before the Texas legislature: "I live within walking distance of two other women who had babies with this problem."[143]

Limited though it was, she felt that she had the data to prove her case. At a press conference urging lawmakers to authorize a birth defects registry, Andis displayed a stack of note cards detailing the deaths of seventy-five Houston-area infants, hers among them. "This is my birth defects registry," she explained. She had gathered the data when, following a newspaper account of her story, mothers began phoning her, contributing the details of their own children's deaths.[144] Angry about how easy it was to dismiss birth defects as a problem of poverty, Andis stressed, "It is not just something that happens to poor women who don't have plumbing."[145] "I think it's happening more than people realize."[146] Her personal registry was a dual effort at inspiring both awareness and fear among a particular constituency: "Fear will help us to get the studies we need to deal with this."[147]

This time the Texas legislature responded swiftly. In 1993 Republican Kevin Brady, proclaiming Andis a "heroine," introduced a bill on the House side.[148] Democratic senator Carlos Truan, who represented the heavily Hispanic Lower Rio Grande Valley, also championed the effort to establish pilot programs in Houston and along the border.[149] Truan, who represented the Cameron County parents, touted the registry in universal terms: it "will enable us to prevent the tragedy of infants being born with serious and sometimes deadly birth defects, and will save the state's taxpayers millions of dollars in expensive medical treatment for children with birth defects."[150] Cost containment would be one of the major new justifications for birth defects surveillance in the 1990s.[151] The MOD would, however, continue to emphasize research. "It can lower the number of birth defects because it can identify them more quickly," said Dianne Bynum, a representative of a Texas chapter of the MOD. "Once a pattern is established, intervention can take place. Without this information our hands are tied."[152]

Despite the fact that undocumented immigrants, who had interests in protecting their identities from officials, were central to many of Texas's surveillance programs—including immunization status, HIV, and birth defects—privacy was never raised as an issue in Texas. In part, this was because the emphasis was on identifying the causes of birth defects, not parents or "defective" children. In addition, the type of cluster under investigation affected the political discussion. The importance of determining the causes of a condition such as anencephaly and trying to save other parents from similar grief seemed self-evident. And there was no dispute over whether anencephaly or other neural tube defects should be defined as birth defects. But anencephaly was, in some respects, unique among birth defects. It was one of a variety of neural tube defects in which the spinal cord and brain fail to develop correctly that was invariably fatal. While children with anencephaly propelled development of the registry in Texas and other states, these children would not have to face the stigma of being "labeled" with a birth defect. All would die within days, if not minutes, of their births. Moreover, as evidence linking neural tube defects and folic acid became solid in the early 1990s, the public health response was structural: pregnant women were not merely exhorted to consume the recommended forty milligrams of folic acid per day; in 1996, after ardent efforts on the part of the MOD, the FDA ordered enriched cereal-grain products to be fortified with folic acid by January 1, 1998.[153] Surveillance proved critical in documenting the success of the mandatory fortification program.[154] Here then was a resounding success story with no villains, no stigma.

But one of the lessons of *Whalen* was that stigma could be a powerful force in parental objections to surveillance. In that 1977 Supreme Court case, one mother of a hyperactive child had testified that prescription surveillance would leave her son "branded for life."[155] Fear of the record, she and others had argued, presented an insurmountable barrier to treatment. Efforts to challenge abortion surveillance in the wake of *Roe v. Wade* were also grounded in the argument that fear of the record raised barriers to a woman's right to choose. The Supreme Court would never accept the threat of stigma as a justification for overriding surveillance activities. In *Planned Parenthood of Central Missouri v. Danforth,* for example, the Supreme Court recognized the "important and perhaps conflicting interests affected by recordkeeping requirements" in the case of abortion surveillance. Such requirements, wrote Justice Blackmun for the court, "while perhaps approaching impermissible limits," were "not constitutionally offensive in themselves. Recordkeeping of this kind, if not abused or overdone, can be useful to the State's interests in protecting the health of its female citizens."[156] But while stigma could not provide the basis for a constitutional challenge to surveillance activities, it would provide powerful political motivation to those who feared the development of disease registries.

The mother and father could both be targets for blame because of public perceptions that parental—but especially maternal—behavior increased the risk of birth defects.[157] In 1971 smoking was identified as damaging to the fetus: "The mother who smokes," wrote Surgeon General Jesse L. Steinfeld, "is subjecting the unborn child to the adverse effects of tobacco and as a result we are losing . . . and possibly handicapping babies."[158] It was not long after that fetal alcohol syndrome would be described, charting a meteoric rise in the medical literature between 1973 and 1981. The surgeon general recommended that women even considering pregnancy abstain from drinking, making fetal alcohol syndrome a threat not only for the child of the chronic alcoholic but also the social drinker.[159] In 1983 New York City became the first locale to require businesses selling alcohol to post warning labels, and in 1989 federal law required warning labels on individual bottles of alcohol stating, "Women should not drink alcoholic beverages during pregnancy because of the risk of birth defects."[160] It was also in the 1980s that concerns about maternal drug use and its impact on newborns were given renewed attention with alarming reports of "crack babies."[161]

THE CHALLENGE TO SURVEILLANCE IN A LIBERAL STRONGHOLD

Although in many states, like Texas, birth defects surveillance would not draw critical challenge, this was not always the case. In 1996 a University of Minnesota and Environmental Protection Agency study found elevated rates of birth defects in rural and agricultural regions of the state. The risk was particularly high among children exposed to pesticides.[162] The Minnesota department of health developed recommendations for creating a birth defects monitoring system that included both a research and services component. But when a year later they sought authorization for implementation, health officials in this deeply liberal state found themselves subjected to overwhelming and unexpected public challenge.[163] Although both the department of health and the MOD had felt certain of victory, the birth defects proposal became conflated, in the minds of both privacy advocates and state legislators, with separate proposals for an immunization registry and the development of a unique patient identification number, proposed as part of a health care reform initiative.[164]

Prominent in the attack on all three measures was the Citizens' Council on Health Care (CCHC), which described itself as an "independent, nonprofit, free-market health care policy organization" founded in response to what it took to be the threat to patient choice and confidentiality posed by increasing health care consolidation.[165] Its president, Twila Brase, was a public health nurse. The organization was libertarian and antagonistic to any claims about the primacy of the public welfare.

Tapping into wide-scale social anxiety about intrusions in the "information age," the CCHC warned that "patients en masse would become unconsenting research subjects."[166] Beyond such concerns were those posed by the proposed registry's service arm. With an echo of debates that had excited physicians almost a century earlier, the CCHC raised fears that health officials would be "getting in their face" unnecessarily. Its members believed that health care providers, not the state, should coordinate services for patients. In assuming such a role, the state would be intruding into the doctor-patient relationship.[167]

In the CCHC's campaign, birth defects registries were portrayed as particularly "onerous" because they represented "government inventories of citizens." Birth defects registries carried the added burden of being a "comprehensive directory . . . of so-called defective citizens."[168] The group thus argued that surveillance "labels children forever as defective." Brase underscored her group's fear that "we are slipping precipitously toward eugenics in America even as we abhorred it in Europe. This is not how we should be treating our children." It saw the effort to prevent birth defects that motivated legislative lobbying in Orwellian terms: "How can [registration prevent birth defects]? By denying care to a mother who refuses an abortion for her birth defective child? By denying marriage licenses to those with less than desirable genetic tendencies? By denying insurance for pregnancy coverage to those at risk for defective children?" The very protean nature of the concept "birth defect" was an invitation to coercion. "There is nothing in the bill limiting the expansion of a birth defect to eventually include anything that makes a person less than perfect. Once a registry exists, we believe researchers will try to expand it to adults, to mental illness, to Attention Deficit Disorder, to anything that it not socially desirable," argued Brase.[169] Thus the CCHC played on privacy concerns that had historically been raised in the arena of reproduction, drawing on a history of eugenic thinking that only intensified with advances in the human genome project.[170]

The invocation of pre–World War II conceptions of eugenics to thwart surveillance was not new.[171] More than a decade earlier, when New Jersey, with its long history of registering crippled children, sought to expand its system, it encountered public resistance for the first time.[172] Although a bill enhancing birth defects surveillance received broad support, it drew a challenge from anti-abortion groups and religious conservatives. The New Jersey Right-to-Life coalition was alarmed that public awareness about birth defects and the rise of amniocentesis, maternal serum alpha-fetoprotein screening, and high resolution ultrasonography were contributing to a rise in therapeutic abortions.[173]

The New Jersey Coalition of Concerned Parents, a group that described itself as being informed by a "Biblical Perspective," also expressed concerns that the legislation would give "the Commissioner of Health too broad a power to determine what is a birth defect" and called the registry "nothing more than malevolent eugenics."[174] As the threat envisioned was inconsistent with the softer trajectory of eugenics in America in the latter half of the twentieth century—which involved primarily genetic counseling, population control, marital counseling, and even environmental conservation as opposed to more apocalyptic measures[175]—these protests had virtually no impact on the shape of New Jersey's birth defects surveillance program.[176]

The story in Minnesota was very different: the opposition invoked the fear of eugenics and also framed privacy as a good in and of itself. Minnesota's legislators were receptive to the concerns of opponents and began to express consternation about how birth defects legislation would label children and follow them throughout their lives. Opponents of the bill managed a late-night hearing from which advocates of surveillance were excluded. When asked to defend the registry proposal by clearly defining the problem it was designed to resolve, however, the health department, remarkably, found itself insufficiently prepared. Because the health department was unable to make clear the compelling public health need that required a registry, the intrusions on privacy and the threat to children and families seemed gratuitous.

In the absence of a strong justification for the registry,[177] an amendment was offered on the floor of the Democratic-controlled Senate requiring informed consent for both immunization and birth defects registration. Rather than yield, public health officials withdrew the measure.[178] The principle of universal reporting, they held, could not be compromised.[179]

But if the politics stalled, defects continued to take their toll. In 2004, at the instigation of parents, the *Owatonna People's Press* began a series of investigative reports regarding a cluster of cases of gastroschisis—a congenital defect of the abdominal wall that allows all or part of the stomach and large and small intestines to extend outside the body—associated with the mothers' employment in a Rochester factory.[180] Still stinging from political defeat in 1997, a health department official could only lament that Minnesota was "flying blind" without a monitoring system comparable to the state's cancer registry: "These are the kind of issues that make it a shame that the Health Department has not been able to get a birth defects registry established."[181]

Against this backdrop, the department of health began to rethink its strategy to reverse the defeat it had encountered. It would first need to make the case to legislators for why surveillance of birth defects was critically necessary. A central element in establishing the scope of the problem was a CDC-funded study that would track three types of "obvious" birth defects that were likely to be the most accurately reported for the entire state: hare lip, cleft palate, and neural tube defects such as spina bifida.[182] The department of health took this opportunity to confront all of the questions it had neglected in 1997 in order "to create a much more comprehensive system, so that the legislature will have a hard time not supporting" birth defects surveillance in the next battles.[183] Significantly, the exploratory initiative was framed as "research," not surveillance, for it was important that the department of health officials were not seen as circumventing the law: if it "look[ed] as if privacy rules have already been broken," it would create the impression that health officials "would not be responsible with future data" and jeopardize any future statute.[184]

The health department also created the Birth Defects Work Group, which began to reframe the "real time benefits" of surveillance, linking any future system to the services that families would need.[185] To connect the idea of surveillance to benefits to families, it would be necessary to build a coalition among various publics. The MOD continued to play a central role in providing that critical link.[186]

But even if legislators and the public could be convinced that birth defects surveillance was essential, the issue of consent would have to be confronted.[187] The Birth Defects Work Group sought to build on the successes of cancer registration to try to make the case that consent would be an impediment to the collection of systematic data.[188] Nevertheless, in a political compromise, it was willing to introduce an opt-out clause into the new legislation to help ease the birth defects bill through the legislature.[189] Parents would be informed, at the time of completing the birth certificate, that data might be retained by the health department. They would also be told of the benefits of surveillance and of their right to remove all identifying information from the record. Parental objection to surveillance would be recorded on a health department form. As a strong disincentive to opting out, parents would be warned that if they chose that alternative, "The commissioner will not be able to inform the parent or legal guardian of a child of information related to the prevention, treatment, or cause of a particular birth defect."[190]

The Minnesota Birth Defects Information System was created in 2004.[191] Minnesota thus followed Virginia and Ohio, which had adopted birth defects surveillance systems in 1987 and 2003 that included provisions for opting out. It was a compromise far more acceptable to surveillance advocates than the Wisconsin alternative, adopted in 2000. There, privacy and right-to-life advocates formed an uneasy coalition in demanding parental written consent before a child's name could be entered into the registry.[192]

Even such compromises were unacceptable to fierce opponents of surveillance. In the wake of the passage of Wisconsin's informed consent legislation, a furious Republican senator said: "You're going to take something very personal and intimate about a baby growing up with a possible birth defect and now you're going to start keeping records on it. I think that it's abominable. It's nobody else's business."[193]

FROM STATE POLITICS TO FEDERAL POLITICS AND BACK AGAIN

Despite such enduring opposition, advocates for birth defects surveillance have, in one way or the other, typically won the day. As of 2004 all but three U.S. states had established a birth defects surveillance program.[194] Although in some instances the impetus to seek a legislative mandate for surveillance came from health officials, it came more frequently from the MOD, which has an office specifically devoted to securing state and federal legislation related to birth defects. Even in states where health officials had the authority to create birth defects registries under already existing public health statutes, the MOD believed it crucial to seek authorizing legislation. While opening the way to a political process posed a risk—as the case of Wisconsin had made clear—it also provided the opportunity to muster communities in defense of measures that could meet the needs of prevention and services and ultimately render birth defects surveillance more secure. Even legally mandated efforts, of course, could later be curtailed, but legislation would "make it very difficult for a state to get rid of a program."[195]

The CDC also had broad authority to support birth defects surveillance without specific congressional authorization. Since 1996 it had been providing funding to states with existing birth defects surveillance systems. But, in the estimation of the MOD, what was needed was a "piece of legislation to rally around."[196] This would come in the form of the Birth Defects Prevention Act of 1998. After several unsuccessful attempts, beginning in the early 1990s, to attach amendments providing funds for birth defects surveillance to the Minority Health Act and then the Health Professionals Act, the MOD decided to pursue a separate bill.[197] The cluster of anencephaly cases in Texas proved to be critical in this effort because it allowed the MOD to gain the support of the congressional Hispanic Caucus.[198] But underscoring how the politics of surveillance could create broad political alliances, the legislative process that began with evidence that minority populations experienced a much higher rate of birth defects reached a successful conclusion when legislators came to believe that birth defects "can happen to anyone."[199]

Strikingly, concerns about privacy were not salient in the politics of birth defects surveillance at the federal level. It was clear that identifiable data about parents and children would remain with the states. There would be no national name-linked registry. But when the Birth Defects Prevention Act came up for reauthorization in 2003, it was opposed by Concerned Women for America, an organization committed to "bring[ing] Biblical principles into all levels of public policy,"[200] because it included a provision that exempted developmental disability surveillance, most notably autism, from the protections contained in the 1974 Family Educational Rights and Privacy Act (FERPA). It allowed health officials access to public school records without parental consent. The CDC argued that because autism and other developmental disabilities did not become apparent until the child reached school-age, records of these conditions were "seldom found ascertained in the clinical setting." Access to school records was imperative, and requirements of informed consent would undermine the accuracy of surveillance data.[201] Granting such access drew the fire of politically and culturally conservative groups opposed to immunization registries and mandatory vaccination. The Eagle Forum's Phyllis Schlafly claimed that allowing CDC access "will undermine and weaken the only privacy law on the books when it comes to the records of school children."[202]

The federal Department of Education, in a memorandum of understanding that was set to expire in 2005, designated the CDC as its "authorized representative." In this way, the CDC was able to support "autism spectrum disorder monitoring programs in 17 states." Many of the state programs were modeled on an Atlanta-based effort in which the CDC was able to access school medical records in all five of the metropolitan counties on which that birth defects registry draws.[203] But the effort failed in some states. In Massachusetts, for example, the Department of Education "determined that releasing records from special-needs programs is significantly restricted." In order for health officials to gain access to children's medical records to assess autism, the Department of Education sent consent forms to parents. Only after consent had been obtained could the children be identified to the department of health.[204] The federal Department of Education followed suit and informed the CDC that "utilizing school records without individual parental consent would not be compliant with FERPA." Efforts to develop a passive consent model did not prove viable.[205] Despite federal recognition of the seeming impasse, the National Autism Association—clearly still stinging from what it considered a failure on the part of the CDC to link vaccination with autism and, further, to share that data with concerned parents—has charged that health department access to confidential educational records continues in some states.[206]

But if efforts at autism surveillance had stalled, if not collapsed, the broader birth defects surveillance effort that the original legislation spawned remained robust. The Birth Defects Prevention Act and its reauthorization resulted in the rapid expansion of surveillance efforts.[207] The 1998 act, which appropriated up to $30 million in 1998, $40 million in

1999, and "necessary" funding for subsequent years, directed the CDC to "carry out through the states, a program to collect, analyze and report statistics on birth defects." It authorized the CDC to create at least five regional centers for conducting applied epidemiological research. In 2005 nine centers were in operation and fifteen states were receiving funding to help conduct birth defects surveillance under CDC cooperative agreements.[208]

The registries that developed as a result of the 1998 legislation were primarily intended to be epidemiological tracking and research tools. The CDC-funded National Birth Defects Prevention Study is "one of the largest [ongoing] case-control studies ever done on the causes of birth defects."[209] The effort has garnered the support of affected parents, which the CDC highlights on its web site: "I can't imagine not participating in this study. . . . Research is essential to learning and if doctors can learn something from my pregnancy, my son's condition, or our family genetics then I feel it is our duty to other families to contribute as much as we can to this study."[210]

But at the state level, as we have seen, given the politics of privacy, the emphasis on research alone could be insufficient to advance the case for surveillance. State legislative battles made clear that, as important as research might be in the quest to prevent birth defects, to be politically viable, birth defects surveillance had to serve the end of caring for children.[211] This was a lesson that the MOD had learned over the course of the 1990s.[212]

Birth defects surveillance had, in a sense, come full circle. In addition to monitoring trends in incidence and mortality, surveillance has increasingly been used to identify children with special health care needs, connect them to programs, and evaluate those programs.[213] The Massachusetts Department of Public Health, for example, asserted in 2000 that "the goal in each state that develops a birth defects system should be to integrate birth defects surveillance into maternal and child health programs and activities in order to create a *seamless system* of data collection, analysis, research, and follow-up interventions."[214]

PART III

Surveillance at Century's End

The Politics of Democratic Privacy

7

AIDS, Activism, and the Vicissitudes
of Democratic Privacy

In June 1981 the Centers for Disease Control reported the appearance in previously healthy gay men of conditions that usually occurred only in individuals with compromised immune systems. The CDC's official publication, *Morbidity and Mortality Weekly Report*, recounted that between October 1980 and May 1981 five young men had been diagnosed with *pneumocystis carinii* pneumonia.[1] By way of explanation, the CDC noted the possibility that some aspect of homosexual lifestyle or disease acquired through sexual contact might be involved.[2] One month later the CDC reported that in the prior two and a half years Kaposi's sarcoma, a malignancy rare in the United States, especially in young people, had been diagnosed in twenty-six gay men in New York and California.[3] These were sentinel cases of an epidemic that would have a profound impact on gay men, intravenous drug users and their sexual partners, and African American and Latino communities in the last two decades of the twentieth century. As the first major infectious disease threat in more than a generation, AIDS would shock the United States and other industrial nations that had come to think of epidemic diseases as a thing of the past. The new disease was all the more stunning because of the youth of those who were struck and the speed with which it claimed their lives.

Early on there would be some calls for rigid separation of the sick, though it soon became clear that the new disease could only be spread through sexual contact, from the sharing of drug injection equipment, by contaminated blood, and from infected pregnant women to their fetuses. That the disease arrived at the very moment when American politics had taken a sharp conservative turn with the election of President Ronald Reagan heightened the concern of those who feared that AIDS would provide the occasion for the wide-scale abrogation of the privacy rights that had gained recognition in the prior decade. Such fears would have a deep and lingering impact on the surveillance activities undertaken in response to the new epidemic threat.

The contours of the struggles over surveillance represented the fullest expression of democratic privacy. Certainly doctors would seek to protect their patients' privacy and would emerge as spokespersons for the men whose sexual orientation, in a society hostile to homosexuality, made the protection of confidentiality so essential. But, drawing upon the skills forged in the early years of the gay rights movement, gay activists and their political allies entered the fray in a manner unmediated by physician advocates. In the struggles that emerged, the democratization of the debates over public health would explicitly and publicly question the appropriate relationship between professionals and laypeople in the shaping of policy. Battles over the scope and goals of surveillance activities took place at CDC headquarters in Atlanta, at the Department of Health and Human Services in Washington, DC, and in almost every state.

REPORTING AIDS CASES

It is remarkable, given the salience of concerns about the privacy of individuals with AIDS, that there was little resistance to initial efforts by state health departments to mandate case reporting by name. Indeed, an assumption that only accurate epidemiological information could unlock the mysteries of the transmission of the new disease led the board of the American Association of Physicians for Human Rights, a gay and lesbian medical group, to propose in 1983 that local health authorities make the names of AIDS cases reportable.[4]

Controversy did emerge, however, when the CDC called upon all local health departments to forward the names and full case reports of those with AIDS to Atlanta.[5] For the CDC, such identified reports were essential if an accurate, unduplicated record of cases was to be developed for the nation as a whole. Although by 1982 the CDC in Atlanta had a list of more than two hundred such names,[6] distrust of the intentions of the federal authorities and anxieties about how such a national list might be misused led gay leaders to oppose such efforts.[7] As a result, some treating physicians and local health departments began to resist the requests to forward name-linked reports to the CDC. New York City, for example, announced in mid-1983 that it would no longer honor the request.[8]

Federal officials responsible for AIDS surveillance were incredulous as they encountered the organized opposition of the gay community, which had gained the support of many local health officials. After outlining the centrality of names for conducting epidemiologic follow-up of cases in outbreak situations, James Allen, the director of AIDS surveillance activities at the CDC, wrote, in language that would be repeated in the surveillance wars over the next two decades, "We are aware of the sensitive nature of the information being collected about patients with AIDS and of the need for meticulous attention to every detail to protect this information from disclosure and to protect the privacy of persons reported as cases. Over the years, CDC has collected sensitive information about patients during a wide variety of epidemic investigations and epidemiologic studies; names and other identifying information about patients with all types of diseases have been protected from public disclosure. . . . Release of information in individual files would constitute a clearly unwarranted invasion of personal privacy." Allen concluded that these protections and public health necessity provided "sufficient justification for collecting names along with other information about persons with AIDS."[9]

Ultimately the CDC was compelled to agree, albeit reluctantly, to reporting by a coding mechanism—called Soundex—that was designed to preclude duplicate reporting without the use of names or other personal identifiers such as Social Security numbers. The agency acknowledged that the compromise would complicate its efforts but asserted, "It's better than the alternative: persons refusing to cooperate by giving inaccurate information. . . . By agreeing to this compromise we can reassure them that we are acting in good faith and won't jeopardize their privacy."[10] Others within the CDC expressed exasperation. "They say the government isn't doing anything, then they accuse us of breaching confidentiality when we try to carry out responsible studies."[11]

Reflective of the deep anxieties of gay leaders in the first years of the AIDS epidemic, even the Soundex compromise appeared insufficiently protective. The Lambda Legal Defense and Education Fund, a gay civil rights and civil liberties group, and the National Gay Task Force pressed the CDC to protect AIDS surveillance data with a federal "assurance of confidentiality"—a legal mechanism that had most commonly been used to secure data acquired during the conduct of research involving highly sensitive matters.[12] Gay advocates warned that codes like Soundex could be broken and the consequences would be devastating given the social context of the AIDS epidemic. "Creating a list of people with AIDS is in effect creating a list of people who are disenfranchised in American society."[13] Gay men were not protected by civil rights legislation. They could lose their jobs if exposed and could be denied child custody rights. Sexual activity between men was a crime in half the states. Irrational fears about contagion had resulted in housing and employment discrimination, even calls for mass quarantines. Additional guarantees were needed if gay men were to cooperate with surveillance activities.[14] Once again, despite initial resistance, the CDC, with support of ASTHO, the CSTE, and other public health alliances, yielded to those pressing the claims of heightened privacy protection.[15]

These initial encounters with the CDC were critically important because they revealed the profound anxiety of gay men over government surveillance activities. None of the privacy protections for intimate relationships that had emerged over the prior decade were given the force of law for gay people, and indeed the Supreme Court would soon dismiss as "facetious" the challenge to Georgia's statute that made homosexual activity between consenting adults a crime.[16] In alliance with civil liberties organizations, gay groups pressed their claim to shape AIDS policies in general and surveillance policies more specifically at the federal, state, and local levels. Their capacity to influence policy was immeasurably affected by the fact that AIDS had struck most forcefully in New York, San Francisco, and Los Angeles, relatively liberal, cosmopolitan cities.

While significant for what they revealed, the encounters over how the CDC should conduct its AIDS surveillance activities were resolved with relative ease. Consequently they provided little preparation for the fierce and protracted struggles that were to emerge in state after state as the question of whether HIV infection itself should be the subject of name-based reporting to state and local health departments was raised.

TOWARD HIV REPORTING:
THE SOLIDIFICATION OF RESISTANCE

HIV was identified as the etiological agent responsible for AIDS in 1984. Soon after, an assay was developed to detect antibody to the virus. The first encounter over a proposal for HIV name reporting took place in New Jersey just a month after the screening of blood donations began nationwide in April 1985.[17] Drawing a sharp distinction between reporting cases of AIDS and the results of the new antibody test with its still-ambiguous clinical implications—Were all those who tested positive infectious? What proportion would progress to full-blown AIDS?—the local gay community denounced the proposal. Challenge came also from the national Federation of AIDS-Related Organizations and the U.S. Conference of Local Health Officers.[18] Confronted with so determined an opposition, the New Jersey Public Health Council deferred to the legislature.[19]

For those who had viewed New Jersey's effort as unwarranted from the perspective of clinical medicine and public health and as a potential threat to the privacy of those whose names would be reported, the deferral was an "important victory."[20] But there was also some trepidation about whether other states would succeed where New Jersey had failed. "We are in the first skirmish," said Tim Sweeney of the Lambda Legal Defense and Education Fund. "This does not mean they will not come back and try again or [that] other states will not try this."[21]

The first successful attempts to mandate public health reporting of HIV antibody test results came in Minnesota, Wisconsin, and Colorado—three states with low-level epidemics and gay communities far less politically potent than those in California and New York.[22] These states would bear witness to the democratization of privacy, underscoring the ways in which the broader culture could shape the politics of surveillance across different domains. The conflict that erupted in Colorado was typical of those that would occur in other states as they attempted to move toward name reporting for HIV.

In August 1985 Thomas Vernon, the executive director of the Colorado Department of Health, proposed that the state require HIV reporting.[23] Drawing upon the evolving scientific understanding of the significance of the HIV test, he noted that positive findings were "a highly reliable marker" for infection and "probably for infectiousness as well."[24] Reporting, he argued, could alert public health agencies to the presence of persons likely to be infected with a dangerous virus. It would allow them to insure that such persons were properly counseled about the significance of their laboratory tests and about what they needed to do to prevent further transmission of the virus. Reporting would also create the possibility of expeditiously notifying the infected when effective antiviral therapeutic agents became available. A failure to extend reporting to this situation would represent a dereliction of professional responsibility in the face of a new deadly disease. Responding to concerns about breaches in confidentiality that could result in social ostracism, loss of insurability, and loss of employment, Vernon and his deputy for sexually transmitted diseases asserted that the system for protecting such public health records had been effective for decades. There was no reason to believe that in the case of infection with the AIDS virus the department's record would be tarnished.

Despite Vernon's belief that his proposal was in the tradition of public health measures, his efforts provoked a sharp response from his opponents in a hearing before the state's Board of Health.[25] The director of public health for Denver warned that reporting would have the counterproductive impact of driving high-risk individuals away from testing, regardless of the health department's pledges to preserve the confidentiality of test results. The director of the gay community–based Colorado AIDS Project asserted that his organization would discourage testing if Vernon's proposal was adopted. The president of the board of Colorado's Civil Liberties Union joined the challenge. In each case, Vernon's opponents underscored their fear that, regardless of the historical and prevailing standards of confidentiality, a repressive turn caused by the hysteria associated with AIDS could well result in social policies that Vernon and his associates would consider anathema. To these concerns Vernon responded with a claim that he was to make repeatedly in the next months: widespread perception that public health officials had failed to do everything possible to control AIDS could foster social anxiety and thus produce the very repression so feared by those concerned with the rights of the infected.[26]

Despite the bitter protests by gay and civil liberties groups as well as the concern of some health officials, one month after Vernon made his proposal the Board of Health unanimously adopted a resolution making Colorado among the first states to require the reporting by name of those testing positive for HIV.[27] To those who continued to stress the possibility that the health department's list of seropositive individuals could be put to ill use, Vernon responded, "The issue before us is the reality of a tragic epidemic of AIDS, not the theoretical risks [that] our confidentiality system will be breached."[28]

In the aftermath of the imposition of mandatory reporting, there was, in fact, a marked downturn in the number of individuals seeking testing in Colorado. To those who had warned of such an outcome, the results only proved how an apparently aggressive public health posture could have counterproductive consequences.[29] To those who defended the new course, the downturn was explained as largely coincidental, paralleling the experience of states that had not adopted a policy of reporting.[30]

To limit the extent to which fears of reporting would deter individuals from seeking testing, health officials made a concession that seemed to undermine their arguments for names. Individuals who appeared at Colorado's test sites would not be asked for proof of identity, making available the option of using pseudonyms. Months later Vernon defended this policy: "Would we require personal identification of those tested? No. The option of not using one's own name has always been available in disease control programs and HIV testing is not different."[31] Some of Vernon's opponents reported that perhaps as many as one-third of those seeking testing used this option.[32] Here then, an option that had characterized VD reporting was repeated, except it was patients rather than doctors who created the code.[33]

In the wake of efforts to require the reporting by name of those infected with HIV, James Mason, director of the CDC, wrote to state health officials, asking them to consider the possibility of requiring "some kind of reporting."[34] Such a move, Mason stressed, would necessitate the existence of confidentiality protections, including legislative shields for health department records against disclosure. But while noting the public health benefits that might follow from the adoption of mandatory reporting, Mason warned that the proposed move might discourage persons from agreeing to anonymous testing. Gay political groups responded to Mason's letter with dismay. When the CDC published its first comprehensive recommendations for broadscale voluntary HIV testing in March 1986, Mason's initial suggestion for HIV reporting had been considerably softened. State and local officials were simply urged to "evaluate the implications of required reporting."[35]

It was not only civil liberties organizations and gay political groups that opposed notification. Many local and state health officials were concerned about the potential impact of Mason's proposed move. In January 1986 the U.S. Conference of Local Health Officers debated the issue of whether testing under conditions of anonymity—the standard at many HIV test sites—was preferable to confidential testing.[36] Anonymous testing would preclude reporting by name. Confidentiality would make it possible. Slightly more than half of the officials rejected efforts to encourage the substitution of confidentiality for anonymity. Most remarkable was what the vote revealed about the early politics of surveillance in the context of the AIDS epidemic. Officials from cities with relatively few AIDS cases supported a more aggressive posture. Those from cities with high caseloads tended to favor a policy that would thwart name-based reporting. Constrained by the need to preserve collaborative working relationships with large and well-organized gay communities and concerned about how reporting would affect willingness to be tested, they could not support a measure that would almost certainly produce alienation with no assured contribution to the public health. Less constrained by such factors, officials from cities with few AIDS cases favored policies that they believed represented merely the application of traditional public health practice to HIV infection.

This pattern was repeated as ASTHO sought to formulate a policy on reporting in 1986. But in this instance the advocates of reporting prevailed. The ASTHO position was particularly distressing to gay leaders who had worked so assiduously to win the support of public health officials in cities like New York and San Francisco. Christopher Collins, who had represented the Lambda Legal Defense and Education Fund at the consensus conference from which the ASTHO recommendations had emerged, wrote in protest that democratic principles should define the course of policy. "I believe credence should be given to the views of those whose states are most affected by the disease. They have had the most experience . . . and should not be 'horse whipped' into having to go along with the views of those health commissioners from states where the disease has not yet reached the extent that it has in New York and California."[37]

Those who believed that reporting by name to state health departments had a potentially important role to play in the public health strategy against AIDS provided a different analysis. In their view, the stance of health officials from areas with large numbers of AIDS cases was not a matter of greater experience. Rather, it entailed an unwise accommodation to the immediate and narrow political interests of those whose primary concern was the defense of "gay rights" and the advance of a "civil liberties agenda."

The depths of anxiety expressed by opponents of name reporting and their sense of outrage at what they took to be the glib dismissal of their concerns by public health officials who repeatedly sought to reassure them by

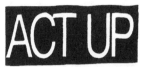

ACT UP / ST. LOUIS
PO BOX 16899
ST. LOUIS, MO 63105
(314) 535-8586

THE AIDS POLICE WANT YOU!

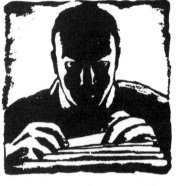

Illustration by Kevin Belford;
Reproduced from the Riverfront Times.

Dr. Baumgartner, chief epidemiologist from the Missouri Department of Health, and Ms. Page, the Surveillance Coordinator of the St. Louis Metropolitan AIDS Program, are attempting an abusive and intimidating search of physicians' private medical records. What are they looking for? **The names and full medical histories of the HIV infected.** Why? **Because they get paid by the head.**

Dr. Baumgartner claims:

1. Name collecting is necessary for the reporting of cases.

2. Name reporting "does allow us to more effectively perform partner notification."

3. Anonymous testing sites were not the Department of Health's idea.

4. Fewer and fewer people are testing at anonymous testing sites.

5. Part of the money received per reported HIV case is used for treatment and prevention.

The Truth:

"We don't have any use for the names," says Chuck Fallis of the CDC.

Contact tracing is an abusive practice proven to be ineffective in stopping the spread of AIDS.

Too bad. It's the law.

That's irrelevant. Without anonymous testing, how many people would not get tested? In South Carolina the number of people getting tested fell by 49% in one year after anonymous testing was no longer available.

Missouri health services for the HIV infected range from the pathetic to the nonexistent. Like any bounty hunter, Baumgartner keeps the cash.

AIDS CARE! NOT AIDS SCARE!

STOP COLLECTING! START PROTECTING!

Figure 21. A decade later, activists continued to resist reporting in some locales. ACT UP poster from a demonstration in St. Louis, July 1991. Original in possession of Marian Moser Jones.

invocations of the honorable history of public health practice must be understood not simply in terms of the broad social climate surrounding homosexuality (fig. 21). Whatever the commitments of public health advocates of surveillance, political forces favoring repressive measures could not be ignored. Just as the director of the CDC and other public health leaders were signaling their interest in the option of HIV case reporting, a furious battle over AIDS policy was taking shape in California which was, with New York, an epicenter of the unfolding American epidemic. The battle was to touch not only on matters of privacy but on the full range of rights of those infected with HIV.

THE SPECTER OF REPRESSION

It was not only those seeking to protect the interests of people with HIV who took advantage of the democratization of public health policy formation. In October 1985 the attorney general of California was notified by officials of the National Democratic Policy Committee—the political arm of Lyndon LaRouche's extremist movement—that they intended to submit a proposition on AIDS to the electorate in the November 1986 election.[38] Under their leadership, the Prevent AIDS Now Initiative Committee (PANIC) began its remarkable effort to obtain the 400,000 signatures needed to qualify for a place on the ballot.

Critical of the refusal of public health officials to adopt harsh measures to control AIDS, LaRouche called for mass testing and quarantine. "In order to insure that the rapid spread of AIDS is halted, nothing less than universal screening and then, under full medical care, 'isolating' or 'quarantining' all individuals who are in the active carrier state" was required.[39] In cities and states across the country, adherents of LaRouche's movement pressured local school boards to remove schoolchildren with AIDS from the classroom and demanded the screening of all food handlers and teachers so that those who showed signs of antibody to HIV could be barred from work that, they asserted against all evidence, would place others at risk.[40]

The proposition ultimately drafted by PANIC bore none of these strident elements in its text. Instead, California voters were to be asked to support a series of ambiguously framed amendments to the state's health and safety code.[41] The proposition required that both AIDS and HIV be defined as infectious, contagious and communicable. Both were to be listed by the Department of Health Services among the reportable diseases and conditions covered by existing relevant state statutes.[42] By the summer of 1986, PANIC had succeeded in obtaining 683,000 signatures for what would be officially termed Proposition 64.[43]

Opposition to the referendum came from the medical establishment: the California Medical Association, the California Nurses Association, and the

California Hospital Association. A statement to voters stressed the irra-
tionality of a proposal that assumed the existence of casual transmission of
HIV in schools, the workplace, or restaurants. Only those who were expert
in the scientific and clinical dimensions of AIDS were qualified to fashion
public health policy, not those driven by politically motivated "partial truths
and falsehoods." Asked the medical community, "Would you let a stranger
with no medical training or no medical background diagnose a disease or
illness that you have? Would you let a political extremist dictate medical policy?" Their answer was straightforward: "OF COURSE NOT."[44] Underscored
here were the complex ways in which scientific evidence and expertise
would play a role in the politics of democratic privacy with its emphasis on
lay participation.

On election day close to seven million voters cast ballots on Proposition
64. Seventy-one percent opposed it; 29 percent favored it.[45] Though this was
a stunning defeat for PANIC, it was a hard-won victory for those who had
mobilized against the proposition. Still, just fewer than two million voters,
almost one in three, had been persuaded to support an initiative linked to
one of the most extreme political movements in America. The referendum
demonstrated the existence of a popular base that could be mobilized for a
repressive turn in public policy. The specter of California's proposition
would leave an indelible mark as AIDS activists encountered proposals for
HIV case reporting in the next years.

NAME REPORTING AND THE REASSERTION OF
CONVENTIONAL PUBLIC HEALTH CONTROL

While the victorious alliance of gay leaders, civil liberties advocates, and
public health officials and medical practitioners was able to hold off the
pressure for name-based case reporting in populous states with large epidemics, there were indications as the 1980s drew to a close that the political climate was shifting. This change was driven, in part, by more optimistic
assumptions about the role of early clinical interventions. Public health
officials increasingly saw the value of adopting conventional approaches to
disease control and viewed the enumeration of AIDS cases as a poor measure of current patterns of HIV infection.[46] Furthermore, clinicians evinced
a growing interest in returning AIDS to the "medical mainstream." In short,
across a range of policy issues, the exceptionalism that characterized the
response to AIDS in its first years was under challenge. In mid-1988, when
only thirteen states had adopted name reporting for HIV, Ronald Reagan's
Presidential Commission on the Human Immunodeficiency Virus Epidemic
recommended that all states adopt case notification for HIV.[47] That decision
was all the more distressing to opponents of reporting since so much of the
commission's final report contained proposals applauded by liberal critics

of the Reagan administration's failure to commit either sufficient resources or political leadership to the struggle against AIDS.

Ultimately more significant were the fissures that had begun to appear in the alliance opposing reporting in those states where the prevalence of HIV infection was high and where gay communities were well organized. In a June 1989 address that was met with cries of protest, Stephen Joseph, commissioner of health in New York City, told the attendees of the Fifth International Conference on AIDS that the prospect of early clinical intervention necessitated "a shift toward a disease control approach to HIV infection along the lines of classic tuberculosis practices." A central feature of such an approach would be the "reporting of seropositives" to assure effective clinical follow-up and the initiation of "more aggressive contact tracing."[48] Joseph's proposals opened a debate that was only temporarily settled by the defeat of New York's mayor Edward Koch in his bid for reelection. Newly elected David Dinkins, New York's first African American mayor, selected Woodrow Myers, formerly commissioner of health in Indiana and also an African American, to replace Joseph. Myers's appointment was almost aborted, in part because he had supported named reporting.[49] The festering debate was ended only by a political decision on the part of the mayor, who had drawn heavily on support within the gay community, to stand by his appointment while promising that there would be no named reporting in New York.[50]

Change was occurring at the national level as well. In 1989 the House of Delegates of the AMA endorsed a resolution calling for HIV reporting, explicitly linking such notification to the need for contact tracing.[51] Among the most avid proponents of the new position was the president elect of the Arkansas Medical Association. In addressing the delegates, he inveighed against the exceptional treatment of AIDS. The failure to adopt standard public health reporting measures had resulted, he said, in sixty-five thousand deaths. "How many more lives have to be lost before we take a stand that, every physician in this country knows, should have been taken several years ago?"[52] Writing in the *Journal of the Arkansas Medical Society*, he was more direct in pointing the finger of blame. The AMA delegates had embraced name reporting, he argued, because "the silent majority was fed up with being intimidated and mesmerized by the vocal civil libertarian–homosexual advocate minority with its self-centeredness and calloused disregard for the health of others."[53] Without endorsing either the substance or tone of such denunciations, the Board of Trustees of the AMA, its highest policy-making body, recommended name reporting in December 1990.[54] But the vitriolic language of some of the most avid proponents of reporting would not be lost on those who sought to forestall such measures in the states.

At the CDC, whose director had signaled its sympathy for HIV reporting, important efforts were made to bring some coherence to the pattern of name reporting that had emerged in a number of states. In a 1989 consultation, a common state reporting form was adopted, and in 1990 the CDC began to receive such reports encoded by Soundex.[55] This move provoked an angry response as AIDS advocates mistakenly came to surmise that the CDC wanted a list of the names of all people with HIV infection. A spokesperson for the National Gay and Lesbian Task Force declared, "First comes the national registry, then come the boxcars, then come the camps for people with AIDS."[56]

THE LIMITS OF REPORTING

While the initial moves on the part of the CDC would, in a short time, set the stage for a formal call for states to adopt HIV name reporting, there was some skepticism about the function of such notification among those responsible for surveillance activities at the federal agency. Although she acknowledged that case reports could improve public health planning and direct needed prevention services, including partner notification, Ruth Berkelman, chief of the Surveillance Branch, candidly noted, "Their epidemiologic usefulness is more limited. HIV infection reports are not representative of all HIV infected persons. . . . Rather, HIV infection reports represent only those within the infected population who are tested and reported."[57] When CSTE, which both served as an advisory body to the CDC and as a forum for considering the recommendations of the federal centers, first adopted a resolution supportive of name reporting in 1989, it underscored the need for each state to make its own reporting determination based on resources and other local "circumstances." The emphasis of CSTE was on how such notification might facilitate interventions with those diagnosed with HIV. The role of reporting as a measure of the epidemiologic burden was clearly of secondary significance.[58]

In fact, some years earlier, in the fall of 1985, just as Minnesota, Wisconsin, and Colorado were preparing to initiate name reporting, officials at the CDC came to believe that an alternative form of surveillance was crucial to tracking the prevalence of HIV infection. Systematically testing blood samples drawn for other purposes at sentinel institutions across the nation was necessary.[59] Stripped of personal identifiers, such samples would not, held the CDC, require informed consent, and the ethicists who considered the matter agreed. The Office for the Protection from Research Risks declared that "since patient identifying information will not be linked to HIV test results, informed consent will not be required."[60] Such anonymous samples would pose no threats to privacy. But the very process of eliminating identifiers would preclude the possibility of notifying those who were infected. Hence the epidemiological strengths of unlinked anonymous serosurveillance limited it as a tool for public health efforts at the individual level.

BROADENING SUPPORT FOR HIV CASE REPORTING

Despite the limitations of HIV case reporting for purposes of epidemiolog-ical surveillance and the centrality of blinded surveillance for monitoring the epidemic's presymptomatic stages, an increasing number of states adopted case notification. Twenty-six states, including New Jersey, with its relatively high prevalence, had done so by 1992.[61] California, Florida, New York, and Texas, with large epidemics, had resisted the trend. Those states that had adopted case notification did so with the support of the CDC.

The CDC, fully alert to the treacherous political terrain in high preva-lence states, recognized the need to act in ways that might not rupture its own relationship with gay communities or imperil collaborative relation-ships between those groups and state health departments. Describing a meeting on reporting sponsored by the AIDS Action Council that brought together health department officials from a number of states and AIDS activist groups, two CDC officials wrote, "It became clear that there was a lack of trust in government at almost every level in dealing with HIV issues. . . . The words of . . . the Act-Up representative summarized the view of many of those representing nongovernmental organizations at the meet-ing. 'First you don't exist, then you're on The List'" (fig. 22). Based on these observations, the CDC was urged by its own representative to consider the potential costs of promoting case reporting: Would the benefits in improved surveillance actually outweigh the predictable negative reactions on the part of some organizations, important constituencies, and the perceptions of those most at risk? Would the CDC increase anger and mistrust of HIV/AIDS activities at the federal, state, and local governments? Would state health departments reduce anonymous testing services as a direct result of HIV name reporting? How likely was it that the presumed benefits of name reporting would be realized and how likely was it that the negative reactions would occur?[62]

For the AIDS Action Council, the meeting provided an opportunity to reinforce not only its long-standing concerns about privacy—it called on the CDC to establish a privacy standard for the states, the violation of which would jeopardize federal AIDS surveillance funds—but to underscore the importance of bringing to bear fresh thinking on the problem of surveil-lance activities. Aware of the power of convention in shaping the activities of state health departments and convinced that careful analysis would reveal that name-based reporting would be counterproductive from the perspec-tive of public health, the council called upon the CDC to sponsor two new research initiatives. The first would be a systematic empirical study of the impact of name reporting on the willingness of individuals to undergo HIV testing and enter early care for AIDS-related conditions. Second, the coun-cil called upon the CDC to investigate the option of using unique identifiers

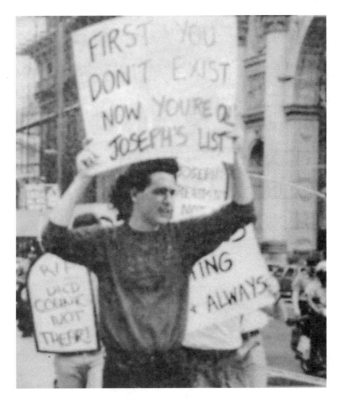

Figure 22. ACT UP demonstration at the Fifth International AIDS conference in New York following a *New York Post* cover story that New York City health commissioner Stephen Joseph planned to begin HIV reporting and abolish anonymous testing. Cover of *ACT UP Reports* 4, June 1989.

rather than names for reporting purposes. Such an approach would achieve the goals of reporting but would do so "by reducing the fear of breaches of confidentiality" and would avoid the risk of inhibiting testing so crucial "to our understanding of the extent of HIV infection."[63]

Aware of the depths of resistance with which it had to deal and the extent to which the battle over names was impeding the task of extending surveillance activities beyond AIDS case reports, the CDC commenced in early 1993 a series of broad-based public consultations. In part, such efforts were essential to conveying the impression that decision making regarding AIDS policy was both transparent and democratic—a rejection of the authoritarian traditions of public health. But as important, such sessions were designed to determine how best to narrow the grounds of disagreement—participants yielded ground on matters such as the ways in which the security of surveillance data could be protected from breaches of confidentiality and assured that case reports could be used solely for legitimate public health purposes—without giving way on the central commitment to name-based notification to state health departments. Democratic participation, in this instance, was not synonymous with popular rule.

The accounts of these sessions provide a remarkable barometer of the concerns and shifting strategic positions of the stakeholders within the gay community, other AIDS activist organizations, and health departments. Cornelius Baker of the National Association of People with AIDS spoke of his fears as an African American. The activities of public health officials were, he asserted, "often in fact discriminatory."[64] In his view, the public health record was far from exemplary. History showed that the burdens of intervention most often fell upon those at the social and political margins of American society. The passage of a statute in Illinois, which some feared would permit state health department officials to notify patients when treated by infected health-care workers, was also cause for alarm. It was precisely the passage of such legislation that underscored for AIDS advocates that the record of health departments in the past was no guarantee about how they might choose—or be compelled—to act in the future.[65]

At the same time at least some AIDS activists were beginning to understand that their capacity to slow the advance toward name reporting was limited. They began to make a strategic argument: since reporting could enhance referrals to needed services, the CDC should take on the responsibility of advocating for the care of people with HIV, an increasing number of whom were black and Latino. While underscoring her strong preference for a unique identifier system, Theresa McGovern of the HIV Law Project, a strong advocate for women with AIDS, acknowledged that confidentiality was not a primary concern of her clients.[66] More important was the question of whether reporting would lead to better prevention and care. She was, however, profoundly skeptical about whether case reporting would give those she represented the attention they deserved. More startling, Jeff Levi, who as director of government affairs for the AIDS Action Council was a stalwart for unique identifiers, declared that if health care were guaranteed for people with HIV, "80–90% of the objections to named reporting would disappear."[67]

THE CASE DEFINITION OF AIDS: EXPANDED SURVEILLANCE, SOCIAL GOODS, AND PRIVACY

The complex political relationship between the claims of privacy and the social and health care needs of individuals and communities most at risk was revealed in the nominally technical debate over the case definition of AIDS.

The CDC had proposed to expand its definition of AIDS to include anyone with HIV infection with a significantly compromised immune system, indicated by a CD4 count—a white blood cell key to immune function—of 200 or less.[68] Such an expansion was necessitated by the need to achieve a better assessment of the "magnitude of morbidity associated with HIV disease."[69] But there were pressures of a very different sort on the CDC as well. AIDS advocates argued that the extant set of clinical signs that triggered an AIDS diagnosis, while reflecting the experience of the disease among gay men, failed to capture the pattern of conditions afflicting drug users and women with HIV. As a consequence, the surveillance definition undercounted women and drug users with AIDS, groups that were primarily African American and Latino. Further, because disability payments under Social Security were linked to an AIDS diagnosis, the most disadvantaged had been deprived of the financial support they needed and to which they were entitled.[70]

Strikingly, then, while AIDS advocates were resisting efforts to expand the list of people held in state health department records through HIV reporting, they were pressing to expand the list through a broader definition of AIDS itself. But abiding concern about privacy rights informed this controversy as well. It was reflected in the intense opposition to proposals that would permit laboratories to report the names of individuals with CD4 counts of 200 or less directly to state health departments.[71] Such reporting would trigger follow-up inquiries with clinicians to determine if those who had been so reported were also infected with HIV. Such a system would replicate the well-established practice of laboratory-based reporting in the instance of TB and syphilis.

A year-long battle ensued. The CSTE supported laboratory-based CD4 reporting but opposed the inclusion of cervical cancer and pulmonary tuberculosis in the case definition because they were insufficiently indicative of AIDS. AIDS advocates rejected the direct reporting of individuals with low CD4 counts but demanded that cervical cancer and pulmonary tuberculosis be among the conditions included. When the CDC finalized its case definition it included medical conditions that AIDS advocates had so forcefully advocated for, but it also refused to bar lab reporting of low CD4 counts.[72] In commenting on this turn of events, a coalition of AIDS advocacy groups applauded the extension of the AIDS case definition but lamented the failure to respect the privacy interests of people with HIV infection. Advocates would therefore be "forced to fight this battle on a state by state basis." The stakes went far beyond the issue of CD4 counts. "Introduction of lab-based name reporting of CD4+ counts may well be the *immediate* precursor to lab-based name reporting of positive HIV antibody tests in the 23 states that have not adopted this approach. This is particularly critical because these remaining states are generally those with the highest prevalence of HIV-positive individuals. *Thus the loss of the CD4$^+$ name reporting issue may foreshadow the advent of more aggressive, invasive surveillance technique—and may ultimately lead to HIV-name-reporting nation-wide.*"[73] Having sounded the tocsin, the coalition urged advocates in every state to demand that when CD4 tests were ordered, individuals be informed that such assays could lead to an AIDS diagnosis and a listing on their state's AIDS registry.[74]

As the debate unfolded, there was a studied silence on the implications of the controversy over CD4 reporting for AIDS reporting itself. Unlike the dispute over asymptomatic HIV infection, this controversy had obvious relevance for AIDS case notification. Virtually all advocates for the use of unique identifiers chose to leave untouched the name-based registry for AIDS. Only ACT UP was willing to seize the matter. "While it is true New York has always had a names AIDS registry, the time has come to question this. . . . The greater length of time spent on a named list increases the likelihood of a PWA's (Person with AIDS) public disclosure."[75]

CODED REPORTING IN MARYLAND AND TEXAS

In January 1992 the AIDS Administration of the Maryland Department of Health submitted a bill to the legislature mandating HIV reporting, the policy already adopted by twenty-two other states. Not surprisingly, AIDS activists fiercely opposed the act. Sympathetic legislators told the activists that they would have to provide some alternative, since resistance to all forms of HIV case reporting was in the long run an untenable position. Ultimately, the proposed legislation was amended, charging state health officials with the responsibility for developing a non-name-based approach to HIV case reporting.[76] Thus began the saga of advocacy for unique identifiers as an alternative to name reporting. The mandate would set the stage for a struggle over scientific authority between AIDS advocates and their political allies on the one hand and health officials on the other.[77]

From the start, state health officials sought to thwart what they viewed as a mistaken political intrusion by legislative leaders. In a letter to William Roper, the director of the CDC, the secretary of Maryland's Department of Health and Mental Hygiene sought to elicit a clear statement that a unique identifiers system would not meet the standards of accuracy required by the federal agency.[78] Roper obliged by writing, "One goal of the Centers for Disease Control's HIV and AIDS surveillance system is to prevent duplication in case reports. . . . Identifying individual case reports by name not only provides a means of eliminating duplicates, but also allows for follow-up and referral of HIV infected persons for medical and social services. . . . A surveillance system that is unable to eliminate duplicate case reports is of limited public health benefit."[79] After a review of technical dimensions of how unique identifier reporting would function and with Roper's letter, the

AIDS Administration finally informed the state legislature that it was not feasible to design and implement a non-named system that would make possible a duplicate-free registry.[80]

In the next legislative session the AIDS Administration again pressed the
case for name reporting, submitting a bill that would have repealed the
prior year's unique identifier enactment. Once again the administration was
rebuffed, and the legislature directed that work proceed in the development of a laboratory-based system of non-name HIV case reporting. When
it did so, after acrimonious meetings of a special advisory committee, it proposed a fourteen-digit code involving birthdates and the last six digits of the
social security number.[81] The code outraged AIDS advocates who viewed it
as little more than a clever subterfuge: it was so closely tied to identifiable
data elements that it would fail to protect the privacy interest of people in
the registry.[82] An open hearing on the proposed code gave opponents an
opportunity to voice their outrage. Representatives of AIDS Action and the
Baltimore Mayor's Advisory Council, among others, spoke of their sense of
betrayal. Most bitter was the testimony of a man who identified himself as
having AIDS. "We have been fighting and struggling and resisting . . . for a
long time. But now they think, once again, we're fools enough that they can
slip underneath the door the unique identifiers that provides names, but
does not write names."[83]

But challenge to the proposed unique identifiers reporting system came
not only from those who viewed it as insufficiently protective of privacy but
from those who, in alliance with the health department itself, believed that
such an approach to surveillance was fundamentally mistaken. The society of
local health officers was joined by the large HMO Kaiser Permanente and the
Medical and Chirugal Faculty of Maryland (Med Chi), the state's medical
society. The medical association described the unique identifiers system as
"unwieldy, time consuming and burdensome," requiring personnel in clinical settings to obtain information that they did not "normally have access to"
such as Social Security numbers and racial or ethnic group identity. "Med
Chi firmly believes that HIV should be treated the same as every other infectious disease. . . . This can only happen if there is name reporting."[84]

Remarkably, it was not such opposition that defined the course of events
but rather the alliance of those pressing for Maryland to blaze the trail for
unique identifiers. When, in 1994, Maryland's governor once again submitted
a bill to repeal the legislature's unique identifier act, defeat was not unexpected. Based on the experience of the prior year, the AIDS Administration
had crafted a code acceptable to AIDS advocates. Unique identifier reporting
was to begin by mid-1994. As she prepared to leave her post as director of the
AIDS Administration after years of bruising controversy, Kathleen Edwards
wrote, "The Legislature directed a system which the Department consistently
felt was less efficient than another available system of reporting."[85]

Of fundamental importance to the implementation of and commitment to the unique identifier reporting system was the appointment of Liza Solomon to the directorship of the AIDS Administration in mid-1995 by a newly elected Democratic governor who had depended upon the strong support of the gay community. Solomon was a well-known AIDS advocate. She had fiercely resisted case reporting of HIV infection and only when threatened by the prospect of name reporting seized upon the idea of using unique identifiers. For her, there was no question that the interest and concerns of the AIDS advocacy community had to shape the course of policy. "We moved to a unique identifying system because we had a very clear history in Maryland that names reporting was not what our community wanted. It was a very bloody fight. A very passionate fight, one that discredited the agency that I now work for."[86]

For Solomon, it did not matter that Maryland's approach to surveillance might be less than perfect. "If one looks to a surveillance system to give basic epidemiological information on populations . . . then some slight over or under-counting will not have a significant impact. . . . In order to plan services, prevention activities, and target programs, it is important to have a good, although not exact, idea of the number of individuals involved. Public health programs are usually targeted at populations and affected communities. Knowing each person's identity is not necessary to accomplish these goals."[87] Indeed, for Solomon there was no obvious reason that partner notification programs had to be linked to state AIDS or HIV registries. In her conception of the role of surveillance as an epidemiologic tool and in her rejection of using state registries for interventions at the individual level, Solomon exposed the deep fissure that would inform future debate. Solomon's commitment to the values of privacy and the needs of the community with which she identified called into question the centrality of case reporting for public health. In fact, she thought of AIDS reporting by name as "an historic relic" that existed in tension with the underlying philosophical assumptions of relying on unique identifiers.[88]

The account of the embrace of unique identifiers in Texas can be told much more briefly because it shares some essential elements with the Maryland story. Where the two differed was in the political context within which they unfolded. In 1987 the Texas legislature made HIV infection reportable at a time when only six other states had done so. The Board of Health, which retained the authority over what information was collected for reportable conditions, chose what turned out to be a useless anonymous system involving only the reporting of age and gender. By design there was no ability to determine whether reported cases were duplicates of already reported instances of HIV. In 1991 the board expanded the number of reported items to include race or ethnicity, county of residence, and the date of the HIV test. That modification also proved futile for surveillance purposes. One year later the health department proposed the use of name-based surveillance, which evoked resistance from the gay community and civil liberties groups. Ultimately, a special work group recommended the use of unique identifiers. Such reporting commenced in 1994. As had been the case in Maryland, the proposal to use unique identifiers was imposed on a reluctant health department.[89] David Smith, the commissioner of health, was an advocate of name reporting. "We listened," he said, "to build rapport and trust." But Smith assumed from the start that the system would fail.

Indeed, in that regard he shared the views of CDC officials who would in 1998 yoke Texas and Maryland in a common critical evaluation of unique identifiers. But while officials in Maryland sought to neutralize what they saw as the name-reporting bias of the federal authorities, those in Texas viewed the influence of the CDC as salutary.[90] In the end, the difference was revealed in the response to the final report from the CDC evaluating the performance of the Maryland and Texas surveillance systems. Liza Solomon struggled to shape the tone, language, and thrust of the analysis, which she viewed as reflective of its bias for name reporting. Her efforts bore little fruit. "The evaluations of Maryland and Texas indicated that the use of unique identifiers limits the performance of an HIV surveillance system and complicates efforts to collect risk behavior information," wrote the CDC in *Morbidity and Mortality Weekly Report*.[91] Texas accepted the analysis and moved enthusiastically to a name-based system. In fact, health officials there saw the evaluation as "premeditated" and intended to use the document to bolster the case for names.[92] Maryland rejected the CDC conclusion as premature and used the opportunity of the evaluation to take steps to strengthen its own system.[93] Solomon would become the public face of the argument for why states should and how they could resist the pressure of the CDC.

THERAPEUTIC TRANSFORMATIONS AND THE CASE FOR HIV REPORTING

The clinical context of the initial debates about HIV surveillance was grim. Since it was first identified, AIDS represented a diagnosis with an almost certain fatal outcome. While progress had been made in managing the opportunistic conditions that afflicted those with HIV and in prolonging the lives of those with AIDS, efforts to attack the underlying disease process had borne little fruit. An attitude of therapeutic despair prevailed.

Then, in 1994, the first breakthrough occurred. A clinical trial with the antiretroviral drug AZT in pregnant women demonstrated the possibility of reducing transmission from mother to fetus by two-thirds, from 22 percent to 8 percent.[94] In 1995 even more startling results demonstrated that a new class of drugs—the protease inhibitors—when used in combination with other antiretroviral agents could reduce viral burden in infected individuals to undetectable levels and could have a dramatic impact on the clinical course for those with HIV. The year 1996 witnessed the first decline in reported cases of AIDS and AIDS-related deaths in the United States since the epidemic's onset.[95]

These therapeutic advances profoundly affected the debate on surveillance. Since the new therapeutic paradigm suggested the importance of early identification of people with HIV, it became more crucial than ever to encourage wide-scale testing and the referral of those with infection to appropriate clinical services. For advocates of name reporting, it was clear that now case notification was required to help save lives. Opponents saw the situation very differently. Case reporting by name would almost certainly scare people away from testing and thus pose a danger to those who could benefit from effective treatment. Further, anything that placed in jeopardy the publicly funded anonymous testing sites created in the mid-1980s for those who wished to shield their identities—in some states HIV case reporting went hand in hand with the closure of such centers—had to be resisted.

But about one issue there was little dispute: AIDS case reporting could no longer serve as an adequate measure of the state of the epidemic. Since the new therapies delayed the onset of AIDS-defining illnesses by years, AIDS case reporting revealed a pattern of infection increasingly remote from current patterns of HIV infection. Just as improving therapeutic prospects made HIV case reporting seem more urgent, it served to undercut unlinked seropositive surveillance, particularly among childbearing women.

Since it had become clear that the birth of babies with HIV infection could be radically affected by the use of AZT during pregnancy, strong voices, including the AMA, began to argue for mandatory screening to identify women who could be offered treatment.[96] Others called for unblinding anonymous surveillance, which they believed deprived women of knowledge, so that they might *choose* whether to undergo treatment. For such critics, surveillance activities that failed to notify the infected bore a resemblance to the notorious Tuskegee syphilis experiment conducted under the aegis of the PHS. The Black Caucus in the U.S. House of Representatives challenged the CDC's funding of anonymous surveillance. The CDC desperately tried to convince its liberal critics that there was a radical distinction between the ethics of case finding, focused on identifying individuals for purposes of clinical intervention, and the ethics of surveillance, focused on apprehending the contours of an epidemic on a population basis. But it was a distinction that critics could not or would not see. When, in May 1995, it became clear that Congress was prepared to unblind such surveillance, the agency bowed to political pressure. The unlinked surveillance of childbearing women that had done so much to provide a window on the patterns of infection among heterosexual women and that had revealed the vast difference between the rates of infection in white women and women of color was brought to a halt.[97]

The loss of a core element of surveillance activity intensified the commitment of the CDC to moving the states toward what it perceived as the only accurate system of case reporting for HIV: name-based notification. The political turmoil that such efforts had thus far produced made clear that bringing the struggle over HIV case reporting to a successful conclusion would necessitate much more than evidence about the technical superiority of name-based reporting. Profound fears about the use of names required that the CDC do everything possible to persuade hostile constituencies that it was committed to a surveillance approach that did not place those with HIV infection at risk for discrimination; that it took seriously the issue of privacy; and that it would act to protect the confidentiality of AIDS and HIV registries from malicious or inadvertent disclosure.

Because of concerns that state health departments might be compelled by law or administrative determination to use HIV or AIDS surveillance registries for purposes that had nothing to do with the public health and that might entail a breach of confidentiality, the CDC forcefully reproved those who engaged in what it considered a misuse of federal surveillance funds. Since surveillance at the state level was dependent on such resources, the CDC had considerable leverage. For example, when Missouri enacted a notification law requiring that information on infected children be released to school officials, the CDC warned the health department that the measure was "outside the scope of the intended use of federal funds. . . . No CDC-supported personnel, activities, or data collected through HIV/AIDS surveillance may be used to carry out the provisions of the school notification law."[98]

Since the CDC placed such great emphasis on protecting surveillance data from misuse, it readily acceded to a call by privacy advocates—concerned about whether the patchwork of state laws on privacy was adequate to the challenge of HIV/AIDS—to sponsor a systematic, state-by-state study of confidentiality protections. We turn to the findings of that study and the proposed remedial legislation in the last chapter. Here it is only necessary to note that what was found confirmed the worst fears of those opposed to HIV name reporting: "Extant laws concerning public health information privacy are inconsistent, fragmented, and inadequate."[99] As a result, the CDC embraced the idea of drafting a model state privacy act that would reflect contemporary understandings about the conditions under which public health surveillance ought to occur.

Whatever such initiatives by the CDC might have done over the long run to assuage concerns about the confidentiality of state HIV and AIDS registries was overshadowed by a single event that seemed to validate the deepest fears of those concerned about protecting the vulnerable from surveillance-associated harm. In September 1996, less than four months before it was to begin HIV name reporting, Florida experienced a dramatic failure in the security surrounding its AIDS registry.[100] A health department official from Pinellas County had reportedly shown a list containing four thousand names of people with AIDS to patrons in a Tampa gay bar. Computer discs containing the names were then sent to local media by someone who claimed that the health department worker had dropped his computer file while drunk. Newspaper headlines captured the sense of disquiet: "AIDS Patients' Fears Confirmed: Names Disclosed"; "AIDS List Is Out."[101]

Florida health officials moved swiftly to control the damage. The state's chief health officials declared, "With this breach, not only was the law broken, but the public trust was broken. . . . We are deeply concerned about this breach and will handle it with all seriousness. . . . We will not rest until we are certain that confidentiality is protected."[102] For the CDC, the Florida events threatened to undo everything officials had done to build the bonds of trust. After conducting an investigation of what lapses permitted the disclosure to occur, the federal agency concluded that while Florida had been in compliance with federal confidentiality requirements and that an individual had violated the standards, measures should be taken to "tighten security systems."[103]

For health officials, both local and federal, what happened in Florida was an extraordinary event that only placed into relief the otherwise unsullied record of those responsible for protecting surveillance records. For many AIDS advocates, it was a defining moment, revealing that name reporting placed individuals at risk no matter what the law dictated and officials promised. In the next years, as the CDC pressed ahead with the goal of HIV name-based case reporting, proponents of unique identifiers would repeatedly invoke the Florida episode.

RAISING THE CURTAIN ON A NEW ACT

With therapeutic advances, the struggle on the part of public health officials to reimpose elements of the tradition of infectious disease control appeared to be drawing to a successful conclusion.

As the prospect of HIV case reporting loomed, fissures began to emerge in the alliance that had so steadfastly resisted such a move. A consultative session convened by the CSTE and the CDC in mid-1997 provided the occasion for those divisions and shifts in opinion to be made public.[104] Placing the new alignment into bold relief was an exchange between two veterans of the surveillance wars: Neil Schram, a gay physician who had headed the American Association of Physicians for Human Rights in the epidemic's early years and who had steadfastly opposed HIV reporting for more than a decade, and Jeff Levi, who, as head of the National Gay Task Force in the

1980s and a senior official at the AIDS Action Council, had given voice to the primacy of privacy for gay men. At the consultation Schram explained why the gay and bisexual community would never support name reporting, especially when linked to partner notification.

Levi took a fundamentally different position. It was no longer possible, he said, to speak of unanimity on the issue of reporting in the gay community. While acknowledging the persistence of American homophobia, he believed that "we are in a different place than we were when we first had the discussions 15 years ago." Both the "science and sociology" of the epidemic had undergone a fundamental change. How, he asked, could AIDS advocates press government to expand the range of social and medical services to people with HIV and at the same time oppose name reporting because of a lack of trust? Then, echoing a perspective that had characterized many African American AIDS spokespersons who were more concerned about access to life-saving care than privacy, he noted: after HIV testing patients ideally would be referred to primary care, possibly in a public clinic with services covered by Medicaid, "and they have your name, your address, your Social Security number, your entire medical history, your HIV status, your CD4 count, your viral load. . . . So we trust the government to have everything there is to know about us when it comes to care."[105]

If the changed clinical, social, and political context of AIDS had provided the conditions for sharp divisions to emerge among formerly allied AIDS activists on the issue of name reporting, that was not so clearly the case with one of the central rationales for such surveillance: partner notification. For years, advocates of name reporting had argued that it would permit health departments to contact the sexual and needle-sharing partners of those who were infected, replicating a practice central to sexually transmitted disease control programs.

At the consultation, Jeff Levi acknowledged that some forms of partner notification—those that were truly voluntary and protected the identity of the index patient—were acceptable. But other advocates did not. Cornelius Baker, of the National Association of People with AIDS, was willing to concede the issue of case reporting, "I think part of the fear that the community has always had, at least from my perspective, is that we open the door and the flood rushes in. That we start with name reporting, and then we're talking about partner notification, and then we're talking about contact tracing, and then we're talking about quarantine."[106] The history of initiatives linking partner notification and case reporting—the LaRouche referendum years earlier and then congressional legislation proposed in 1996, 1997, and 1998 by conservative Oklahoma representative Tom Coburn—served to underscore the malevolent intentions of those who advanced such a "public health" agenda.[107]

It was on this terrain of shifting perspectives that the CSTE finally moved to call definitively for name reporting.[108] The CSTE made clear that efforts on the part of AIDS advocates to press for the adoption of the unique identifiers, enthusiastically pioneered by Maryland, would face professional resistance. Unique identifiers were inadequate to assure the accurate epidemiological characterization of the epidemic and were deemed unacceptable because they posed difficulties for follow-up referrals to social and clinical services.

In September 1997 the CDC formally announced that it would call upon all states to adopt a system of HIV case surveillance.[109] Support could be anticipated from the all-important medical community. The AMA had long supported HIV name reporting, and in 1997 the prestigious *New England Journal of Medicine* editorially took the same position.[110] To demonstrate the broad-based support for change, John Ward, a senior surveillance official at the CDC, joined with Lawrence Gostin, a Georgetown University law professor with a history of advocacy for civil liberties, and Cornelius Baker, an African American AIDS activist, to coauthor an article published in the *New England Journal of Medicine.* "We are," they asserted, "at a defining moment in the epidemic. . . . Unless we revise our surveillance system, health authorities will not have reliable information about the prevalence, incidence, and future directions of HIV infection. . . . We propose that all states require HIV case reporting."[111]

But the aura of inevitability and consensus could not mask the persistence of bitter opposition to name reporting. The American Civil Liberties Union brought its considerable intellectual and political resources to the fray. "There may come a time when HIV is so unremarkable a part of our social landscape, and care for it is so routinely available to those who need it, that no one will reasonably fear being identified as a person with HIV. But we are nowhere close to that time yet. On the contrary, the best evidence we have suggests that those who most need HIV testing are afraid of name reporting because they fear discrimination. Moreover, we know those fears are not groundless."[112]

As the CDC began what would ultimately be a more-than-two-year process of developing a set of recommendations for states on HIV case reporting, it was faced with divisions among its senior personnel.[113] Those involved directly in surveillance activities were firmly convinced that only a name-based system would be effective. By contrast, among those primarily engaged in prevention activities, where direct, ongoing contact with at-risk communities defined the work environment, there was much greater sympathy for fears about the dangers of stigmatization and discrimination. Even when such personnel did not themselves think the threats credible, they believed that respecting community fears was crucial for purposes of sustaining their all-important working relationships.

But such internal disagreements did not determine what the CDC would be permitted to recommend. Rather, officials at the Department of Health and Human Services, within which the CDC was administratively housed, had come to the conclusion that the fears of activists in the AIDS community warranted consideration. DHHS could see little advantage in antagonizing a constituency that was an important part of the Democratic Party's base. When the chief of the CDC's AIDS Surveillance Branch told his superiors in Washington that the CDC planned to call on all states to adopt name reporting without the option of using unique identifiers, he was simply told, "That won't do." Recalling the impact of that clear directive, Kevin DeCock noted, "We technical people work within a hierarchy. The best that could be achieved was to *recommend* names, with strong performance criteria" established for all reporting systems.[114] It was such criteria, the CDC believed, that would ultimately compel states to give up their enthusiasm for unique identifiers, which might meet those standards only with great effort and the expenditure of considerable resources.

As the CDC crafted national recommendations, it had to confront two questions that had haunted the discussion of HIV case surveillance. Would state health departments be able to secure their records in a way that could dispel the specter of the Florida breach in confidentiality? And even if they were successful in securing HIV case reports, would the legacy of Florida and the more generalized anxiety about confidentiality serve as deterrents to HIV testing among drug users and their sexual partners, gay and bisexual men, and others at increased risk?

While underscoring the protective functions of the federal privacy act and the exemptions to the Freedom of Information Act and Certificates of Confidentiality, the CDC acknowledged that there was "no uniform law on the privacy and security of HIV/AIDS surveillance information that applied across all settings and situations." To remedy this situation, stringent security standards were developed.[115] By mid-1998 the CDC notified those responsible for HIV/AIDS surveillance at the state level that receipt of federal funds for their efforts would be conditional upon a demonstration that its standards had been met by the year 2000.[116]

Since the first steps toward name reporting occurred in Colorado and Minnesota almost fifteen years earlier, there had emerged a large, if uneven, empirical literature on whether HIV case reporting by name had a negative impact on the willingness to be tested. Early studies appeared to suggest that it did. But of what relevance were such investigations, undertaken in an era of relative therapeutic impotence, to the latter part of the 1990s, when effective antiretroviral therapy served as a powerful inducement to testing as a prelude to treatment? For the CDC, nothing was of greater importance than an accurate answer to that question.

In 1999 a CDC-funded investigation reported that while the potential benefits of HIV case reporting in assuring access to care or enhanced partner notification appeared to be smaller than proponents of reporting had long suggested, the negative impacts of reporting on the willingness to undergo testing were also far less clear than opponents had warned.[117] Despite the fevered rhetoric about driving the epidemic underground, "most participants did not know their state's HIV reporting policy."[118] Reporting was not associated with test avoidance, although for some intravenous drug users it might have contributed to a delay. This study, as well as others undertaken directly by the CDC itself, merely confirmed what the CDC advocates for name reporting had long believed. They would deploy this evidence in the struggle unfolding in states that had yet to adopt any form of HIV case reporting in the next years.[119]

The most significant of those encounters occurred in New York, which accounted for almost 40 percent of the AIDS cases in the United States. For years a powerful alliance of AIDS activists, public health officials in New York City, and the leaders of the Democratic Party with important links to the gay community had been able to thwart serious consideration of HIV case reporting. In 1997 changes in the AIDS epidemic contributed to the beginning of the first sustained discussion of HIV case reporting. The state health department's AIDS Advisory Council created a working group on HIV surveillance. At a public meeting of the group, the divisive issues that had characterized the debate for almost a decade and a half were plain. A columnist for the *New York Times* wrote, "Fervor and near theological certitude were everywhere."[120] When the committee, composed of privacy advocates, community-based organizations, and local and state health officials, issued its report, the divide was not only unbridged but clearly exposed. A majority rejected both the use of names and the use of unique identifiers that incorporated any elements of the Social Security number.[121]

A dissent signed by nine committee members, including its co-chair, was scathing. They denounced the majority for its failure to consider the scientific evidence and challenged the composition of the group as "unbalanced." Made up of public health officials on the committee, the minority embraced what it considered the lessons of confronting threats to the community's health: "HIV name reporting is an essential tool for planning the fight against HIV."[122] Such reporting, argued the dissenters, should be linked to partner notification, which would save lives.

The committee's failure to reach agreement paved the way for action in the legislative arena. In June 1998, in the waning hours of the legislative session, the Democratic-controlled state assembly voted overwhelmingly for a bill that would mandate name reporting and a more vigorous approach to partner notification. In so doing, it joined the Republican-dominated state senate, which had already passed the bill.[123]

To advocates of name reporting in other states and at the CDC, it would have been hard to overstate the significance of the New York decision. But whatever the symbolic importance of the decision in New York, efforts in other states made clear that the CDC would confront resistance as it pressed to have name reporting adopted as the standard of public health practice.

In the winter of 1998, Massachusetts joined Maryland in adopting a coded reporting system.[124] In the state of Washington a compromise unfolded that sought to achieve the positive end of name-based reporting while acknowledging the concerns of those who feared that such notification would create state-held lists of infected people who could be expected to live for years because of the effectiveness of the new therapies. A "name to code" approach was made state policy in mid-1999.[125] Under this compromise, new HIV cases would be reported by name. Local health departments would then have three months to follow up in order to complete case reports, determine if they represented duplicates, and undertake partner notification or other interventions. At the end of the three months, the name would be expunged and converted to a code to be held by both local and state health departments. To its advocates, such an approach avoided the problems posed by unique identifier systems while providing the assurances deemed so essential by those concerned about privacy. While the compromise satisfied some, others remained troubled and angry. A spokesman for HIV-positive patients in Seattle, King County, said, "I feel like we've really been sold down the river."[126]

TOWARD UNIVERSAL CASE REPORTING

In December 1998 the CDC issued its long-awaited draft guidelines.[127] They bore the imprint of the compromises that emerged out of the tortuous political process that had pitted public health officials against AIDS advocates and their political allies over the prior years. In short, they illuminated the complex interplay of empirical evidence and the politics of privacy. While strongly recommending that states adopt the name-reporting system—the gold standard of AIDS surveillance since the early 1980s—and noting that the experiments with unique identifiers in Maryland and Texas had proved that such approaches were problem ridden, the draft guidelines left to each state the determination of how to undertake HIV case surveillance. Stringent performance criteria for the completeness of each reported case and the ability to eliminate duplicate case reports would be, the CDC assumed, easier for name-based systems to attain. States were to be given time to meet those standards. But if they failed to do so they would risk losing federal funds for their surveillance activities.

In a striking bow to those who had rested their claims on the adequacy of unique identifiers systems and to AIDS advocates who had so forcefully sought to sever the relationship between surveillance and public health measures such as partner notification, the proposed guidelines asserted that the primary purpose for surveillance activities was the collection of timely epidemiological data. It was for the states to determine whether and how case reporting could be used for other public health purposes. Less surprisingly, the draft guidelines strongly supported the preservation of anonymous testing, where permitted by state laws, and emphasized the centrality of security and confidentiality for case surveillance registries.

The response of public health departments to these draft recommendations only served to underscore how deeply divided the nation still was. Thirteen states that had adopted name reporting rebuked the CDC for leaving open the option of case reporting by unique identifiers.[128] Officials in Texas, which had, in response to the CDC's own evaluation, scuttled its unique identifiers system, all but suggested that the CDC had capitulated to political pressure, ignoring "the best available data."[129] Kentucky, which was required by state law to collect data using patient initials, expressed disappointment that the CDC had not taken a stronger position in favor of name reporting because that would have enhanced the ability of the state health department to press for legislative change.

The effort to distinguish surveillance from public health interventions also drew the ire of a number of states, including Colorado and Minnesota, that had pioneered name reporting almost fifteen years earlier. Colorado stated that intervention to prevent and control disease was the primary public health and statutory purpose for collecting HIV surveillance data. It was that conception of surveillance that set the terms for the state's voluntary partner notification system. Missouri's health department was more forceful. "Local and state partnerships exist to ensure daily efficacious sharing of surveillance data with [sexually transmitted disease] investigators and HIV case managers to verify diagnoses, link patients with early HIV care, and solicit partner infected individuals for notification, counseling and evaluation."[130] Among states with long-established name reporting systems, only New Jersey supported the CDC position on the relationship between surveillance and partner notification.

The final CDC recommendations, published one year later on December 9, 1999, were essentially unchanged, although some cosmetic modifications were made in response to the outpouring of commentaries.[131] In the two years that had elapsed since the CDC first signaled that it would be preparing national HIV case surveillance guidelines, nine states had adopted or begun the implementation of such notification. Demonstrating the resistance to the CDC's own predilection for name-based reporting, five states had chosen some variant of a coded system. The events of the next three years would only serve to reveal the preeminence of local considerations in the politics of surveillance.

More powerful as an impetus for change than the CDC's guidelines was the action of Congress. The Ryan White CARE Act, first passed in 1990, provided federal funds for treatment and care to localities that had borne the brunt of the AIDS epidemic. With broad congressional support, the act represented a singular commitment to providing a safety net for the most vulnerable people with AIDS. Inevitably, concerns emerged about the adequacy of the funding formulas to truly reflect the social burdens created by the epidemic. Did the resources reflect current AIDS needs, or did they unfairly advantage those metropolitan areas where the epidemic had first struck? Were the needs of women and minority members being addressed?

In 2000, as the act was being reviewed for reauthorization, the adequacy of formulas based on AIDS cases became a focus of attention. Representative Tom Coburn, a Republican from Oklahoma who had long argued for HIV name reporting, now pressed the need for a shift to HIV case reports. "Those with HIV are too often not figured in, in the components for care."[132] The chair of the House Subcommittee on Health and the Environment, Michael Bilirakis, stressed the need for "reliable data on HIV prevalence" for meeting the act's purposes.[133] But the use of HIV surveillance was also supported by California Democrat Henry Waxman, a liberal representative closely aligned with AIDS advocacy groups, many of which had begun to rethink the univocal opposition to HIV reporting.

In the end, the reauthorized CARE Act directed that the formulas for the allocation of funds to state and "eligible metropolitan areas" incorporate data on reported cases of HIV infection. Such data was to be used in allocations as early as fiscal year 2005 if the secretary of health and human services determined that the data was sufficiently accurate for resource allocation purposes.[134] Technical assistance to the states would be provided to assure that case reporting met acceptable standards. The deadline for attaining the requisite level of proficiency was 2007. Congress remained silent on whether name reporting was more likely to serve the purposes of the act. With billions of dollars in aid at stake, it was not surprising that it would provoke a move to case reporting in those states that had yet to embrace HIV surveillance.

Most important was California, which had followed a byzantine course to HIV surveillance.[135] Case reporting based on unique identifiers began in California on July 1, 2002. The system was certainly more costly and difficult to implement than would have been the case had names been used. But it was a system responsive to the political claims of those who deemed privacy a value too precious to be compromised. (In 2006, however, California scuttled its coded reporting and adopted a name-based system.) Nine other states and the District of Columbia had elected either coded or name-to-code approaches. When Georgia, in December 2003, became the last state to adopt HIV case reporting, it was one of only two that had chosen name-based systems since January 2000.

In pressing the states to adopt HIV case reporting, the CDC had made a strategic determination to emphasize the significance of such surveillance for mapping the contours of the epidemic. The role of reporting for facilitating public health interventions like partner notification had been deemphasized, even minimized. In some states, those responsible for HIV case reporting systems, either name-based or coded, asserted that the sole function of the databases they oversaw was epidemiological. Such a position not only represented a radical break with the historical understanding of the role of case reporting, it also stood in sharp contrast to the conclusions contained in two reports prepared by the Institute of Medicine (IOM), a branch of the National Academy of Science that advises the government on health issues. In its study *No Time to Lose,* published in 2001, the IOM underscored the limitations of both AIDS and HIV reporting for tracking the epidemic.[136] For the purpose of guiding prevention efforts, resource allocation, and policy at national, state, and local levels, the IOM recommended a surveillance system that relied on blinded seropositive surveys and studies capable of identifying recent HIV infections. Three years later, when called upon by congressional mandate to evaluate the potential role of HIV reporting for allocating Ryan White CARE Act funds, the IOM concluded in *Measuring What Matters* that while case reporting could well serve some public health ends, alternatives to AIDS or HIV reporting had "the potential of providing estimates that are more accurate, more timely, and more consistent across jurisdictions than complete enumeration."[137] Only by fully apprehending the ways in which the politics of privacy and the politics of public health have played out in the context of the AIDS epidemic over the course of close to twenty years can we understand the ironies surrounding the ultimate form HIV case reporting assumed at the end of a very public, very extended, and very political series of struggles.

8

Counting All Kids

Immunization Registries
and the Privacy of Parents and Children

As the list of vaccines recommended for routine administration to children grew from just one (smallpox) in 1900 to almost a dozen by 2000, immunization achieved almost mythic status among public health interventions for its ability to control and even eliminate formerly endemic scourges such as diphtheria and whooping cough. Surveys showed that overwhelming numbers of parents favored having their children receive doses of all recommended vaccines.[1] That such registries would raise concerns over privacy and confidentiality might seem unlikely, given the broad public support vaccination enjoys.

At a time of increasing concern about the extent of health information held in government and private sector databases, immunization registries extended surveillance from sick people to healthy ones, primarily children (though some systems tracked adult immunization as well). An immunization registry, which contains records on all children in a defined area with information on which vaccines they have received, serves multiple purposes. Since many children receive their vaccinations in several different clinical settings and parents frequently misplace their children's records, clinicians may use a registry during a patient encounter to determine which immunizations have been given and which are still needed. The information in registries can trigger "reminder and recall" interventions such as letters and phone calls urging parents to bring children in for boosters or additional vaccinations. Registries also enable planners and policy makers to identify patterns of vaccination coverage in a population, pinpoint areas of low rates, and target the "pockets" of unprotected children who served as reservoirs for the spread of infectious disease.

Because they must be capable of tracking multiple encounters in different locations over the course of several years, immunization registries are a daunting technological undertaking requiring sustained financial support. The CDC and state and local health departments made repeated attempts beginning in the 1960s to set up computer tracking systems for immunizations, but technological hurdles and fiscal constraints stymied their efforts. It was not until the 1990s that an infusion of philanthropic and public funding enabled the nationwide development of registries to move forward.

Because enhancing patient care was a central goal of immunization registries, anonymous reporting was never an option—such systems depended on the use of a name, age, and some amount of medical history. The target population for inclusion in an immunization registry was not just a small group of people defined by their experience with an illness but the entire birth cohort of a city, state, region, or—according to the most ambitious visions—the whole country. Even for those with an expansive view of the state's role in tracking health information, the idea of a database with records on all children gave pause. For those who held antistatist views or who mistrusted the safety of vaccines—an increasingly vocal constituency at the turn of the twenty-first century—the penetration of the eyes of government into the lives of healthy people triggered a visceral opposition, which they channeled into political advocacy at the local, state, and national levels to block the implementation of registries.

The concerns about the confidentiality of immunization registries were of a piece with the broad themes that characterized the democratization of privacy: suspicion of the judgment and integrity of the public health establishment, mistrust of government bureaucracies more generally, and fear that a small and disfavored minority group—in this case, parents whose children were inadequately vaccinated—would be subject to persecution because of the information contained in the database. Efforts to record and monitor immunization status also drew opposition from many clinicians, though for reasons that reached back to the era of paternalistic privacy. Doctors, especially those in private practice, tended to look warily upon the use of registries. The proposed systems required integration into a practice's existing system for charts and billing and ongoing time and effort from office staff. Health officials used both persuasion (repeated office visits to promote the benefits of registries) and compulsion (laws requiring the reporting of all immunizations) to overcome this resistance.

IMMUNIZATION TRACKING IN THE PRE-COMPUTER ERA

In the nineteenth century, the use of cowpox to prevent infection with smallpox, first developed by the English physician Edward Jenner in 1796, was the only vaccination, one of the few effective interventions medicine had to offer. A handful of jurisdictions in the United States mandated physician reporting of the procedure. The purpose of this surveillance was to verify compliance with the compulsory vaccination laws on the books in some cities and states. "Boards of health often make wholesale vaccination upon the population of large districts, institutions, schools, the employees of corporations, etc., without even a slight record of the names . . . of those who have been vaccinated," complained a Massachusetts physician in 1902.[2] Vaccination provoked both active and passive resistance from those who doubted the practice's safety and efficacy, and in this context the record of a successful vaccination "is often of very great value in settling disputed cases" over whether someone had complied with the law. The filing of a report with the person's name, age, and sex and the date of vaccination was a common requirement in European countries but rare in the United States. As with other forms of surveillance during this period, compliance with these laws was inconsistent at best.[3]

Around the turn of the twentieth century, advances in bacteriology led to new attempts to control the spread of disease through prophylactic injections. Haltingly during the first half of the century and then with increasing rapidity following World War II, vaccines transformed the public health landscape by controlling diseases that had once been responsible for the majority of illness and death in infants and children. Vaccines for diphtheria, tetanus, and pertussis (also known as whooping cough) came into use in the 1920s, even though the evidence of their efficacy was sometimes contested.[4] Initial public acceptance of these preventives was far from universal, but they grew in popularity as parents increasingly relied on the guidance of pediatricians and child-rearing experts.[5] Vaccine development accelerated amid the postwar boom in scientific medicine. In the 1950s the nationwide testing and subsequent licensing of Jonas Salk's polio vaccine was a media sensation and brought unprecedented public acclaim for immunization. Dramatic advances in virology and immunology led to the licensing of vaccines against measles, mumps, and rubella in quick succession in the 1960s.[6]

As use of vaccines became commonplace, public health officials sought more systematic knowledge about coverage levels in neighborhoods, cities, and states. They considered such data to be an important marker for whether children were receiving needed care in the first years of life and a more general indicator of the overall health of the community.[7] But the practical value of this information was less clear. The concept of "herd immunity," first formally articulated in the 1920s, was poorly understood in the middle decades of the century. While health officials intuitively knew that higher levels of coverage meant lower rates of disease, no one knew the exact percentages that had to be attained in order to halt the spread of disease. One of the few communitywide studies of herd immunity was conducted early in the century in Baltimore, where the city health commissioner tracked the incidence of measles over several years and calculated the ratio of susceptible children to those were immune because they had had the disease (the study predated the development of the measles vaccine). Evidence from Baltimore suggested that when immunity to measles was higher than 55 percent, outbreaks of the disease were kept under control.[8] But what percentage might be needed to forestall the spread of other diseases in other populations remained uncertain.

Even were such a precise target to be identified, the physician rank-and-file rarely took the time to report the shots they gave. Record keeping, wrote one health officer in 1932, was "the pet aversion of the physician."[9] As a result, public health officials typically had only the most general idea of what percentage of their population had been vaccinated against a given illness. As the number of routinely given vaccinations increased to four—smallpox, diphtheria, pertussis, and tetanus—in the 1940s and 1950s, it became even less feasible to expect full reporting of the vaccinations that physicians were giving. "With rare exceptions," wrote a county health commissioner in 1960, "physician reporting [of immunization] is too incomplete to be used as a basis for statistical purposes. Practicing physicians are just too busy, and the paperwork incident to present-day medical practice is just too overwhelming, to expect consistent reporting when it does not contribute directly to the well-being of the individual patients involved."[10]

In 1958, as part of an effort to increase use of the recently licensed polio vaccine, the CDC's Epidemic Intelligence Service began regular monitoring of vaccinations in 125 U.S. cities using a sampling method in which a proportion of residents within individual city blocks were surveyed. For data analysis, the surveyed blocks were grouped into four socioeconomic classes based on census data; one of the principal motivations for such surveillance was concern over the socioeconomic gradient in vaccination status that had been observed in some smaller-scale parental surveys.[11] These surveys were the first systematic source of data about the country's levels of vaccination coverage, but they represented at best an incomplete picture.

THE VACCINATION ASSISTANCE ACT OF 1962

The CDC's ongoing monitoring of coverage levels was significant because it was one of the first steps toward greater federal involvement with immunization. Like many public health activities in the United States, immunization programs were marked by considerable geographic variation; decisions about who should be targeted and how vaccination should be promoted were made at the local or state level according to the needs and priorities of different communities. That began to change with the passage in 1962 of the Vaccination Assistance Act. The CDC, hoping to leverage the increased public support for immunization in the wake of the recent triumph over polio, devised a plan to create a permanent bureaucracy within the PHS to support the delivery of shots for infants and children. The infectious diseases of childhood had been on a steady decline for several decades, and CDC officials believed that as the rising incidence of chronic conditions such as cancer increasingly preoccupied city and state health departments, vaccination campaigns would languish without federal support.[12] The idea for a dedicated funding program found a receptive audience in the Kennedy administration, which advanced the act as part of its efforts to reform the health care system.

Flush with financial support, CDC officials provided grants to states to help promote the use of routinely recommended vaccinations. The agency had high hopes for the eventual role that registries might play in the nation's efforts to control infectious disease. "To picture an ideal situation, perhaps in the rather distant future," said CDC chief James Goddard in 1964, "the capabilities of electronic computers for storing and retrieving information could greatly facilitate our immunization programs. Computers could be used to store information with regard to the immunization given each individual, automatically print out a listing of those due repeat or booster immunizations, and manipulate data to compute the preventive effects of immunization."[13]

Goddard looked ahead to a system that would enable "efficient national follow-up of births for maintenance of immunization levels."[14] His optimistic forecast reflected a sense of limitless possibilities about immunization that prevailed during the 1960s. The annual incidence of polio, which had numbered in the tens of thousands during the pre-vaccine era, declined to near zero; on the heels of this triumph, scientists announced in 1963 the creation of a vaccine against measles, one of the most common childhood scourges. In the fall of 1966 the CDC launched a national campaign to eradicate measles with the same confidence that animated Lyndon Johnson's Great Society programs and the federal war on poverty. The sanguine view of the role of immunization registries was strikingly at odds, however, with the growing anxiety among the lay public about computer databases.

While Goddard and other public health officials envisioned databases with sophisticated tracking capabilities, most of the programs undertaken around the country with CDC support were not dedicated immunization registries that could follow individual children over time. Instead, most grantees grafted a simple reminder function onto their existing system of birth certificate records, which virtually all jurisdictions collected, often in computerized databases.

The idea of using the vital records systems to boost immunization rates was an old one. New York City, for example, instituted a reminder system in the 1930s in which a letter was sent one year after a child's birth encouraging parents to have their children protected against diphtheria. This system had no capacity to follow up on whether the immunization ultimately took place, and even its reminding capabilities were limited: approximately one-

Dear Parents,

Now is the time for your new baby to be receiving protective vaccine against Diphtheria, Whooping Cough, Tetanus, Smallpox and Polio.

To let us know about your baby, please fill in the following information and mail this card today. NO STAMP IS NEEDED.

Please check (✓) one box only:

☐ My baby is already getting protective vaccines

☐ My baby will be getting protective vaccines soon

Estimados Padres,

Ahora es el tiempo para que su nuevo bebé esté recibiendo las vacunas para la protección contra la difteria, tos ferina, tetano, viruela y polio.

Para nosotros saber de su bebé por favor llené la planilla o continuación y ponga la tarjeta en el correo hoy mismo. NO NECESITA SELLOS.

Marque así (✓) en sólo una de los cuadritos:

☐ Mi bebé ya comenzó a recibir vacunas de protección

☐ Mi bebé va a recibir vacunas de protección, pronto

6-139185 1 1

Name of Doctor or Clinic

▓▓▓ EAST 7 ST BKLYN
BROOKLYN, N Y   11218

Nombre del Médico o Clínico infantil

Your Name

IF NAME OR ADDRESS IS INCORRECT,
PLEASE CHANGE
120M-1 1/60031 (60)

Su nombre

CORRIJA SU NOMBRE Y DIRECCION
SI ESTÁ EQUIVOCADO

Figure 23. New York City's Immunization Reminder System used birth certificate records to generate and send a postcard ninety days after each child's birth. Courtesy of the New York City Municipal Archives.

third of the letters were returned to the health department with the addressee "not found."[15]

Federal funding through the Vaccination Assistance Act enabled new or more technologically sophisticated systems to be established. For its Immunization Reminder System, begun in 1967, New York City upgraded from stenographers to a computer mainframe that could generate reminder cards to the parents of the approximately eleven thousand babies born each month in the city. The cards, printed in Spanish and English, were mailed ninety days after the child's birth and asked parents to indicate whether their children had received the recommended vaccines and to return the card to the health department. Those who failed to return a card after one month were sent a second reminder card, and, if necessary, a third (fig. 23).[16]

One of the most successful reminder/recall programs was instituted in Rhode Island. Using information from birth certificates, a computer program generated a series of mailings to all parents of newborns. The first letter, urging parents to have their child vaccinated, included a return card to be signed by a physician once the immunization series was administered. If no response was received within thirty days, a second mailing was sent; the follow-up appeal was more emotional in tone and included a picture of a young boy wearing leg braces as a result of having been stricken with polio. Finally, if the second appeal was unsuccessful, public health nurses made home visits to the unresponsive parents. The nurses were instructed to be "doggedly persistent in their efforts" to get parents to accept vaccination, according to a report on the program.[17]

There was little hard evidence for how well such systems worked. But even some proponents questioned whether the results achieved were commensurate with the expense, time, and effort that were necessary. North Carolina, which sent reminder letters to all parents in their child's thirteenth month, determined that just 6 percent of children received any vaccine in the month following the parents' receipt of the letter.[18] And while computerization made the systems more efficient than they had been in the past, the follow-up activities remained costly and labor intensive. "Most [local] health departments viewed this as the state's program and they would have no involvement in it," lamented one North Carolina official, "particularly when there were costs to them in terms of staff time, travel and postage."[19] Rhode Island found that its program cost about $42 per child immunized as a result of the follow-up; while the program was especially helpful at boosting rates among poor children, it was less cost effective for middle- and upper-class parents.[20]

It is uncertain whether parents ever objected to home visits urging immunization, but even the seemingly modest forms of mail outreach reminder systems could draw protest. In New York a representative of Catholic Charities complained to the city health commissioner after receiving reports that unmarried mothers who had placed their babies up for adoption were getting the reminders. Some of these young women had taken trips away during their pregnancy in order to give birth in secret, leaving their families unaware they were pregnant—until the open-faced immunization reminder postcard arrived at their home.[21] Health departments in other cities reported receiving angry responses from grieving parents whose children had died soon after birth.[22]

The most advanced system for tracking which vaccines were administered to a given child over time was established in Delaware in 1973 in all public health clinics. At a baby's first immunization, the physician or nurse delivering the shot recorded on a paper form the baby's full name, birth date, place of birth, and current address. The form was then sent to the state health department in Dover where the information was entered into a central computer database. On subsequent visits, clinicians could call a toll-free number to learn what immunizations were needed if the parent had misplaced the child's records. The system was able to generate a quarterly report for all participating providers of their own patients' immunization histories, with "incompletes" flagged with an asterisk. The report also included the statewide percentages of fully immunized children so that individual practitioners could compare their rates to other participating providers (figs. 24 and 25).[23]

Delaware's system was atypical in its completeness and capabilities. Despite the presence in Atlanta of a permanent bureaucracy supporting local and state immunization efforts, the development of systems for tracking the immunization status of children proceeded in fits and starts. The collection of data remained variable and largely incomplete, the state of

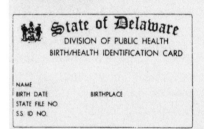

YOUR CHILD'S IMMUNIZATIONS ARE BEING RECORDED IN DELAWARE'S IMMUNIZATION REGISTER.

☕tate of Delaware
DIVISION OF PUBLIC HEALTH
BIRTH/HEALTH IDENTIFICATION CARD

NAME
BIRTH DATE   BIRTHPLACE
STATE FILE NO.
S.S. ID NO.

WHEN YOUR CHILD STARTS SCHOOL, THE RECORD WILL BE TRANSFERRED AUTOMATICALLY.

TO FIND OUT MORE ABOUT THE IMMUNIZATION REGISTER AND YOUR CHILD'S RECORD,

CALL 1-800-282-8672

TOLL-FREE FROM ANYWHERE IN DELAWARE.

Figures 24 and 25. In 1973 Delaware created a tracking system for infant immunization in all public health clinics. When the first shots were given, parents received an information packet and an identifier card for the baby (*above*). The physician or nurse delivering the shot recorded the baby's name, birth date, place of birth, and address on a form (*below*) that was then entered into a state health department database. The department provided a toll-free number clinicians could call to learn what immunizations were needed. Photo courtesy of Centers for Disease Control, from U.S. Department of Health, Education, and Welfare, *14th Immunization Conference Proceedings.* Atlanta, 1979.

computers was relatively primitive, and the systems required a substantial investment of time and money. Federal immunization funding was block-granted along with other public health dollars during the Nixon administration. Many states, facing health problems they considered more pressing than childhood infectious diseases—all of which had dwindled to insignificant numbers—chose to spend their federal health dollars on other programs.[24] As a result, few of the immunization reminder or tracking programs undertaken in the 1960s and 1970s were sustained.[25] Meanwhile, the measles eradication campaign petered out, along with much of the optimism that had animated it, amid the realization that infectious diseases—like poverty, racism, and other social ills targeted by Great Society programs—were far more intractable than they had seemed.

In the hangover of the failed eradication effort, immunization programs languished during the 1970s. The incidence of childhood illnesses began to inch back up after declining for years. Federal funding was erratic and, in the eyes of most public health officials, inadequate.[26] The reputation of the CDC suffered in 1976 when the largest mass vaccination program in the country's history—a campaign to protect against a feared epidemic of swine flu—collapsed into a quagmire of lawsuits and negative publicity. The predicted epidemic never materialized, and the vaccine was linked to the development of Guillain-Barré syndrome, a rare neurological disorder, in some recipients, leading to thousands of tort claims against the federal government, which had assumed liability for the huge program after the vaccine manufacturers' insurers balked.[27] Officials at the Department of Health, Education, and Welfare were alarmed that public acceptance of other vaccines might decline as a result of the debacle.

At this low point, immunization programs and the development of registries got a political boost from the change in presidential administrations. Betty Bumpers, the wife of Arkansas Democratic senator and former governor Dale Bumpers, had championed the cause of childhood vaccination when she had been the state's first lady. Bumpers was a friend of Rosalyn Carter, and when Jimmy Carter took office at the beginning of 1977, Betty Bumpers convinced the first lady that the issue should be elevated to the top of the nation's health priorities. The Carters requested that Joseph Califano, the new secretary of Health, Education, and Welfare, undertake a national immunization campaign.[28] Califano, eager to repair the damage done by the swine flu affair, announced an initiative to boost childhood immunization rates in 1977. One component of the plan was the Childhood Immunization Follow-Up System (CIFS). It was to be based on the birth certificate data that was collected by all states on the three million children born each year in the United States. The CIFS would involve, in the words of a CDC program manager, "routine data sharing systems within health departments, and among many organizations and individuals who provide childhood immunizations."[29]

Societal anxieties about privacy had steadily increased since the mid-1960s, and this new proposal sparked concerns that had largely been absent when the CDC had first raised the idea of tracking vaccinations. Speaking to a national conference of immunization providers in 1979, John Fanning, a legislative coordinator with the Department of Health and Human Services who had a long involvement in matters of privacy, warned of the potential violations that might occur in a system linked to birth certificate records. "The purposes of this tracking are clearly good," Fanning asserted, "but it is tracking by the government nonetheless." He went on to describe the decisions that would have to be confronted. "One possibility is to track every child who is born in the State or other jurisdiction. That has overtones of the universal, all-seeing government, checking every last family to be sure that its health status meets the government's standards. The other approach is to identify certain children, using carefully drawn selection criteria. . . . That has overtones of labeling and categorization. . . . If the criteria include factors like number of years of [parental] education, or worse, legitimacy status, the system really does have the potential for harming individual families."[30]

In Fanning's view, it was essential to implement registries in ways that respected family autonomy and assured political support, including obtaining buy-in from community groups and parent organizations.

Secretary Califano's 1977 initiative rekindled some of the hope of the previous decade that a national tracking system might some day be realized. But the challenges of technology and labor proved greater than expected—backlogs of millions of birth certificates had to be entered just to get the systems up and running—and only two years after the CIFS was announced, a pessimistic summary of progress conceded that the system was proving "costly and difficult to implement."[31] Devising an efficient and cost-effective way of tracking children's immunization status seemed to present an insurmountable challenge: at the beginning of 1980, when the monthly newsletter of the American Academy of Pediatrics asked all members to forward their ideas for a workable recall system, the association received not a single response.[32]

The CDC scaled back its plans and began to focus on smaller-scale, more incremental systems. In 1980 the agency supported pilot projects in three states, Arkansas, New Hampshire, and New Mexico. Each system ran on a single desktop computer. Information on children—name, birth date, parent's name and address, dates of vaccination, health care provider, and vaccine lot number—were entered from birth certificates and records submitted by providers as the children received their immunizations.[33] Over the next decade, the CDC piloted similar systems in about ten other state and local health departments. Their main function was to provide clinicians with a listing of which vaccines children in their practice needed. Because they were too incomplete to provide useful information about patterns of coverage for children in the state, these systems served as adjuncts to pediatric medicine rather than as tools of population health.[34] At the dawn of the era of personal computers, the speed, efficiency, and storage capabilities of desktop systems left much to be desired. CDC officials noted with frustration that while sophisticated computer systems in the private sector were increasingly common, public health remained a technological backwater.

RESPONDING TO CRISES

The centerpiece of the CDC's 1977 initiative to boost childhood immunization had been an effort to get schools to enforce laws excluding unvaccinated students. This approach proved effective at raising vaccination rates among school-aged youth. But children were supposed to have received the majority of their shots by age two, and rates for the younger age group lagged far behind. In the mid-1980s child welfare activists in the nonprofit sector—who saw the delivery of vaccines as a key indicator by which to judge the country's success at improving the health of infants and newborns—took on the issue of immunization and jump-started the faltering effort for more systematic and comprehensive surveillance.

In 1987 the liberal advocacy group the Children's Defense Fund published the report *Who's Watching Our Children's Health?* which sounded the tocsin about low immunization rates. The group charged that the Reagan administration had cut already limited funds for immunization programs with the result that levels of protection against childhood illnesses had actually declined since 1980. The percentage of children under age two who had been vaccinated against polio, for example, declined from 81 percent in 1980 to 77 percent in 1985.[35] The report garnered extensive coverage in the national news media. "There are many ways to hold down federal spending," declared the *Washington Post*. "Limiting funds for vaccinations is perhaps the worst way to do it."[36] It also caught the attention of congressional representatives interested in immunization and prompted the CDC to redouble its efforts to reach children under two. The agency brought together a panel of experts for consultation about how to improve the rates and what kind of surveillance would enable it to determine whether its efforts were successful. Several members of the panel indicated that a *national* registry linked to existing data systems such as those for birth certificates would be useful.[37]

The efforts of the Children's Defense Fund and the CDC might never have borne fruit had it not been for a deadly resurgence of a childhood infectious disease. Beginning in 1989 and continuing over the next two years, the worst outbreak of measles in decades swept across the United States. Measles had been preventable since 1963, when two vaccines against the disease were licensed, but it is one of the most highly contagious of all infectious diseases. Health officials had been consistently frustrated in their efforts to eliminate it. During the epidemic of 1989–91, cases were heavily concentrated among African American and Latino children of low-income families, a pattern that reflected a larger secular trend in infectious disease, which had become increasingly limited to inner-city and rural poverty areas. During the 1980s only about 10 percent of counties in the United States reported any cases of measles; a large percentage of the cases were concentrated in about twenty counties, mostly urban areas with high population densities and large numbers of African American and Latino residents.[38]

The persistence of measles was widely seen as an embarrassing failure that exposed the inadequacy of existing surveillance, among the many other shortcomings of the immunization system. Aggregate data about immunization coverage at the national or even state level was insufficient: the vaccine-preventable diseases of childhood had declined so greatly that highly targeted surveillance was needed to pinpoint the remaining "pockets" of unprotected children. In the wake of the epidemic, the Children's Defense Fund renewed its calls for more complete and detailed surveillance. The National Vaccine Advisory Committee, made up of physicians and researchers who offered guidance to the CDC, added its voice when it issued a set of recommendations for improving delivery of vaccines. The report, released in 1991 and known as the Measles White Paper, emphasized the importance of reducing barriers of cost, access, and availability.[39] The premise of the recommendations was that children remained without vaccination, not because their parents were ignorant or unmotivated, as had traditionally been assumed, but because the health care system was faulty. Whereas past campaigns to promote the use of vaccines had often placed the onus of responsibility on parents, health officials increasingly called for major systemic changes that would make vaccines more accessible. "Though it is tempting for health care providers to attribute low immunization uptake to consumer apathy," noted one analysis, "much evidence points to correctable deficiencies of the health care system."[40]

In fact, the health care context in which children received their immunizations was less a "system" than a labyrinth of unconnected clinical settings and payment mechanisms. About half of U.S. children received their shots in the private sector and half in public facilities, such as municipal health departments, community clinics, or public hospitals. Federal monies administered by the CDC and a variety of other agencies covered the costs of about half of public sector vaccinations; the remainder were paid for by state and local government funds, flowing through entitlement programs such as Medicaid. Few private health insurance plans covered routine immunization, so that even parents who had a regular pediatrician often had to go to a public facility for their children's shots.[41] The gaps in continuity of care led to "record scatter"—documentation of a child's immunization history being held at disparate sites—with the result that health care providers often had no idea which injections a child had received and which were still needed. This confusion resulted in missed opportunities to give needed immunizations, and, less frequently, in children receiving unnecessary doses of vaccines they had already received.

This problem was exacerbated by the increasing complexity of the vaccination schedule. In the mid-1980s there were seven universally recommended childhood vaccines, typically given at two, four, six, fifteen, and twenty-four months. Over the next decade the number of recommended shots almost doubled. In 1990 a vaccine against *Haemophilus influenzae* type B, a common childhood infection that could lead to serious complications including bacterial meningitis, was introduced; it was given in a series of either three or four doses. In 1991 three doses of a vaccine against hepatitis B were added to the schedule, the first given hours after birth. Also around this time a second dose of the combined measles-mumps-rubella vaccine was recommended to provide additional protection. Within a few years two more vaccines, against chicken pox and pneumococcal disease, were introduced. The more injections were added to the schedule, the more difficult it became for parents and providers to keep track of whether children were fully protected. Surveys showed that pediatricians tended to overestimate the proportion of children in their care who were up to date.[42] Parents likewise tended to misjudge the extent of their children's protection.[43]

Several authors of the Measles White Paper, recognizing that government policy documents often languished unread, were determined to make it a catalyst for political change.[44] They succeeded in having a summary of the report reprinted in the *Journal of the American Medical Association* and implemented a concerted press strategy aimed at mobilizing political stakeholders who could push through reforms in the vaccine delivery system. The attention the report garnered in the media—newspaper headlines around the country declared that the nation's immunization system needed "a shot in the arm"—helped to galvanize two related policy initiatives. One originated in the philanthropic sector and one was a piece of federal legislation; both aimed to create a national system for immunization tracking.

ALL KIDS COUNT AND THE CLINTON PLAN

As the experience of programs funded under the Vaccination Assistance Act from the 1960s to the 1980s demonstrated, the investment of time and money necessary to establish a registry, including purchase of computer hardware and software, presented an enormous roadblock, especially for cash-strapped public sector health facilities where registries were most needed. The Children's Defense Fund began discussions with officials at the CDC and senior managers at the Robert Wood Johnson Foundation (RWJ), one of the country's largest health-related philanthropies, to determine how the charitable sector could augment federal financial support for the development of registries. In 1991 the RWJ Foundation established All Kids Count, a grant program to spur the development of registries nationwide by making up for the chronic shortages of money that had plagued efforts over the previous two decades.[45]

In preparation for creating the All Kids Count program, Kay Johnson, a policy analyst with the Children's Defense Fund who had co-authored the Measles White Paper, spent several weeks interviewing people at the CDC and public health officials around the country to determine what types of system would be most feasible and desirable and how a national database might become a reality. Wariness about a federally controlled registry was widespread. Officials with the CDC felt the technology was still inadequate and worried that the system would be seen as intrusive. Those who ran state or local registries were enthusiastic about expanding their use and possibly linking them to other city, state, or national systems, but they were cautious about drawing the opposition of privacy advocates such as the American Civil Liberties Union. Even in the case of vital statistics, local officials pointed out, there was no truly "national system"; each state collected data on its births and deaths in its own way and then submitted the information to the CDC.[46]

In spite of these concerns, Kay Johnson remained convinced that a single interconnected system was best. At the 1991 National Immunization Conference, an annual meeting for providers and policy makers, Johnson made the first public call for the creation of a nationwide registry that would track the vaccination status of children from birth.[47] Ultimately, however, RWJ determined that multiple state and local systems would be more feasible and less politically contentious than a central database. In 1993 the foundation funded a dozen grantees, mostly city or county health departments, for four-year periods to develop fully operational registries containing the records of all the children within a defined area (city, county, region, or state). The foundation devoted some $9 million to the program in its initial round of awards; at the same time a coalition of five other foundations with an interest in health care funded an additional nine projects.[48]

It was during the creation of the initial All Kids Count request for proposals that the idea of linking immunization registries to other child health data indicators began to gain currency. Although measles had propelled the issue forward and immunization was to be the initial focus of the All Kids Count program, RWJ envisioned from the outset that the registries would eventually expand to include other data on child health, such as blood lead levels and hearing and vision tests, that many public health entities collected.[49] But there was disagreement about how far beyond immunization the registries should extend. Some experts worried about "data creep."[50] Only one grantee, the Rhode Island health department, started off with the explicit intention of creating a database that tracked a range of child health data in addition to immunizations. Parents in Rhode Island had complained in focus groups about having to give the same personal information repeatedly to different units of the health department and wanted greater coordination of efforts.[51]

The second major boost for registries, on the heels of the creation of All

Kids Count, came again from a new presidential administration. At the time the first round of All Kids Count grants were awarded, many activists viewed the chaotic delivery system for immunization as symptomatic of much more far-reaching problems with the nation's health care system. A sense of crisis about the growing numbers of people without health insurance gained prominence in the 1992 presidential campaign, when Bill Clinton made health care reform a defining issue. At the time of his election, polls showed that an overwhelming majority of Americans believed there was a health care crisis in the country.[52] In the first weeks of the new presidency, as a task force convened by First Lady Hillary Clinton, who had chaired the board of the Children's Defense Fund, was developing a plan for health care reform, the administration sent Congress a $1 billion plan to overhaul the way the country provided immunization. The initiative, the cornerstone of which was a program to purchase and distribute vaccine free to providers, included a national computer database for tracking children's immunization status.

The Clinton administration viewed the childhood immunization program as a trial run for the broader effort at health care reform it would soon undertake.[53] Foreshadowing the problems that plagued its plan for universal health insurance, the administration made several political missteps. It failed to court key allies who would have helped shepherd the plan through Congress, such as Arkansas senator Dale Bumpers, whose wife, Betty, had played a key role in the nation's last major immunization initiative.[54] The pharmaceutical industry was alienated by charges that high vaccine prices were responsible for poor vaccination rates of low-income children.[55]

Especially problematic as the bill faced congressional scrutiny was that it proposed a universal purchase program, under which even children of the wealthy would receive free vaccine. Secretary of Health and Human Services Donna Shalala defended the proposal by arguing that to structure the plan otherwise would require means testing. Using language that resonated with proponents of universal health care, Shalala declared that full immunization was "a basic right" for all children.[56] The disagreement over the value of universal purchase hinged on a fundamental question: What was really responsible for the nation's low immunization rates? Senator Nancy Kassebaum, a moderate Republican, laid the blame for poor coverage levels on lack of parental education about the importance of vaccination, over-burdened public health clinics, and failure of private physicians to accept Medicaid because of low reimbursement rates. She contended that the president's initiative "misdiagnoses the causes of the problems and prescribes a remedy that is likely to be ineffective and perhaps wasteful."[57]

Nonetheless the bill predictably drew support from a broad spectrum of child welfare and health organizations, including the Children's Defense Fund, the American Academy of Pediatrics, and the ASTHO. But there was uneasiness about the idea of a national registry even among those who supported the overall intent of the bill. Health officials in Mississippi and Minnesota, which already had registries, testified before Congress that a single national system was technologically unfeasible and would lack the flexibility to meet varying local and regional needs.[58] Concerns about the scope of the information contained in the registry were also voiced by the American Civil Liberties Union's Privacy Project. Already involved in contentious battles over HIV case reporting, the ACLU conceded the importance of immunization but worried that "the temptation to use information for some other purpose could become overwhelming once it's in there."[59] This position underscored the recurring tension in American liberalism between advancing social welfare goals and protecting individuals from state intrusion.

When a much-scaled-back version of the Clinton immunization initiative was ultimately passed in mid-1993, it was no longer a universal purchase program and plans for the national database had been jettisoned. Nevertheless, the initiative did provide substantial funding, administered through the CDC, for development of local registries.[60] While the monetary investment of the CDC in immunization registries over the next several years dwarfed that of the All Kids Count program—some $200 million, compared to about $30 million from RWJ—the foundation took a more visible public role in supporting and publicizing registries. The political fiasco of the Clinton health care overhaul had sparked an antigovernment backlash that, coupled with a new wave of concern about computer privacy and pervasive fear of "Big Brother"–type databases, forced the CDC to take a low profile.[61] RWJ would go on to launch a second round of All Kids Count funding in 1998 to help the most advanced registries meet various operational standards, such as completeness of coverage and ability to generate reminders and recalls. Registries in nine states, two counties, two multi-county regions, and three large urban areas (New York City, Philadelphia, and Baltimore) received funding; together they served approximately one-fifth of the nation's annual birth cohort.[62]

As registries proliferated with private and public support during the 1990s, they were affected by a growing social movement that caused reverberations throughout the world of vaccines in the 1990s: parents who questioned the safety, efficacy, and necessity of routine childhood immunization.

CHALLENGES TO THE VACCINATION ORTHODOXY

Antivaccination sentiment has had a long history in the United States and many European nations. Activist groups arose in the nineteenth century to oppose smallpox vaccination and laws that made it compulsory.[63] The antivaccination movement experienced a heyday in the first three decades of the twentieth century, when a heterogeneous assortment of individuals and organizations advanced political, religious, and scientific arguments against the practice. Activists' protests against smallpox vaccination and health officials' efforts to reassure the public that it was safe and effective represented fundamental conflicts over the status of elite scientific knowledge in a liberal democratic society.[64] But as additional vaccines were developed, as vaccination became accepted as an uncontroversial scientific orthodoxy, and as the medical profession grew in cultural authority, opposition to vaccination waned. It remained a fringe movement until after the dawn of the patients' rights era. A small but highly vocal activist movement, which asserted that vaccination was a dangerous procedure whose risks frequently outweighed its benefits, questioned the integrity of health officials charged with securing high rates of immunization coverage. It looked with dismay upon plans to establish large databases to track the receipt of childhood vaccines.

The contemporary movement against vaccines arose in the 1980s amid an often acrimonious series of public debates over the safety of the vaccine against pertussis. The controversy began when an article in the British medical journal *Archives of Diseases of Childhood* suggested that the vaccine—typically given as one component of the trivalent DPT (diphtheria-pertussis-tetanus) shot—could in rare instances cause severe brain damage in infants.[65] The report, which attracted mainstream attention in the United States in a 1982 television documentary, galvanized a small but committed core of parent activists who believed their children had suffered a range of harms, including learning disabilities, seizures, severe brain damage, and death from the DPT shot. These parents accused pharmaceutical companies and the health establishment of turning a blind eye to vaccine-related harm and failing to ensure that vaccines were as safe as they could be. Led by a national organization called Dissatisfied Parents Together, these activists succeeded in pushing through Congress landmark legislation to provide compensation for the small number of children who were inevitably harmed by vaccine adverse events.[66]

Though they would come to oppose immunization reporting because of the threat of coercion, Dissatisfied Parents Together demanded another type of surveillance that took a page from occupational disease reporting: instead of tracking either the incidence of naturally occurring disease or the delivery of vaccination, they wanted mandatory reporting to a national database of all injuries and deaths thought to result *from* vaccines. Such a system was established in 1988 as the Vaccine Adverse Events Reporting System, jointly operated by the CDC and the Food and Drug Administration.[67]

Plans that got underway in the early 1990s for widespread government tracking of immunization did not immediately draw the fire of antivaccination parent activists. The national compensation system that had been established in 1986 was working through a backlog of cases. Dissatisfied Parents Together devoted its limited resources to advocating for parents who feared the system would not assess the cases fairly.[68] Thus program officers at RWJ never heard from activists during the initial round of All Kids Count grant making.[69] But there were soon signs that a vocal minority of parents stood ready to oppose any programs that might make it easier for the government to enforce compulsory vaccination. During the congressional debates over the Clinton immunization initiative, several members of Congress reported hearing from constituents concerned that a plan for universal distribution would lead to compulsory vaccination. Democratic senator Ron Wyden of Oregon, for example, said that the telephones in his office "rang off the hook" with parents wanting assurances that the legislation would not lead to compulsory vaccination for all children.[70]

The growing unease among some parents about childhood immunizations was exacerbated by new additions to an already crowded vaccination schedule. By the end of the 1990s, a typical child received a total of eleven vaccines in a possible twenty injections, depending on which combination vaccines were used, by the age of two. This expansion fueled an increasingly vocal backlash against what was sometimes termed the "pediatric pincushion" phenomenon.[71] As the schedule grew during the 1990s, a variety of theories began to surface that vaccines were responsible for a wide range of chronic and acute child health problems, including sudden infant death syndrome, multiple sclerosis, and autism. The spread of these theories was accelerated by the growth of the internet, which served as a powerful force for democratizing information about medicine and health care.[72]

Activists suspicious of the safety of vaccines saw doctors, government health officials, and pharmaceutical companies as tainted by a web of financial conflicts of interest and rejected the very premise of paternalistic privacy: that members of the health care establishment could be trusted to serve as gatekeepers for personal information. A particular source of animus was the compulsory nature of immunization. Laws in all states required children to be immunized before they could enroll in school or licensed day care facilities, and in some cases charges of neglect had been brought against parents who failed to immunize their children.[73] These sanctions gave special urgency to the claims of privacy. Barbara Loe Fisher, a cofounder of Dissatisfied Parents Together and one of the country's most visible opponents of compulsory vaccination, warned that registries "could be used to discriminate against and economically or socially punish loving, conscientious parents and their children if they do not conform with every government recommended health care policy."[74] Fisher, like many activists opposed to universal vaccination, had personal reasons for fearing the intrusion of the government: her son Chris suffered from learning disabilities and attention deficit disorder, which Fisher believed were caused by the DPT shot he received at age two and a half.

Opponents further argued that automatically including all children in a registry without the express permission (or even knowledge) of their parents violated the principle of informed consent, which had, since the 1970s, become enshrined in clinical practice and biomedical research. Adopting the language of privacy rights activists and placing it in the service of an antigovernment stance, they insisted that tracking individual children was the first step down the slippery slopes of coercion and total surveillance. "If the State can tag, track down and force citizens against their will to be injected with biologicals of unknown toxicity today," Fisher warned on her organization's web site, "there will be no limit on what individual freedoms the State can take away in the name of the greater good tomorrow."[75]

COURTING PARENTS AND PROVIDERS

The rising mistrust of the vaccination orthodoxy dovetailed with increased public concern about the confidentiality of electronic information, especially health data.[76] Immunization registries typically included sensitive information such as address, parental marital and employment status, and sometimes family income, so a key first step in setting up a system involved effort to win the support of—or at least neutralize the opposition of—civil liberties groups and privacy rights organizations active in a given area.[77]

During their start-up phase, All Kids Count grantees made great efforts to engage local communities and gain the buy-in of local stakeholders. Even parents who had no objections to vaccination were worried about privacy and confidentiality. "When we started, the biggest concern we heard from parents is would the state be able to take kids away from parents or be punitive toward parents if they found out the children were missing immunizations," recalled Amy Zimmerman-Levitan of the Rhode Island health department, which was one of the original All Kids Count grantees. "Could anyone get addresses from the system? Could courts get information for custody fights? There were concerns about Big Brother, big government."[78]

Recognizing that the linked concerns about vaccine safety and medical privacy could fuel resistance that might endanger the implementation of registries, the CDC in 1996 held a series of public meetings intended to gain community support. At the meetings, a wide range of groups and individuals expressed concerns about the scope of the information contained in the registries, who would have access to the data, and improper use. "There was a strong, consistent message from those testifying," noted a report on the meetings, "that narrowing and focusing the scope and use of registry information would best protect patient privacy and confidentiality."[79] At another public hearing in 1998, CDC officials heard testimony from the

CCHC, the libertarian grassroots organization based in St. Paul, Minnesota, that had led the successful campaign against the state's proposed birth defects registry. The CCHC's president insisted that any proposed registry adopt an "opt-in" procedure for participation, in which parents had to actively consent before their children's information was included. The group saw this feature as especially urgent in light of the stated intention to link the information about immunizations with other child health data systems. "If there is no requirement for informed and voluntary consent," the group warned, "it should be clear that this seemingly harmless breach of medical confidentiality will be used to support further breaches of confidentiality with information much more sensitive."[80]

In 1998 the CDC also held twenty focus groups around the country to gauge parent attitudes and identify areas of concern. Most parents in the groups supported the idea of registries, generally viewing them as a helpful public service rather than as an invasion of privacy. While only a few indicated that they would not wish to participate, many expressed concerns about who would have access to the information, with health insurance companies being the object of particular mistrust. "It could be used against you," cautioned an African American parent who envisioned an insurance company executive saying, "Ethnic people are not getting their well baby shots, so let's up their premiums." Another parent worried that health officials might "do a query on all bad parents who didn't have their children immunized, and they'll go . . . forcefully and take them away from their family. I'm worried about any governmental centralized databases."[81] Parents disliked the idea that children would be automatically included in the registry and felt that laws should require the explicit written consent of parents to include their information.[82] About half of the registries operating at the time drew information directly from birth certificates.[83]

Those who opposed registries, though small in number, were well organized, politically astute, and ready to tap into the organizing power of the internet to mobilize a core of committed allies. The political influence that activists could wield was vividly demonstrated in Texas, which created an immunization registry in 1996 with state and federal money. Within two years, records on some three million children who received their vaccinations in the state's public clinics had been entered into the system. The records were drawn, without parental consent, directly from birth certificates. But in 1997, when legislators drew up plans to expand the registry to include children seen by private sector providers, it ran up against a grassroots political movement of parent activists.

The movement was led by Dawn Richardson, a Houston mother who had chosen not to have her children vaccinated after coming to believe that because of genetic susceptibilities they were at heightened risk of having an adverse reaction. Richardson became disillusioned with the medical establishment after pediatricians reacted with hostility to her decision not to vaccinate her children. When the Texas health department's plans for expanding the registry became public, the news galvanized Richardson to form Parents Requesting Open Vaccine Education (PROVE).[84] The group began with a core group of about twenty supporters and some two hundred more connected through an email distribution list. PROVE took its case to the Texas state legislature, where the group found a receptive audience for the argument that parents should have to give active, informed consent before having their children included in the database. "The government," commented one sympathetic legislator, "already has too much information on citizens."[85] PROVE's arguments were also well received by a new state commissioner of health, Reyn Archer, who believed in natural immunity and refused to have his own children vaccinated.[86]

As a result of PROVE's lobbying, state law was changed to require an "opt-in" procedure through which parents had to give active consent prior to their children's records being included. In the wake of the change, the registry was forced to purge almost seven hundred thousand records, and the number of providers reporting to the registry dropped by almost two-thirds because of the requirement of obtaining active consent. Reporting to the state legislature in 2003 on challenges created by the "opt-in" procedure, officials noted that the requirement had led to confusion among providers and third-party payers over who had the responsibility for obtaining and documenting consent—neither group wanted the additional responsibility or had systems to track it. The law's new strictures on who could gain access to the data also created problems. Grandparents or foster parents were not allowed to view the immunization records of children under their care; records were inaccessible to third-party payers, pharmacists, community-based organizations that held immunization clinics, and state child welfare agencies.[87]

The Texas controversy vividly illustrated the extent to which immunization registries had come to serve as a lightning rod for much more wide-ranging antigovernment sentiment. "You are about to read a chronological account of a bureaucracy out of control," began the account of the controversy on PROVE's web site. "These events will shock you and underscore how important it is for concerned citizens to stay on top of government agencies and to keep their legislators informed."[88]

Mistrust of "big government" was also a leitmotif running throughout the effort in Minnesota to establish a statewide registry. Immunizations there were tracked through independent registries that had been established in the mid-1990s by several cities and health maintenance organizations. After a public task force was formed to investigate the possibility of combining these stand-alone databases into a unified statewide system, the proposal became a magnet for critics who objected to what they saw as the state's intrusion into a private parental concern.[89] The state had one of the most stringent sets of laws on medical privacy, and when the health department sought to join the databases, it needed to change state law to allow the health commissioner expanded access to the data. In an unfortunate coincidence, the 1998 legislative session also saw bills to create a birth defects registry and establish a "health ID card" for state residents. The timing of the three proposals, as noted in the previous chapter, set off alarms among a range of individuals and organizations who were concerned about threats to health privacy and overreaching government. A popular right-wing radio talk show host mocked the idea that government bureaucrats should assume responsibility for keeping track of children's shots, while the CCHC warned about compromising citizens' confidentiality.[90]

Just as they did on the birth defects front, the vituperative public objections caught the health department off guard. "We thought we had a motherhood and apple pie thing, but we were wrong," recalled Aggie Leitheiser, an assistant commissioner. Instead, she said, "we went down in flames."[91] The bill on the immunization registry failed to pass the legislature, and the health department got neither the funding nor the enabling language it had sought. In response, proponents adopted a more modest set of goals for developing the capacities of the existing regional registries, which would remain separate entities.

Leitheiser saw the battle over the immunization registry as emblematic of a much broader statewide shift to the political Right. Despite the state's long-standing reputation as a liberal bastion, by the time the three health-related bills were being considered in the 1998 legislative session, it had a Republican governor and the Democrats' majority in the state legislature was shrinking. "It used to be Minnesota's motto that 'we can do it better than anyone else.' But gradually the anti-tax/small government folks have become more influential," Leitheiser said. "Now the feeling is, 'Why does Minnesota have to be first [with health care innovations]?'"[92]

Across the country, an even greater challenge than reassuring suspicious parents and their elected representatives by ensuring stringent privacy and confidentiality procedures was gaining the cooperation of health care providers on the immunization front lines. Whatever benefits a tracking system might promise in terms of better patient care, an additional layer of administrative procedures was a hard sell to busy pediatric practices already overburdened with paperwork related to insurance coverage through managed care and other third-party payers. A 1999 survey of pediatric providers in the Seattle area found that lack of completeness of the databases presented a catch-22 for their creators: "Registries are only as complete as providers make them but providers are reluctant to use them until they are more complete."[93] The most receptive attitudes toward registries were found in public clinics, where there tended to be greater confusion about a child's immunization status; young people seen in these sites were most likely to lack a "medical home," a continuous source of all their care. The systems offered less benefit to private practices, which were more likely than public sector facilities to see a stable population of children whose immunization records were all in one place.[94]

The challenges registries had to overcome were evident in the position paper on the issue by the American Academy of Pediatrics in 1996. Offering a tepid endorsement of registries only "insofar as they benefit children," the organization laid out several conditions that it believed should be met for all registries: preserving the confidentiality of both the children and their health care providers; ensuring that all information in the system be available to providers at all times; and ensuring that data would not be used to sanction health care providers whose rates of immunization were low. The organization also sought to protect its members from unnecessary burdens the system might impose: it stipulated that providers would not have to purchase specialized hardware or expensive software, and—in a reprise of claims made one hundred years earlier when physicians were asked to take the time to report cases of tuberculosis—that they should be reimbursed for any costs related to providing data to the system.[95]

One option for gaining the participation of providers was to require it by law. Soon after the first round of All Kids Count funding had been awarded, Mississippi had in 1994 become the first state to require that all physicians report immunizations to a statewide registry.[96] Several other states soon followed suit.[97] But others judged that securing voluntary cooperation, while more labor intensive, was more politically palatable. When Rhode Island registry officials interviewed doctors around the state, they heard conflicting feedback from providers about compulsion: some physicians contended that a mandate would be the only way the state would achieve the participation of private providers, while others warned that practitioners would resent another reporting requirement and fail to comply. In spite of a state law already on the books that would have allowed the health department to require immunization reporting, the department decided to keep the procedure voluntary. But convincing providers to participate required time- and labor-intensive outreach by registry employees making personal visits to doctors' offices. In Rhode Island the health department hired dedicated staff members whose job was to make the rounds doing provider outreach and education. "We modeled ourselves after pharmaceutical company representatives," the program manager recalled. "We tried to be in their offices as much as possible."[98] This approach recalled the efforts of many health officials to win physician cooperation for venereal disease reporting in the 1960s and 1970s.

In Illinois a move to make reporting to the registry compulsory drew opposition from doctors who feared they might be sued for disclosing children's immunization information to third parties without the permission of parents. During hearings on a bill that would mandate physician reporting, the Illinois State Medical Society sought to gain immunity from such lawsuits—an effort the state's trial lawyers association forcefully opposed. One solution to the liability issue was to have all parents sign explicit consent forms allowing sharing of the records, but state health officials worried such a system would make operating the registry cumbersome and inefficient.[99] A stalemate ensued, and reporting remained voluntary.[100]

LET A THOUSAND FLOWERS BLOOM

Over the course of the 1990s, as state, county, or regional databases proliferated around the country, the idea of a single national system was abandoned. The prevailing stance at both the CDC and RWJ was "let a thousand flowers bloom": whatever might be lost in terms of uniformity or accessibility of data would ultimately be outweighed by the greater political acceptability of multiple smaller-scale databases.[101] This pragmatic concession was born in part of the increased expectations for medical privacy that had taken hold. As one assessment of registries noted, parents "often become confused or anxious when they hear about an information system being developed by a government agency that will 'track' their children's health information wherever they are." Those setting up programs should thus use "terms such as 'national network of registries' rather than 'national system' to reflect the fact that registries are community- or state-based and should only share information with other systems when necessary."[102]

The public health officials and child welfare advocates who had fought to advance an expansive vision of immunization surveillance had learned hard lessons during the decade in which foundation and federal money had poured into registries. Most of all, they had "underestimated the cost and complexity" of their task, according to a 2004 evaluation of programs around the country.[103] Involving providers, parents, and other stakeholders at every stage of planning; learning to make a strong case for the systems' concrete benefits, and managing the technological intricacies of hardware and software all proved daunting challenges. To be sure, there had been much progress. By 2003 information on some 44 percent of U.S. children under age six was contained in an immunization registry; about three-quarters of public vaccination sites and a third of private sites contributed data to a registry. But there was a long way to go: *Healthy People 2010,* the decennial blueprint for health in the United States, set a goal of increasing the proportion of children nationwide participating in immunization registries to 95 percent of children under age six. Nine of the fifty-six CDC-funded registries in 2003 had met that target for their service area while an additional eight were nearing attainment.[104]

9

Panoptic Visions and Stubborn Realities
in a New Era of Privacy

As the twentieth century drew to a close, concerns about the erosion of privacy in medicine and other realms focused attention on the need for federal measures to secure health records. These concerns were not new. For almost forty years there had been repeated expressions of anxiety about intrusions into the world of privacy. But in the 1990s the political context had changed, making the time ripe for comprehensive federal regulation designed to protect medical records from misuse on the part of those who wielded either public or commercial power. At the same time, however, there were moves to extend the scope and functions of public health surveillance. Some reflected new visions about how expanded reporting could enhance the prospects for interventions that might limit the impact of disease and assure that those most in need of care received it. As important were concerns about bioterrorism and national security that informed proposals designed to invigorate the capacities of public health departments to monitor the presence of pathological threats, whether their sources were domestic or foreign. It was at the crossroads of the competing urges to protect privacy and radically augment surveillance efforts that the politics of public health reporting unfolded in the late 1990s and opening decade of the twenty-first century.

THE MODEL PUBLIC HEALTH PRIVACY ACT:
THE LIMITS OF DEMOCRATIC PRIVACY

During the two-decade-long battle over HIV surveillance, public health officials had repeatedly asserted that by convention, law, and regulation the disease registries they maintained were secure and that a commitment to confidentiality would protect the rights of those whose names had been reported to them. It was thus troubling news when a CDC-commissioned review revealed the problematic nature of legal protections for disease registries in the 1990s. Anxious to bring the HIV reporting controversy to a conclusion and to provide a firm statutory basis for the protection of surveillance efforts, the CDC asked Georgetown law professor Lawrence Gostin to draft the Model State Public Health Privacy Act, which would embody contemporary understandings about the conditions under which disease reporting ought to occur and the legal protections that ought to be afforded to the personally identifiable data thus accumulated. Such statutes could, the CDC believed, safeguard confidentiality, preclude the possibility of future controversies, and advance the cause of public health surveillance.

The model act was originally intended to provide privacy protections for HIV surveillance data. But the CDC feared that limiting a statute to AIDS-related efforts would draw the antagonism of social and political conservatives and was weary of the exceptionalism that had shaped AIDS policy. It therefore decided to broaden the legislative scope and address the challenge posed by the acquisition and use of all personally identifiable public health information. Nonetheless, AIDS-based concerns would dominate the effort, informing every element of the drafting process. It was as if the history and practice of surveillance more generally had little to contribute to the understanding of the problems to be resolved and the interests to be accommodated.

To provide input into and an imprimatur for the drafting process, the CDC convened a diverse group in 1998, the Privacy Law Advisory Committee (PLAC). More than a third of its members represented the U.S. Department of Health and Human Services, state and local health officers, and the CDC. Others were elected officials and professionals from medicine, law, and the worlds of AIDS and privacy advocacy. The PLAC thus brought together many who in recent years had viewed each other as antagonists. And they would, in fact, engage in a struggle during the consultative process to impose their mark on the proposed act. While nongovernmental participants were thus fully engaged, demonstrating the extent to which privacy advocates had gained the right to meet with public officials as partners in a process of democratic consultation, the CDC made clear from the outset the limits to such participation: "The PLAC will be influential but not absolute."[1]

In preparing an initial legislative draft, Gostin believed that he had struck a balance that would begin to bridge the ideological gulf that had separated privacy advocates and public health officials during the AIDS debates. Drawing on the three-decade-old Code of Fair Information Practices, the draft would have prohibited the secret acquisition of personally identifiable information and required agencies to make public the types of lists and registries involving personally identifiable data that they held.[2]

Privacy advocates were quick to assert that the proposed draft, like the old code, did not go far enough. Reflecting the deep concerns of those who were still embroiled in the struggle over the issue of HIV name reporting, Chris Anders of the ACLU asserted that individuals had to be told that the results of their medical examinations would be reported and could be disclosed by health officials. Such personal notification was, for him, "an important part of whether something's secret or not secret."[3] Anders received support for his assertion from John Fanning, a privacy specialist in the DHHS: "The fair information practice ideal is that people should be informed up front of what will be done with information that's collected from them."[4]

The representative of the CSTE, Christine Moore, voiced skepticism about the relevance of the fair information standard. Personal notification would impose an insuperable burden on public health officials and clinicians given the number of reportable conditions.[5] Public health officials also objected to the modest limits the act would have placed on the uses of surveillance data—that they be related to "legitimate public health purposes compatible with and directly related to the purposes for which the information [was] collected."[6] There was an uneasy sense that the draft represented the first stage of a capitulation to the views of a group committed to privacy that had dubbed itself the "Gang of Three": the representatives from the ACLU, the AIDS Action Council, and the Lambda Legal Defense and Education Fund.[7] In a broadside challenge to Gostin's efforts, the three had jointly written that the model act was "entirely inappropriate for protecting the confidentiality and security of the names of persons whose HIV status has been reported to public health authorities."[8]

Reflecting the political dimension of what some viewed as a purely technical question, the three emphasized that surveillance was a statistical enterprise appropriate *only* for epidemiological ends: "We understand that the reason that certain public health officials support name reporting is their belief that such data will result in better statistics to track the HIV epidemic," they wrote. "Our expectation was that any model statute would focus solely on how a state may collect and track—but otherwise hold secure—identifying public health information, and avoid disclosing such information to anyone except under the most narrow and clearly defined circumstances. The draft blueprint goes well beyond that limited objective by authorizing disclosures for reasons which have no relationship to surveillance."[9] In arguing that access to identifiable data should be given only "for the purpose for which the information was originally collected," these advocates sought to ensure that surveillance data could be used for only broad policy formation, resource allocation, and perhaps some research functions.[10] Anything beyond those functions had to be treated as an exception that was clearly defined, rigorously justified, and very narrowly circumscribed. Most important, the Gang of Three vehemently objected to the notion of leaving the determination about what represented "legitimate public health practice" to state public health officials.[11]

The CDC had, in the context of the HIV debates, suggested that surveillance was centrally concerned with epidemiologic monitoring, not intervention. But no such formulation could be acceptable to state public health officials, who viewed such a narrow definition of surveillance as representing a fundamental misunderstanding of the scope of their work and the mandate under which they operated. Guthrie Birkhead, director of the New York State Department of Health AIDS Institute and a member of the CSTE, stressed the importance of maintaining a broad conception of the appropriate uses of surveillance data: "One important use of surveillance data at the state and local level that we may want to reflect in the document is for public health officials to identify other persons ('contacts') who are at risk or may have been exposed to disease, and to try to reduce their risk, provide preventive therapy and/or get them into early treatment. This is probably the original purpose of collecting surveillance data 100 years ago. Back then, quarantine and other similar preventive measures were all we had to apply. Today, public health officials routinely contact persons exposed to TB, meningitis, and other possibly life-threatening illnesses."[12]

An additional source of contention centered on the extent to which surveillance data collected by health departments could be shared among departmental subdivisions and among health departments across jurisdictional boundaries. Once again concerns that had taken hold in the concurrent debates about HIV reporting were brought to bear on the question of surveillance more generally. While those centrally committed to privacy sought to impose a very high bar on data sharing, public health officials insisted that such exchanges were essential to confronting disease outbreaks that respected neither bureaucratic nor political boundaries.

In the end, both sides brought together in the PLAC saw in Gostin's draft a threat to their central values and interests. Public health officials believed that it would hamper their capacity to do their legally mandated work, while privacy advocates saw the specter of rights violations wrapped in the mantle of rights protections. Timothy Westmoreland, who for years had served as a senior congressional staff member and played a critical role in trying to thwart measures that might have harmed the rights of people with HIV, concluded that the model act "will be conveying authority in the guise of conveying privacy."[13]

Despite his belief that reaching an acceptable middle ground was possible, Gostin found the conflict intractable. In an effort to neutralize the opposition of privacy advocates, he proposed in a second draft of the model act that name-linked surveillance reports be relied upon only when public health purposes "cannot otherwise be achieved as well or better with non-identifiable information."[14] And, in a major concession that was bound to provoke the opposition of state health officials, he now proposed that no identifiable data be collected without individual notification.[15]

Having won a signal victory in the matter of personal notification, privacy advocates turned their attention to what they considered the unacceptable standards that would guide the disclosure of surveillance data within and among health departments and other "appropriate federal agencies"—"a term to drive a truck through," according to Robert Gellman, a privacy expert on the PLAC. What, he asked, were appropriate federal agencies? "The CIA? Any federal [inspector general] who happens to ask? The Army?"[16] But even a clarification that would have limited disclosure to public health agencies was insufficient. Steven Scarborough of the Lambda Legal Defense Fund warned, "Once identifiable information is 'in the door' of any public health agency, it can be sent down the hall, to another municipality, or across the country whenever a public health official expresses a coherent reason for desiring it."[17]

Finally, those concerned with what they took to be overly permissive standards expressed dismay about the circumstances under which identifiable records might be used for research. Despite the fact that the draft would have subjected such uses to review by Institutional Review Boards, the critics characterized the legislative provisions as inadequate. Health officials, doing their work under the cover of law, would not have been subjected to such ethical oversight. There was a more general failure to require the informed consent of each individual whose record would be used. This was, of course, a long-standing matter of contention involving record-based epidemiological studies, and there were federal guidelines specifying the circumstances under which consent could be waived.[18] Nonetheless Lambda's Scarborough characterized opposition to his stance as troubling: "Concern for privacy in the research context is portrayed as an extremist's fixation on individual rights." In his view, "The current draft seems to value researcher-convenience and administrative efficiency over protection of names. . . . Surely this choice reflects skewed priorities, as it threatens to codify in all the adopting states a broad intrusion on individual autonomy that is not even linked to a current, specific public health need."[19]

Gostin's next formulation reflected the degree to which state public health officials and those at the CDC had become dissatisfied with the turn of the discussion and the concessions entailed in the second draft of the proposed act. Virtually all of the provisions designed to meet concerns of privacy advocates were gone or had been modified. Most notably, the proposal for individual notification about reporting had vanished. Weaker standards for defining the acceptable uses of data were now in place. Despite these changes, Gostin believed that he had demonstrated to those most concerned about privacy that what he was proposing was in their interest and represented an advance over the inadequate patchwork of state legislation that prevailed. He was thus stunned to discover that Lambda, the ACLU, and the AIDS Action Council had addressed their concerns directly to Secretary of Health and Human Services Donna Shalala, who in turn instructed her subordinates to reopen the discussion about the proposed act. Indeed, officials at the DHHS would play a critical role in the process of final revision. What emerged was more compatible with the worldview of privacy advocates. The requirement of individual notification of reporting was not, however, reincorporated. Rather, the final proposal required that health agencies make public their intentions to acquire, store, and use "protected health information."[20]

In the end, the imbroglio provoked by the model act was more important because of what it revealed about the deep ideological fissures that characterized the debates over public health surveillance than because of its policy impact. By 2001 legislatures in only three states considered bills based on the model act.[21] They passed in none. The model act was clearly too restrictive to gain the support of state health officials. Democratic privacy had its limits. While democratization could open the way to consultation and discussion, it could not guarantee an outcome that would be welcomed by those for whom privacy interests were preeminent.

The proposed act was also overshadowed by the ongoing discussion of the privacy regulations being considered by the federal government pursuant to the Health Insurance Privacy and Accountability Act of 1996. Indeed, some privacy advocates believed that whatever the virtues of the model act, it had been a misconceived effort to address a matter that required a federal solution. "Having separate health record legislation for every department in the world that has health information," wrote Robert Gellman, "makes no sense. It will only contribute to the patchwork quilt nature of privacy protection, and it will make it more difficult to pass legislation that is more important."[22]

HIPAA: PRIVACY AND THE PUBLIC HEALTH "CARVE-OUT"

The conflict engendered by the model privacy act and the bitter state battles over HIV case reporting were embedded in a broader context of anxiety about medical privacy in the 1990s. Despite such popular sentiment and the concerns that had surfaced in the 1960s and 1970s that had led to the Privacy Act of 1974, there had been no progress in enacting stringent national privacy legislation.

What protection existed at the state level, ironically, had emerged as a consequence of public health disease surveillance. Georgetown University's Health Privacy Project noted that state laws had been enacted "on the back end of laws requiring doctors and other health care providers to report to state officials patient data related to certain illness and conditions." Whatever the law's limits—and there were many—those concerned about privacy argued that they needed to be extended beyond public health records and applied to providers, hospitals, and insurance companies holding similar information.[23] It was this set of circumstances that served as a prod for federal privacy legislation.

In 1993, as President Bill Clinton proposed universal health insurance, privacy advocates expressed consternation about whether medical records would be protected as the management of health care became increasingly centralized. In the wake of the defeat of Clinton's proposals, a broad bipartisan coalition in Washington retained its commitment to the matter of health privacy. The Health Insurance Portability and Accountability Act of 1996 (HIPAA) that resulted was part of a broader effort at administrative simplification for computer-based communication for the health care and insurance industries. Once again the promise of computers was viewed as requiring protections against the threat that they could pose.

The passage of HIPAA set the stage for a complex political process that would extend over six years as Congress struggled with the act's mandate to craft a medical privacy statute. The act called upon the secretary of health and human services to provide Congress with recommendations regarding what such legislation should entail. If Congress failed to pass a privacy law within three years, the secretary would be charged with issuing federal privacy regulations.

Despite the enormous significance of the passage of HIPAA and the many issues that the act placed on the congressional agenda, it was unambiguous about the nearly sacrosanct status of public health surveillance. The salience of privacy and the urgency of moving to protect patients against intrusions that threatened the confidentiality of their medical communications could not undermine state requirements that physicians, laboratories, and health care institutions report by name those affected by notifiable conditions. And so a public health "carve-out"—all the more striking given the contemporaneous conflicts over other kinds of surveillance—was central to Secretary Donna Shalala's guidance to Congress as it began to consider privacy legislation: consent would not be sought for acquiring personally identifiable information or sharing such data within and among state and local health departments. Those recommendations mirrored the explicit intent of Congress. "Nothing in this part," declared HIPAA, "shall be construed to invalidate or limit the authority, power or procedures established under any law providing for the reporting of disease or injury, child abuse, birth or death, public health surveillance or public health investigation or intervention."[24]

The text of Shalala's proposals incorporated sweeping language about the importance of both privacy for democratic life and surveillance for the protection of the welfare of society. Citing President Clinton's concerns—"technology should not be used to break down the wall of privacy and autonomy free citizens are guaranteed in a free society"—the secretary deplored the prevailing legal structure that "did not effectively control information about individuals' health." At the same time she termed public health surveillance "the single most important tool for identifying infectious diseases that are emerging, [or] are causing serious public health problems."[25]

For advocates of privacy who had long labored for national standards to protect medical records from inspection by law enforcement officials, researchers who had not secured informed consent, or marketers who sought to troll medical records for potential customers, the political opportunity opened by the passage of HIPAA was one that had to be seized. In testimony before a congressional committee, the Health Privacy Project's Janlori Goldman, a stalwart of the medical privacy movement, declared in language that echoed the concerns of Alan Westin three decades earlier: "Over the course of a person's lifetime, the record of one's life collected through . . . largely unregulated networks can make real the 'womb to tomb dossier.' . . . If people continue to lose control over the ability to choose when, what, and to whom to divulge personal sensitive information, they will be unwilling to step forward and fully participate in society, fearing unwanted disclosure, judgments, discrimination, surveillance, stigma, and loss of jobs, credit, housing, or family. . . . A new framework is needed that intertwines the values of protecting patient privacy and fostering health care initiatives." Hoary assumptions about a tension between privacy and public welfare had to be abandoned, Goldman claimed. Securing privacy was not antithetical to good research, good health care, and public health. Rather, privacy served as the foundation for such goods. What subverted privacy would subvert such goods.[26]

In the ultimately fruitless effort of the Congress to craft privacy legislation in the three-year period specified by HIPAA, a plethora of bills were drafted. In all but two the public health carve-out remained virtually intact. Only in a bill sponsored by Vermont senator Patrick Leahy and in a companion bill sponsored by twenty-two Democrats in the House was there an indication that the concerns of privacy advocates had made an impact. Echoing the views of those who had sought to shape the Model State Public Health Privacy Act, these bills rejected the assumption that public health surveillance always required the use of names to be effective. Only when there was evidence that "de-identified" reports could not serve the ends of public health were names to be used.

With the failure of Congress to meet its own deadline for the passage of privacy legislation, Shalala issued comprehensive guidelines in 2000 for public comment. More than fifty thousand responses were received. Strikingly, the regulations covering public health surveillance drew relatively little hostile attention. Even those organizations that might have been expected to use the occasion of the formal comment period to underscore concerns about how public health surveillance compromised the right to privacy chose not to do so. In fact, the ACLU raised objections to a proposed provision that would have permitted the release of health records to government health data systems involved in policy, planning, and management functions, but it did not challenge to the public health "carve out."[27] Despite its fierce opposition to reporting during the discussions of the Model State Public Health Privacy Act, the Lambda Legal Defense and Education Fund never mentioned public health surveillance in its formal comments. It focused instead on issues bearing on law enforcement, prisoners, and administrative proceedings.[28] A strategic decision had been made that the HIPAA privacy regulations were not the context within which to wage a battle over public health surveillance.[29] That was a struggle to be pursued in those states where name-based reporting for specific conditions was still a matter of dispute and where specific constituencies could be mobilized to confront disease notification requirements.

Advocacy organizations for people with particular illnesses vigorously defended the traditions of public health surveillance. In so doing they revealed that however important the protection of privacy was, it was not always preeminent. As the American Cancer Society underscored the importance of cancer registries, it warned about dire consequences if potential subjects of name-base reporting were able to opt out.[30] The March of Dimes noted that while "de-identified" information might be appropriate for some public health functions, the failure to collect names in birth defects registries would subvert the critically important ability to undertake necessary follow-up investigations. "While the individual has an interest in maintaining the privacy of his or her health information," said the MOD, "public health authorities have an interest in the overall health and well being of the entire population."[31]

The final privacy regulations were published on March 27, 2002. Despite lingering concerns about gaps in the new protective regime, many privacy advocates saw the moment as a milestone. A year earlier in testimony before a congressional subcommittee, Janlori Goldman said, "Americans should be proud of what Congress set in motion with HIPAA and with the thoughtful and deliberate way in which [DHHS] carried out its Congressional mandate."[32] At a juncture when there was consternation that the administration of George W. Bush might attempt to substantially modify the proposed final regulations, Goldman and her allies sought to hold the line with the achievements already secured.

Despite the explicit shielding of public health surveillance activities from the requirements of HIPAA, considerable confusion about what was permissible surfaced in the period immediately following the promulgation of the privacy regulations. The CSTE conducted a survey of its members in 2003 that revealed the extent of the uncertainty. Twenty-five percent asserted that there was a "significant problem" for those who were required to report disease. One state epidemiologist commented, "We have almost weekly examples of people refusing to give us routine or outbreak related surveillance data, citing HIPAA concerns as their reasons for refusal." In South Carolina, epidemiologists in two health districts noted that between 20 and 30 percent of their investigations of disease had been obstructed. Physicians, according to the CSTE, said, "this is my license at risk" as they justified their reluctance to report notifiable conditions.[33]

Problems existed with reporting to immunization registries as well. Many states had opted for a voluntary system as a way of sidestepping the politics of mandatory reporting. Physicians interpreted the HIPAA carve-out as applicable only to reporting that was required by law. Hence they were reluctant to maintain cooperative relationships with immunization registries. Although some states were able to negotiate with providers to continue reporting, the confusion provided an impetus for new legislation to make such reporting mandatory.[34]

In California, differing interpretations of the HIPAA regulations triggered an extended standoff between the state cancer registry and major universities. At issue was a procedure known as "rapid case ascertainment," in which researchers reviewed, very soon after diagnosis, the case records of people with rapidly progressing cancers such as those of the lung and pancreas. In response to the new federal privacy rule, the University of California directed all of its researchers to stop providing rapid access to cancer records. Concerned that cancer patients might receive the first word of their diagnosis when contacted by a researcher, the university ordered a lag time of several weeks after diagnosis. Many major hospitals in the state took comparable action. Researchers countered that not having timely access to patient records would cripple critical studies. An agreement was finally brokered between the university and the state health department that allowed continuing access to the records but required researchers to wait six weeks from diagnosis before contacting a patient about enrolling in a clinical trial.[35]

Faced with such impediments to surveillance, the CDC and the DHHS worked assiduously to dispel what they asserted were misinterpretations of and unwarranted apprehensions about the surveillance-limiting consequences of the new privacy regulations. Although they were ultimately successful, the challenge to effective public health surveillance in the new century had deeper and more extensive roots.

THE SPECTER OF FAILURE:
THE STATE OF PUBLIC HEALTH SURVEILLANCE

Looking back on the twentieth century, those concerned about the fate of privacy have sometimes viewed the halting but seemingly inexorable extension of public health surveillance activities as a grave threat. Even when acknowledging the benign intent of health officials and the potential benefits that disease notification might make possible, they have been seized by concerns rooted in a broader narrative. They have seen the expansion of disease notification as inseparable from other threats to privacy and warned that it might be placed in the service of a surveillance more ominous in nature.

Public health advocates, in contrast, have been haunted by a different set of concerns. For them it was the prospect of failure that loomed: diseases spreading uncontrolled because health authorities lacked critical information to guide their efforts. Despite the existence of laws and regulations mandating reporting for a wide range of illnesses in every state, physician resistance and apathy persisted and financial support to carry out the work was lacking. In the 1990s a series of reports from officials committed to surveillance as the cornerstone of public health sounded the alarm. Commenting on the state of affairs at the CDC, a senior official said the National Center for Infectious Disease "was sometimes referred to as the unfunded infectious disease center."[36] In 1994 CDC scientists asserted, "Our ability to detect and monitor infectious disease threats is in jeopardy. . . . There has been no federal financial support to states for the notifiable disease systems and many state health laboratories receive no federal support."[37] An analysis from state health officials working with the CSTE echoed these concerns: the "foundation upon which public health decisions are based is threatened."[38]

A report to the DHHS in 2000 reflected the continuing sense of concern: "Current capacity for infectious diseases surveillance is a product of a century of piecemeal investments. . . . Much of the investment has been categorical, resulting in uneven capacity depending on disease."[39] Despite the fact that states bore legal responsibility for determining which diseases should be reportable, they contributed only about a quarter of the resources for surveillance activities.[40]

Within the realm of infectious diseases, HIV/AIDS surveillance was by far the most robust. As one CDC official explained, "There's AIDS, and then there's everything else."[41] A 1992 assessment found that 46 percent of federal infectious disease surveillance resources went to HIV/AIDS, and 85 percent went to HIV/AIDS, tuberculosis, sexually transmitted infections, and vaccine-preventable diseases.[42] In some instances, the only epidemiologists in a locale were those funded by the CDC to conduct HIV/AIDS surveillance.

The impact of funding was clearly shown in the rates of completeness of reporting for infectious diseases. The average for high-profile and relatively well-funded surveillance systems covering AIDS, tuberculosis, and sexually transmitted disease was significantly better (79 percent) than for all other diseases, where less than 50 percent of cases were reported.[43]

Surveillance of chronic and noninfectious conditions lagged far behind that of contagious illnesses. In 2000 the Pew Environmental Health Commission issued a stinging report on the state of surveillance. "The federal government tracks many things all the time," the commission noted. "It knows how many women dye their hair every year . . . but has only rough estimates of how many people have Parkinson's Disease, asthma, or most other chronic diseases that cause four of every five deaths in the U.S. each year."[44] The report recommended a nationwide system for tracking chronic disease and environmental pollutants. In spite of the interest in cancer surveillance over the past two decades and the federal support from both the CDC and the National Cancer Institute, state-level cancer surveillance activities—like public health work in general—remained variable, inadequately funded, and vulnerable to economic and political vagaries.[45] A 1999 editorial in the *Columbus Dispatch* lamented that Ohio's cancer registry "has limped along understaffed and underfunded, using its limited resources to collect data no one can afford to analyze."[46] Many other states were similarly lacking resources.

The state of birth defects surveillance was also wanting. Two evaluations of birth defects registries gave high marks to only eight state-based registries. A full third of the states received "failing grades" for having no registry. Two-thirds of states failed to "explore any possible links between birth defects and environmental exposure information, or other state registries such as cancer registries."[47] The CDC lacked sufficient funding for all state-based birth defects surveillance programs.[48] Reliant on a patchwork of funding, any piece of which was potentially at risk, registries faced uncertainty. Iowa, for example, boasted one of the best state-based surveillance systems. Yet it received only $50,000 a year from the state, which was enough to fund one staff position. The remainder of the funding came from the CDC and the University of Iowa, which was, in turn, reliant upon grant funding from the National Institutes of Health and other sources.[49] Many states have struggled to move beyond an unfunded mandate to conduct birth defects surveillance.[50] Despite the patina of progress, the state of affairs remains "woefully inadequate."[51]

Environmental and occupational health surveillance was in an even more parlous state. If, as 1984 congressional hearings concluded, occupational disease surveillance was "70 years behind infectious disease surveillance and counting," then in 2004 occupational disease reporting was arguably ninety years behind that of infectious disease. The $6 million spent on the federally funded occupational disease surveillance system—SENSOR—had remained virtually unchanged since 1998, in spite of limited state involvement, rising costs, and growing awareness that conditions such as musculoskeletal disorders accounted for as many as 34 percent of all nonfatal illnesses and injuries.[52] States, too, have seen falling interest in occupational disease surveillance. More than three-quarters of states reported that they had minimal capacity for occupational health surveillance or none at all.[53]

BEYOND SILOS: INTEGRATED SURVEILLANCE

Confronted with the gulf between what was legislatively mandated and what they realistically could do, public health officials nevertheless aspired to a robust surveillance that would require resources far beyond what history suggested they could command. As early as 1965, even as privacy concerns were mounting, some began to imagine an "electronic future" in which centralized medical records "will form the basis of a continuing, up-to-the-minute health profile of the entire country." The appeal of such a vision was broad. Media titan David Sarnoff imagined that "any trends that may affect the public health will be noted without delay and their meaning swiftly interpreted." The idea was exhilarating not only because it held the possibility of sounding a "warning prelude to an epidemic," but also because "the correlation of vast quantities of data would facilitate definitive research not only on specific diseases but on possible relations between air pollution and cancer" or other diseases.[54]

But Sarnoff's grand vision might have been labeled a grand illusion. In the mid-1990s the CDC, in collaboration with the CSTE, embarked on a significant project to expand and integrate surveillance.[55] The CSTE described the National Electronic Diseases Surveillance System (NEDSS) as "one of the cornerstones for disease surveillance and reporting for state and local public health departments and health care settings."[56] The CDC was charged with continuing the ground-breaking work to "integrate" surveillance systems—creating data standards to assure vital information collected could be easily shared among programs, across county lines, and among states. When the General Accounting Office, a nonpartisan oversight unit of the Congress, examined NEDSS at century's end, it found the system wanting. In 2004 only four states had fully adopted the system.[57]

Limited achievements also characterized the effort to create integrated surveillance systems for monitoring environmental threats to health. In 1992 the CDC created the National Environmental Public Health Tracking Program, aimed at building a nationwide network for studying exposures to environmental hazards. A decade later, representatives from the American Lung Association and Health-Track, a public education project, joined the call for a "comprehensive and coordinated network to track and monitor diseases such as birth defects and asthma, and potential environmental exposures that may be linked to those diseases."[58]

By 2002 Congress had allocated funds to help create a system that linked hazard exposure and disease data. By 2004 the CDC had announced funding for twenty-one local health departments and public health schools to help move toward a national environmental public health tracking system.[59] Nevertheless, in 2005 the Trust for America's Health was still urging an integration that had failed to materialize. "For a fully-functioning national health tracking network to be realized, it is critical that the various components of health tracking—birth defects surveillance systems, chronic disease registries, environmental health hazards, occupational influences, lifestyle, behavioral, and other health-related factors—be systematically integrated and adequately funded."[60]

The attempts to integrate surveillance of environmental hazards were paralleled by efforts focused on children's health. Here there had been some discernable progress, albeit slow and with many setbacks. Undaunted by problems encountered while establishing immunization and birth defects registries, the most ardent advocates of child health began to set their sights on creating databases that would gather together information on a range of health indicators. Health departments around the country routinely collected information derived from various infant and newborn clinical procedures: birth registration; dried blood spot screening for inborn errors of metabolism; birth defects surveillance; hearing screening; blood lead level screening; data from programs for children with special health care needs; patient billing records; and enrollment information from Women, Infants, and Children, a federal assistance program.[61] But, reflecting the fragmentation and duplication that characterized the U.S. health care system, this information tended to reside in "silos." The ability to link data could offer a comprehensive clinical picture of each child, enabling follow-up and treatment when needed.

Beginning in 2001 the RWJ Foundation devoted $5 million to a three-year program, Connections, to foster linkages among child health data systems. The new effort was shepherded by the Task Force on Child Survival and Development, an Atlanta-based nonprofit organization that had served as the national program office for All Kids Count, the foundation's initiative that fostered immunization registries. The endeavor was also supported by DHHS's Health Resources and Services Administration, which, in 1999, began funding a program to foster linkages between newborn screening for genetic defects and other maternal and child health services.[62]

By 2003 twelve states and large metropolitan areas were establishing integrated child health data systems, and another six were planning to do so. In the initial phases, most of these programs concentrated on linking data on four procedures: vital registration, newborn dried blood spot screening, immunization, and early hearing detection and intervention. These four were selected because all were universally recommended (and mandated in most states). All were conducted in the newborn period, and for all a delay in carrying them out could result in adverse health outcomes.[63] Among the most advanced of these systems was Rhode Island's KidsNet, which combined data from nine public health programs to create a child health profile, and Utah, where the health department developed CHARM (Child Health Advanced Records Management), a web-based interface that provided access to information stored in several stand-alone databases.[64]

BIGGS REDUX?

The efforts on the part of the New York City Department of Health, beginning in 2005, to extend the scope and functions of surveillance would underscore the tension between two visions of the state: as a provider of service and protection on the one hand and as an intruder in the clinical relationship on the other. Under the leadership of Commissioner Thomas Frieden, the department of health proposed new surveillance programs for diabetes and HIV. His effort harkened back to Hermann Biggs's bold moves to control tuberculosis a century earlier.

In July 2005, with the fanfare of a new public health campaign, New York City health officials described the dual epidemics of obesity and diabetes. With levels of self-reported diabetes more than doubling between 1994 and 2003, the disease, said Frieden, was "the only major health problem in this country that's getting worse and getting worse quickly."[65] It had accounted for some twenty thousand hospitalizations in 2003.

As a first step in controlling the epidemic, the health department put forward a bold proposal for electronic laboratory-based reporting of hemoglobin A1C tests, an indication of blood sugar levels. Never had a city or state health department initiated ongoing, systematic diabetes surveillance for an entire population.[66] In justifying the new surveillance effort, the health department underscored its legal mandate to prevent and control chronic, as well as communicable, disease. Registries for cancer, dementia, and congenital malformations provided well-established precedents for diabetes surveillance, the department claimed.[67] But more than epidemiological surveillance would come to be involved in the city's plan. Most radically, the health department proposed to use its authority to contact both doctors and patients when A1C levels suggested the need to review the clinical picture and even to modify the course of treatment if needed. It was that dimension of the proposed effort that would become the object of the most sustained debate.

As the department began to develop its registration plan, officials consulted with the CDC, the Americans with Diabetes Association, major city hospitals, clinicians, and patients with diabetes. Remarkably, they did not initially consult the county, state, and national medical associations. Given the sensitivity of surveillance surrounding HIV case reporting, it is likewise striking that privacy advocates were not included in early discussions.[68]

In response to concerns about stigma and discrimination,[69] Frieden argued that the privacy protections for the registry would be stronger than those for communicable disease reporting. Confidentiality provisions, the department asserted, would explicitly prohibit sharing that might "make it more difficult for persons with diabetes to obtain or renew a driver's license, health insurance, life insurance, etc."[70] Indeed, even patients themselves would not be able to authorize further disclosure of their registry data.[71]

When the proposal was open for public comment, it attracted scant notice. Those physicians who supported it were all involved in monitoring the quality of care in hospitals. They viewed the surveillance program as an effort to replicate on a citywide basis the system that health care institutions and managed care plans had already put into place. Libertarian physicians' organizations, however, characterized the proposed system as an unwarranted extension of public health authority into the domain of clinical medicine.[72] The Association of American Physicians and Surgeons, an organization opposed to the "evil" of government-based or "socialized" medicine, saw the plan as "replacing individualized medical care with population-based medicine."[73]

Patient proponents of the proposed surveillance effort included those who had experience with voluntary diabetes registries. None who offered comments on the New York proposal felt that their privacy had been violated; all expressed confidence in registry security.[74] Further, they underscored the direct benefits offered by case management. One patient enrolled in the Vermont Diabetes Information System, which had provided the model for the New York proposal, argued that because of registration, "I get letters from my doctor reminding me when to have my blood tests and helping me to decide what to do with the blood tests. This has been a very good service for me."[75] Another noted that, more than once, he had been alerted when he had fallen behind in getting his A1C tests. "Thank goodness for this wonderful program," he wrote.[76]

Patient opposition to the diabetes proposals centered on privacy and intrusions in the clinical relationship. One patient who testified against the proposal said, "As a diabetic I am not a threat to the city's public health, nor do I wish to be treated as one." Said another opponent, "This isn't smallpox." The health department "does not have a compelling interest in the health of an individual that overrides that individual's right to privacy."[77] Another asked, "What is next? Will New York City get the gynecological records of everyone woman and put the ones who don't use proper birth control on a registry too?"[78] She did not need or want the city to "babysit for [her]."[79] What was termed a "Big Brother" approach was denounced by one patient who told the Board of Health, "You're sure as hell not my doctor—my diabetes is well controlled without your unasked-for paternalistic assistance and oversight."[80] Like the American Diabetes Association, those who opposed the plan would have been satisfied only by an informed consent provision.[81]

In the era of democratic privacy, none of this language was surprising given the scope of what health officials had proposed and the history of earlier struggles over surveillance. What was striking was how few opponents came forward. Neither the ACLU, its New York affiliate, nor any of the other groups that had been so engaged in debates about surveillance during the past two decades appeared at the public hearing or submitted formal comments. Nonetheless, the city scaled back its efforts, permitting patients to opt out of health department interventions. Their names, however, would remain in the registry. Further, what had initially appeared to represent a citywide program would begin with a trial in the South Bronx, an impoverished area of the city where diabetes rates were the highest and medical care was inadequate.

Protest broadened only after the Board of Health endorsed Commissioner Frieden's proposals on December 1, 2005. The reaction was fueled in part by city proposals to radically change the scope and function of HIV testing and surveillance. Part of a broader set of moves that included an easing of the informed consent requirements for HIV testing, the HIV surveillance effort sought to give health authorities the ability to intervene with patients whose clinical care appeared to be less than optimal, just as it had proposed to do with diabetes. "We know people are dying," said Commissioner Frieden, but "we are prohibited by law from lifting a finger to try and help" in the same fashion that "we are able to do . . . with every other communicable disease."[82] Of chief concern were patients lost to care, who had "no one responsible, no one accountable" for their medical management.[83] Frieden said that the disparities between whites and people of color infected with HIV represented "a damning indictment of our system."[84] He proposed that when officials became aware of someone whose health required a modification of treatment that the department be able to use the information already in hand to contact patients and consult their providers.[85] Further, the health department argued that it was uniquely positioned to refer newly diagnosed cases to clinical services, contacting the patient directly if necessary, and to help physicians contact patients who had dropped out of care.[86]

A *New York Times* editorial gave a resounding endorsement to the city's proposals. Underscoring the ways in which surveillance could be viewed as a prelude to protection rather than as a threatening intrusion, the *Times* argued that "surely most patients would rather get life-extending treatments than languish in neglect."[87] The Latino Commission on AIDS was similarly supportive, viewing expanded monitoring as representing "a 'third pair of eyes' [that] can only benefit" minority patients in New York City.[88]

But organizations that had long been involved in battles of HIV case reporting moved to thwart the health department. In part, opposition centered over disagreements about how to understand the obvious racial disparities in HIV status. Ronald Johnson of the Gay Men's Health Crisis commented that the problem for African American gay men was not falling through the cracks once they received care, but getting into the system for an initial test.[89] The HIV advocacy group Housing Works asserted, "The very fact that lab work is being done demonstrates that the patient is already in the care of a healthcare provider licensed by the State of New York."[90]

Mirroring the arguments of those who opposed diabetes surveillance, Housing Works—which emerged as the most vocal opponent of the new effort—expressed concern about health officials making contact with patients' health care provider without consent and second-guessing the doctor. The city's plan would "interfere in the doctor-patient relationship of people living with HIV/AIDS. . . . Receiving a call from an unknown bureaucrat questioning the quality of my care and the decisions that my doctor and I are making about my treatment" represents nothing more than "Big Brother watching over our shoulder."[91] The specter of where the new surveillance might lead shaped the views of those who sounded the alarm over erosions of privacy. Said a Housing Works advocate, "Perhaps in the beginning the intrusion will only be advisory. But who knows what future use of this power of intrusion might be put to. Am I going to be coerced into treatment, or sanctioned for being non-adherent?"[92]

To meet the challenge provoked by his proposals, Frieden appeared to modify his stance, as he had in the much less volatile dispute over diabetes surveillance. In contrast to his diabetes program, individuals would have to opt in to the clinical oversight that was at the heart of what he had put forward. "We would reach out to treating doctors, case managers and, *only if there are no viable alternatives,* directly to patients to offer to help link them to existing HIV services." While acknowledging the concerns that such direct intervention would generate, Frieden stressed, "The epidemic demands effective approaches to reach patients who are not in care."[93]

However the controversies of 2005 and 2006 involving surveillance of diabetes and HIV play out, it is clear that Thomas Frieden has begun to write a new chapter in the history of public health—one with clear antecedents in the nineteenth century. Although framed in the language of quality assurance and improvement—processes arising from the influence of managed care and third-party payers that had begun to circumscribe the professional autonomy of doctors[94]—the proposals were reminiscent of earlier efforts when health officials, with teams of nurses and a network of clinics, sought to oversee the management of tuberculosis.

DISEASE SURVEILLANCE AND THE SECURITY STATE

Efforts to yoke public health surveillance to national defense triggered anxieties that dwarfed the concerns provoked by moves to integrate and expand the scope of surveillance systems. The creation of surveillance systems capable of responding to threats of bioterrorism inevitably posed questions about the appropriate relationship of public health to law enforcement and state security.

The danger of bioterrorism gained increasing attention in the late 1990s. Among those who repeatedly sounded the warning were D. A. Henderson, who had been a central figure in the global smallpox eradication effort, and Michael Osterholm, former state epidemiologist in Minnesota, who had been an architect of that state's aggressive campaign against AIDS. In testimony before a Senate subcommittee in mid-1998, Osterholm cautioned that weaknesses in local health departments left the nation vulnerable and would hobble efforts to respond to a bioterrorist attack. Speaking in his capacity as a representative of the American Society for Microbiology, he noted that it was health workers, not soldiers, who would be called on to provide the first line of defense. They would be hampered, he said, by the lack of adequate surveillance. Observing that over the course of his career he had been called upon to confront Legionnaires' disease, toxic shock syndrome, and AIDS, he said, "There is simply nothing that scares me like this issue because the implications are so far reaching."[95] Addressing the same Senate panel, the president of the National Association of County and City Health Officials highlighted the poor state of surveillance and preparedness. Half of the nation's local health departments, he said, did not have electronic mail and at least a thousand of those departments had no on-line computer communication.[96] In 1999 the Institute of Medicine and the National Research Council spoke of a "glaring need" to enhance surveillance capacity in anticipation of a potential bioterrorist attack.[97]

Within the Clinton administration, the sense of alarm had also taken hold. Margaret Hamburg, who had been health commissioner in New York in the early 1990s when it faced a threatening upsurge in drug-resistant tuberculosis and who was now assistant secretary for planning and evaluation in DHHS, noted, "We need to strengthen our nation's public health infrastructure. This means enhancing our surveillance and epidemiologic capacity; our laboratory capacity to support surveillance efforts; and our communication systems to collect, analyze, and share data."[98] There was widespread support for such initiatives, even among people skeptical of the risk posed by bioterrorism and who saw in the campaign to arouse public concern an alarmist threat that could lead to the militarization of public health.[99]

When, in early 2000, the CDC issued a strategic plan for confronting biological and chemical terrorism, it laid out a five-year time frame for rapidly upgrading the capacity for communications among health departments and between the medical care sector and health departments.[100] The CDC noted the need to "integrate surveillance for illness and injury resulting from biologic and chemical terrorism into the U.S. disease surveillance system."[101] Such an effort would necessitate linkages between the CDC and state and local health departments with medical personnel, hospital emergency departments, and poison control centers. Clinicians and health departments had to move beyond the conventional role of serving as a bulwark against naturally occurring threats; they would now be called on to provide a line of defense against enemy assault. This was, of course, not the first time such roles would be merged. The threat of bioterrorism during the Korean War had led Alexander Langmuir to create the CDC's Epidemic Intelligence Service.

The events of September 11, 2001, and the anthrax attack of the following month created a national mood of heightened anxiety.[102] A United States that now saw itself as vulnerable responded with a range of wartime-like measures. The five-year time frame for enhancing surveillance capacity proposed by the CDC only a year earlier seemed utterly out of step with what was required. Some regarded the new roles imposed on the CDC by the claims of national defense with trepidation. As Harold Jaffe, a senior official at the CDC, summarized, "To be told that you are partly responsible for the security of this country is a change for the agency. People are accepting it, but they are not entirely comfortable with it."[103]

In the wake of 9/11, the inadequacy of the nation's surveillance capacity to meet the threat of bioterrorism became a matter of wide public debate. Based on investigations in early 2002, the General Accounting Office concluded, "Existing surveillance systems have weaknesses, such as chronic underreporting and outdated laboratory facilities, which raise concerns about the ability of state and local agencies to detect emerging diseases or a bioterrorist event."[104]

With federal support, several cities also began to develop innovative Early Aberration Reporting Systems (EARS) designed to monitor unusual clusters of illness, such as respiratory or enteric disease, that might suggest a bioterrorist attack.[105] New York City was a pioneer in this syndromic surveillance, which tracked emergency room visits, pharmacy sales, and illnesses among transit workers. At the heart of the system was the monitoring of every 911 emergency phone call. Reports were electronically transferred to the health department, where a computer program spotted anomalies. Michael Osterholm, reflecting the sentiment that surveillance must represent a call to action, likened such systems to a set of smoke detectors, sounding alarms before a disease swept through a community: "If a whole bunch of alarms go off we may need to get to a large number of people with antibiotics or vaccines. . . . We are not here to record history but to change history."[106]

In reviewing such a syndromic surveillance system in Pittsburgh, President George W. Bush evoked memories of cold war threats of missile attacks from the Soviet Union. He compared the Pittsburgh system, the Real Time

Outbreak and Disease Surveillance (RODS) system to the earlier era's DEW line—the Distant Early Warning system of radar installations placed across northern Canada and Alaska—that served as a warning against impending enemy attack.[107] Like other syndromic surveillance systems, RODS looked for unexpected spikes in infectious disease. It did not track disease by patient name. As the RODS developer explained, "When you're trying to find an outbreak, it's not necessary to accurately diagnose every single case."[108] But of course, treatment of the sick or containment of an outbreak of contagious disease might necessitate contact tracing and, hence, the collection of names. In the context of a bioterrorism event, law enforcement officials would undoubtedly press the case for access to names in relevant public health registries. Accordingly, President Bush emphasized the importance of data sharing as well as the ability to identify cases and intervene.[109]

In October 2002 the CDC announced plans for a national syndromic surveillance system as part of the nation's defense against terrorism. Two years later, however, the General Accounting Office concluded that optimism about syndromic surveillance might have been premature. "There are concerns that these systems are costly to run and still largely untested."[110] Similarly D. A. Henderson, who chaired the Council on Public Health Preparedness for DHHS secretary Tommy Thompson, said, "The conclusion a lot of us have reached is that while, in principle, this seemed like a good idea, in reality, it is not very practical."[111]

But it was not simply the technical features of the new public health surveillance efforts that were the subject of increasing concern. It was the fact that such expansion took place against the backdrop of moves to enhance domestic vigilance—the passage of the U.S.A. PATRIOT Act and the creation of the Department of Homeland Security—that led privacy advocates and others concerned about civil liberties to raise urgent questions. Emblematic was their response to a proposal to create a vast, multisectoral surveillance system that could anticipate potential terrorist threats. Total Information Awareness, planned under the guidance of retired Vice Admiral John Poindexter, Ronald Reagan's national security advisor, would have required an amendment to the Privacy Act of 1974. The system would have given intelligence analysts and law enforcement officials access to internet communications, telephone records, credit cards, and banking transactions without a court-approved search warrant. Poindexter saw the need to "break down the stove pipes" that separated commercial and governmental databases. "We must," he said, "become much more efficient and more clever in the ways in which we find new sources of data, mine information from the new and the old, generate information, make it available for analysis, convert it to knowledge, and create actionable options."[112]

This was, to those worried about the fate of privacy, nothing short of an Orwellian vision. In "A Snooper's Dream," the *New York Times* wrote, "The threat of terrorism has created a powerful appetite in Washington for sophisticated surveillance systems to identify potential terrorists. These efforts cannot be allowed, however, to undermine civil liberties. . . . The last thing we need is a vast new system of domestic surveillance engineered by John Poindexter."[113]

Such overarching and penetrating surveillance efforts created an environment in which essential public health initiatives would be viewed with suspicion and hostility, indeed, in which the boundary between national security and public health could become blurred. This was the context within which a furious debate emerged over a CDC-backed initiative to draft a Model State Emergency Health Powers Act. The act would have provided local and state health officials with a template for expanding their powers to confront the threat of naturally occurring disease as well as bioterrorism. The model act enumerated the terms for the declaration of an emergency, the seizure of property, the imposition of quarantines, the compulsory administration of immunizations, and the requirement to undergo treatment. Central to these measures was an invigorated system of public health surveillance. To its drafters—led by Lawrence Gostin, the architect of the Model State Public Health Privacy Act—prevailing restrictions on surveillance thwarted the ability of public health officials to detect in a timely fashion an emergency or disaster. "Current statutes do not facilitate surveillance and may even prevent monitoring. . . . They do not require and may actually prohibit public health agencies from monitoring data in the health care system. . . . New federal health information privacy protections may unintentionally impede the flow of data from private to public sectors."[114]

To face these impediments, the model act would have mandated reporting under emergency circumstances by health care providers, pharmacists, veterinarians, and laboratories within twenty-four hours. Because such reporting was instrumental to the initiation of public health interventions with those thought to be carriers of dangerous pathogens, it was essential that names be used. Since public health emergencies required the cooperation of an array of government agencies, the conventional limits on the sharing of data were to be suspended. "The model act recognizes that exchange of relevant data among lead agencies is essential to assure the public's health and security."[115]

Although many public health officials and legislators embraced the model act in part or in whole, it became the target of fierce opposition from across the political spectrum. George Annas, a prominent liberal figure in public health law, denounced the measure as "the old Soviet model of public health (lots of power and no standards for applying it), hardly a new American model."[116] Georgia's conservative Republican representative, Bob Barr, described the act as an effort to "hijack the constitutional freedoms of Americans."[117] And Barbara Loe Fisher, who had long framed her campaign against compulsory immunization in libertarian terms, said of the act, "It treats us like runaway slaves in need of subjugation."[118] In a reprise of the antagonism toward surveillance given voice more than a century earlier, it was not simply the invasions of privacy that so provoked the opponents of the act, but the direct linkage of expanded surveillance to coercive measures that might be imposed by health officials or the police.

Janlori Goldman, a persistent critic of the model act, said, "The danger here is that the HIPAA privacy regulations' limits on the use and disclosure of personal health information will be overcome by the national security and public health authority encoded in the statutes enacted after September 11th."[119] With endless war against an elusive enemy, "there has been a dangerous absence of public debate over how much information is needed, by whom, and for what purposes to achieve public health preparedness goals."[120] For her, these fears are potentially realized in centralized reporting systems. BioSense, a "near real-time reporting, analytic evaluation and implementation, and early event detection" system, was created by the CDC in cooperation with the Departments of Defense and Veterans Affairs and the Laboratory Corporation of America, which operates some thirty-one labs nationwide. Like other syndromic surveillance systems, Bio-Sense did not use names but instead relied on patient age, zip code, and sex. Although data had been made available to state and local health officials since April 2004, unlike traditional disease surveillance, data was reported directly to the CDC, bypassing departments of health.[121]

Thus, at the turn of the twenty-first century, in the effort to fashion monitoring systems capable of responding to the threats of bioterrorism, which will inevitably entail questions of the relationship of public health to law enforcement, the tensions among surveillance, privacy, and the searching eyes of government will be thrown into sharp relief. No longer will the issues involve the merely metaphorical relationship between health and state security.

Conclusion

An Enduring Tension

We conclude this more than century-long history of public health surveillance by returning to the enduring tension between the claims of privacy and the challenge of securing the public's well-being.

Privacy evokes worlds of intimacy. For law professor Alan Westin, who did so much to chart the vicissitudes of privacy in the 1960s, privacy meets a psychological need, not only for exercising autonomy but also for enjoying opportunities for emotional release and self-reflection.[1] To protect such vital needs, privacy requires a "sanctuary," a means of "prohibiting other persons from seeing, hearing, and knowing."[2] Charles Fried, who served as solicitor general under President Ronald Reagan, writes that privacy is as necessary to "relations of the most fundamental sort as oxygen is for combustion."[3] Privacy thus represents a precious good, valued in and of itself.

But however cherished, privacy is not, at the beginning of the twenty-first century, an absolute value—nor has it ever been. It is "constantly forced into accommodation with other important individual or societal values," as one student of Westin's observed.[4] Nowhere is this clearer than in the context of disease surveillance.

Public health surveillance evokes deep concerns about protection from naturally occurring and socially created threats to well-being and even survival. From the last decades of the nineteenth century, when systematic disease notification was described as the "eyes" of public health, to the closing decades of the twentieth century, when the image of radar was used to describe the role of disease reporting, public health officials and other proponents of surveillance underscored the necessity of limiting privacy in the name of the common good. When challenged by doctors or patients, public health officials argued that the claims of the individual had to yield to the needs of the collective and that protecting communal health, safety, and security was preeminent. They offered assurances that disease registries were not public records, open to general examination, and indeed pressed for laws to shield the identities of those reported. On occasion they were compelled to compromise, agreeing to receive coded reports in lieu of names, as in the case of venereal disease at the start of the twentieth century and, for a period, HIV at its end. Sometimes they compromised the principle of universal reporting by granting individuals the opportunity to remain beyond the scope of a particular registry. This was true both for immunization and birth defects registries.

Although we have centered our analysis on moments of controversy in the history of disease reporting, public health surveillance has, for the most part, drawn little attention. The concerns of those responsible for developing, enhancing, and securing disease registries have centered on technical and administrative matters. What kinds of surveillance could best capture the incidence and prevalence of disease? Was it always essential to have individual, name-based case reports to map the occurrence and extent of disease? Which approaches to surveillance could best assure appropriate public health interventions?

But whether the subject of dispute or not, disease reporting always involves trade-offs among competing social, ethical, and legal interests and values. Whether these tensions become manifest is a matter of historical contingency. If the routinization of surveillance tends to mask these fundamental conflicts, moments of controversy illuminate them. What explains the extent to which surveillance has sparked political debate and determined the duration and intensity of encounters over its limits?

Most critical has been the extent to which surveillance might trigger public health interventions and the way such interventions have been viewed as either threatening or potentially beneficial. Fears that those identified through surveillance would be the targets of unacceptable supervision, control, or coercion energized opposition to name-based reporting. In the late nineteenth century, physicians resisted tuberculosis notification because they sought to protect their private patients from intrusions on the part of public health officials. In the 1990s gay men and other AIDS advocates resisted efforts to require name-based reporting of HIV because of fears of how public health registries could be used to foster discrimination in employment, housing, and insurance. Moreover, some feared the possibility that such lists could be used as a prelude to the imposition of quarantines.

In contrast, the consequences of notification have sometimes been viewed as beneficial. In those cases, the subjects of surveillance have been willing to compromise their own privacy for the sake of some other good. Labor advocates thus supported occupational disease reporting because it could represent a first step to state protections from hazardous work site conditions. For public health labor reformer Alice Hamilton, the state was not an "invading hostile power." She asserted, "What is the federal government? It is ourselves—ourselves organized."[5] Similarly, cancer and birth defects activists regarded disease registries as crucial to much-needed research that could lead to more effective prevention and treatment. Thus the terms of the trade-off have been affected by persistent patterns of social inequality in America. The needs and preferences, when they could be given voice, were different for the relatively privileged and those made vulnerable by race or class. Minorities often had to trade privacy for basic health care services. Those for whom access to health services was not a problem traded privacy for advancements in research, which could lead to more-sophisticated or effective therapies.

The invocation of the claims of privacy by powerful entities could set the stage for dispute. Labor and its allies, for example, saw the efforts of large employers to thwart surveillance by the NIOSH as nothing other than a subterfuge, an effort to shield records that would make clear how workers were endangered. But the articulation of an exacting standard of privacy did not always reflect such narrow interests. When citizens in Illinois and New York sought data from the states' cancer registries as part of their grassroots efforts to understand the environmental risks posed to their communities, health officials demurred, asserting that their legal duty to protect privacy required that they prohibit access to de-identified data when there was even a remote risk of disclosure. The impulse was not to withhold information from the public but to fulfill a mandate to protect the public.

Resistance to surveillance could be especially intense when socially stigmatized conditions became the object of reporting proposals. Physicians refusing to report venereal diseases, patients objecting to a registry of prescriptions for psychoactive medications, gay men fighting HIV reporting—all defended the right to remain beyond the scope of the searching eyes of government. To be sure, they expressed alarm about what might be done to them because they were socially vulnerable. But they also gave voice to a very different concern: their "medical secrets" could be viewed by those not directly involved in their care, which was a violation, even if they suffered no subsequent harm. Privacy, under such circumstances, was not simply an instrumental value. It was essential, not be traded or compromised.

The capacity to give voice to claims for privacy or state protection determined the occurrence, scope, and outcome of clashes over surveillance. In the era of paternalistic privacy, doctors had to be informed about surveillance activities since their active cooperation was essential. They relied on their professional associations to negotiate with and influence the decisions of public health officials, and in so doing asserted the sanctity of the doctor-patient relationship. Organization, however, did not assure success, as the long history of failed labor efforts to achieve occupational disease reporting throws into bold relief.

A fundamental change occurred in the era of democratic privacy, when concerns about government and corporate threats to personal information emerged at the very moment a host of social movements had begun to challenge medical paternalism. Indicative of this broad transformation was adoption of the Code of Fair Information Practices in 1973 and passage of the Privacy Act the following year. For the first time, individuals had the right to know when personal information was included in government files. This right, in turn, created the possibility of a broadened public role in determining what records were created, how they were used, and what methods were employed to protect them from unwarranted disclosure. But between the promise and realization of democratization there was a vast gulf. It would take the force of the women's, gay rights, consumer, and environmental movements to set the stage for a new kind of popular participation in public health discussions. The subsequent emergence of a politics of identity centered on diseases—AIDS and breast cancer most notably—would indelibly mark the era of democratic privacy.

But it was not only the efforts of those with disease that served to define the new era. Organizations such as the March of Dimes and the American Cancer Society became forceful institutional advocates for surveillance efforts. Those who were seized by concerns about invasions of privacy or overly intrusive government also joined the fray. They could be hostile to the social welfare functions of the state or committed to civil liberties as vital to a democratic order. Although antagonists on one level, libertarians at opposite ends of the political spectrum might come together around the politics of surveillance. Diverse groups have consistently pushed back against disease surveillance: the ACLU; antivaccination activists; libertarians committed to thwarting a protective role for government, such as the CCHC; and grassroots religious groups concerned that birth defects surveillance could be a prelude to abortion.

However they took form—whether they involved resistance to or demand for more extensive reporting requirements—controversies over surveillance not uncommonly entailed questions about the appropriate relationship between public health and clinical medicine. This was true not only at the turn of the twentieth century, when New York City extended notification to tuberculosis and venereal diseases, but also at the turn of the twenty-first, when the city's health department again sought to chart a bold new course involving the oversight of the care of people with diabetes and HIV. In the period between these two bookends, while public health was at times intimately involved in direct service provision, especially to the poor, it had largely been divorced from clinical care.[6] The debates that have been provoked by New York City's effort raise far-reaching questions not only about whether health officials *could* but whether they *should* take on the challenge of clinical disease management.[7]

If the debates about the relationship between public health and clinical medicine represent questions about the flow of data and authority from doctors to health officials, the threat of bioterrorism represents a challenge posed by the prospect of information flowing from public health departments to other government agencies. In the aftermath of 9/11, the issue has taken on a special urgency.

As they face the recurrence of old debates or fundamentally new challenges posed by surveillance, privacy advocates argue that good public health and the protection of privacy need not be in tension. Indeed, proponents of privacy in the latter part of the twentieth century have invoked instrumental claims when warning of the consequences of intrusions on what they viewed as sacrosanct domains. They have sought to demonstrate that limits on the confidentiality of the doctor-patient relationship would subvert not only clinical care but also the public's health. In the context of anxieties about how national security considerations could narrow the purchase of privacy, Janlori Goldman wrote, "The codification of vague promises that power will not be abused and good judgment will be employed ignore the historical lesson that during a crisis, privacy and civil liberties are given little weight in the balancing of competing law enforcement, national security, and commercial interests. Preserving public health and protecting privacy can—and must—go hand in hand."[8] But her alarm extends beyond the issue of national defense. Goldman worries, too, about efforts to draw clinical medicine and public health into a closer relationship. While arguing for the most stringent protections of surveillance data, she, like other privacy advocates, believes that it is essential to address the question of whether an effective public health program always requires the use of personally identifiable reports. There is no necessary trade-off, in this view, between a robust commitment to privacy and good public health practice.

Our study of public health surveillance brings us to a different conclusion. We believe that it is clear that there is an enduring tension between privacy and public health surveillance,[9] though it has been expressed differently as conceptions of privacy and the scope of surveillance changed over time and played out in different domains. This tension is sometimes expressed in bitter controversies. On other occasions, those who had believed that their needs required greater surveillance themselves decided to trade some degree of privacy.

Enduring tension, then, does not produce either inevitable or unending conflict. Just as the emergence of disputes is historically contingent, so too are their conclusions. On occasion, debates about disease notification have come to an end because one side has triumphed over the other. In other instances compromise has, at least temporarily, removed the source of contention. Finally, conflicts have come to an end when opponents' interests have shifted to what they considered other, more urgent matters such as access to treatment. Thus, for example, the bitterly contested issue of HIV name reporting in California came to a close in 2006 when advocates recognized that they either had to accept the end of unique identifier reporting or lose critically important funding for AIDS programs.[10] But the end of conflict does not foreclose the possibility of renewed debate. Even apparently settled matters involving surveillance may be subject to renewed challenge.

In the end, we have not sought to resolve the conflict between privacy and greater public health surveillance, nor do we think it desirable to do so. The vitality of democratic communities necessitates an ongoing effort to negotiate and renegotiate the boundaries between privacy, society's "limiting principle,"[11] and public health, which at its best has sought to expand the role of government as a guardian against disease and suffering.

NOTES

PREFACE

1. Lawrence Tribe, *American Constitutional Law,* 2nd ed. (Mineola, NY, 1988), 1302.

2. William O. Douglas, *The Right of the People* (New York, 1958), 108.

3. Tribe, *American Constitutional Law,* 1303.

4. Ibid.

5. Gary L. Bostwick, "Comment: A Taxonomy of Privacy: Repose, Sanctuary, and Intimate Decision," *California Law Review* 1447 (1976): 1456.

6. Cited in Janlori Goldman and Deirdre Mulligan, *Privacy and Health Information Systems: A Guide to Protecting Patient Confidentiality* (Seattle, 1996), 5.

7. James C. Scott, *Seeing Like a State: How Certain Schemes to Improve the Human Condition Have Failed* (New Haven, CT, 1998), 4.

8. Michel Foucault, *Discipline and Punish: The Birth of the Prison* (New York, 1979).

9. James Miller, *The Passion of Michel Foucault* (New York, 1993), 220.

10. Alexander D. Langmuir, "Communicable Disease Surveillance," *Proceedings of the Royal Society of Medicine* 64 (1971): 9. Alexander D. Langmuir, "Developing Concepts in Surveillance," *Milbank Memorial Fund Quarterly* 43 (1965): 369–72. Guthrie S. Birkhead and Christopher M. Maylahn, "State and Local Public Health Surveillance," in *Principles and Practice of Public Health Surveillance,* ed. Steven M. Teutsch and R. Elliott Churchill (Oxford, 2000), 253–86. John W. Trask, "Vital Statistics: A Discussion of What They Are and Their Uses in Public Health Administration," *Public Health Reports,* Supplement No. 12 (April 3, 1914).

11. Stephen B. Thacker and Ruth L. Berkelman, "Public Health Surveillance in the United States," *Epidemiologic Reviews* 10 (1988): 164–90. William H. Foege, Robert C. Hogan, and Ladene H. Newton, "Surveillance Projects for Selected Diseases," *International Journal of Epidemiology* 5 (1976): 29.

12. Donna F. Stroup and Ron Brookmeyer, eds., *Monitoring the Health of Populations: Statistical Principles and Methods for Public Health Surveillance* (New York, 2004), 5. World Health Organization, "Terminology of Malaria and of Malaria Eradication:

Report for Drafting Committee," cited in Stephen B. Thacker, "Historical Development," in *Principles and Practice of Public Health Surveillance*, 4. Lorenzo D. Botto et al., "Fostering International Collaboration in Birth Defects Research and Prevention: A Perspective from the International Clearinghouse for Birth Defects Surveillance and Research," *American Journal of Public Health* 96 (2006), 774–80.

13. Thacker, "Historical Development," in *Principles and Practice of Public Health Surveillance*, 1–16. Alexander D. Langmuir, "William Farr: Founder of Modern Concepts of Surveillance," *International Journal of Epidemiology* 5 (1976): 13. Foege, Hogan, and Newton, "Surveillance Projects for Selected Diseases."

14. Alexander D. Langmuir to Lester Breslow, June 28, 1989, Alexander D. Langmuir Papers, Box 2, Surveillance 1989 Folder, Alan Mason Chesney Medical Archives, the Johns Hopkins Medical Institutions, Baltimore.

15. Alexander D. Langmuir Papers, Box 3, COOP Group Vaccines Folder, Notes, October 25, 1992, Alan Mason Chesney Medical Archives, the Johns Hopkins Medical Institutions, Baltimore.

16. Alexander D. Langmuir, quoted in the *Medical Tribune*, January 14–15, 1967, 10. Alexander D. Langmuir Papers, Box 1, Folder 1, Alan Mason Chesney Medical Archives, the Johns Hopkins Medical Institutions, Baltimore.

17. *Houston Chronicle*, August 30, 1993, Discovery Section, 7. *Dallas Morning News*, July 7, 1993, A14. *Washington Post*, September 30, 1999, B2. *New York Times*, March 15, 2003, A5.

CHAPTER 1

1. Laws Relative to Quarantine and Public Health (1858), 34–35.

2. Barbara Gutmann Rosenkrantz, *Public Health and the State: Changing Views in Massachusetts, 1842–1936* (Cambridge, MA, 1972), 110, quoting An Act Concerning Contagious Diseases (March 21, 1884), *Acts and Resolves*, chap. 98, 77–78.

3. J. W. Kerr and A. A. Moll, "Organization, Powers, and Duties of Health Authorities: An Analysis of the Laws and Regulations Relating Thereto in Force in the United States," *Public Health Bulletin No. 54* (1912), 8.

4. Barbara Laslett, "The Family as a Public and Private Institution: An Historical Perspective," *Journal of Marriage and the Family* 35 (1973): 481.

5. Ibid., 485, 486.

6. David H. Flaherty, *Privacy in Colonial New England* (Charlottesville, VA, 1972), 71.

7. Ibid., 60–70, 85–88, 175–79.

8. Ibid., 15, 92–97, 100, 166.

9. Ibid., 170.

10. Ibid., 170–75.

11. Laws Relative to Quarantine and Public Health, pp. 34–35. See also George W. Morton, *Laws and Ordinances Relative to the Preservation of the Public Health in the County of New York* (1860), 36, and Graham Mooney, "Public Health versus Private Practice: The Contested Development of Compulsory Infectious Disease Notification in Late-Nineteenth-Century Britain," *Bulletin of the History of Medicine* 73 (1999): 243.

12. Rosenkrantz, *Public Health and the State*, 21–23. Alexander D. Langmuir, Alexander D. Langmuir Papers, Box 2, Surveillance 1989 Folder, Alan Mason Chesney Medical Archives, the Johns Hopkins Medical Institutions, Baltimore. John W. Trask, "Vital Statistics: A Discussion of What They Are and Their Uses in Public Health Administration," *Public Health Reports*, Supplement No. 12 (April 3, 1914).

13. Kerr and Moll, "Organization, Powers, and Duties," 28. They described the prevention and control of disease as the "primary *raison d'etre* of health organization," necessitating the conference of "vast powers" on boards of health (28).

14. "Letter from Henry I. Bowditch, et al., Members of the State Board of Health, Boston, Commonwealth of Massachusetts, November 1, 1874," *Public Health Reports*, Supplement No. 12 (April 3, 1914): 31. See also Trask, "Vital Statistics," 30–33.

15. Kerr and Moll, "Organization, Powers, and Duties," 11.

16. Laslett, "Family as a Public and Private Institution." Helena Znaniecka Lopata, "The Interweave of Public and Private: Women's Challenge to American Society," *Journal of Marriage and the Family* 55 (1993): 177–78.

17. John Duffy, *The Sanitarians: A History of American Public Health* (Urbana, Ill., 1990). Paul Starr, *The Social Transformation of American Medicine: The Rise of a Sovereign Profession and the Making of a Vast Industry* (New York, 1982).

18. James A. Morone, *The Democratic Wish: Popular Participation and the Limits of American Government* (Princeton, NJ, 1990), 116–17. Robert Wiebe, *The Search for Order, 1877–1920* (New York, 1967).

19. Charles Rosenberg, *The Cholera Years: The United States in 1932, 1849, and 1866* (Chicago, 1987), 154–55.

20. Starr, *Social Transformation of American Medicine*. Kenneth Ludmerer, *Learning to Heal: The Development of American Medical Education* (New York, 1985). John Harley Warner, *The Therapeutic Perspective: Medical Practice, Knowledge, and Identity in America, 1820–1885* (Cambridge, MA, 1986).

21. Charles J. Hailes, *Bender's Health Officers' Manual and Public Health Law of the State of New York* (Albany, NY, 1910), 206.

22. L. L. Boyce, *The Health Officers' Manual and Public Health Law of the State of New York* (Albany, NY, 1902), 234. See also Walter P. Bowers, "Reporting Cases of Tuberculosis," *Boston Medical and Surgical Journal*, 1915, 236.

23. "A Model State Law for Morbidity Reports," *Public Health Reports* 27 (1913): 1323–29.

24. Henry Bixby Hemenway, *Legal Principles of Public Health Administration* (Chicago, 1914), 558.

25. Ibid., 558–59, 597. See also Frank G. Boudreau, "The New Plan of Collecting Vital Statistics in Ohio: How the Physician Can Aid in the Health Campaign," *Ohio State Journal of Medicine* 11 (1915): 308.

26. The move toward the reporting of disease by name to health officials in the United States was paralleled in Europe, driven in part by the cholera epidemics of the nineteenth century. Graham Mooney, in recounting the history of surveillance in Great Britain, argues that "notification was *the* crucial policy development in the move toward the individualization of public health strategies in the later nineteenth century." Intervention "would not have been possible without it." Mooney, "Public Health versus Private Practice," 267. Peter Baldwin's analysis of the state and conta-

gious disease in England and the Continent underscores the linkage of disease notification and what he terms the "neoquarantinist system"—inspection, isolation, disinfection, and surveillance. In 1889 a parliamentary act gave localities the authority
to require notification. By the early 1890s such provisions covered more than 80 percent of the English population. In 1899 the Notification of Diseases Act was passed,
requiring reporting throughout the country. Thus not only did notification make
intervention possible, such intervention provided the justification for notification.
Peter Baldwin, *Contagion and the State in Europe, 1830 to 1930* (Cambridge, England,
1999), 154–55, 162.

27. Richard French, *Antivivisection and Medical Science in Victorian Society* (Princeton, NJ, 1975), 224. Lloyd Stevenson, "Science down the Drain: On the Hostility of
Certain Sanitarians to Animal Experimentation, Bacteriology and Immunology,"
Bulletin of the History of Medicine 29 (1955): 1–26. Nicholas A. Rupke, ed., *Vivisection
in Historical Perspective* (New York, 1987). R. M. MacLeod, "Law, Medicine and Public
Opinion: The Resistance to Compulsory Health Legislation 1870–1907," *Public Law*
(1967): 107–28, 189–211. Martin Kaufman, "The American Anti-vaccinationists
and Their Arguments," *Bulletin of the History of Medicine* 41 (1967): 463–78. R. Porter
and D. Porter, "The Politics of Prevention: Anti-vaccinationism and Public Health in
Nineteenth-Century England," *Medical History* 32 (1988): 231–52.

28. Judith R. Walkowitz, *Prostitution and Victorian Society: Women, Class and the State*
(Cambridge, England, 1980).

29. James Colgrove, *State of Immunity: The Politics of Vaccination in Twentieth Century America* (Berkeley, CA, 2006).

30. Judith W. Leavitt, "Politics and Public Health: Smallpox in Milwaukee, 1894–
1895," *Bulletin of the History of Medicine* 50 (1976): 553–68.

31. Trask, "Vital Statistics," 2. P. Johnson, "Social Hygiene and the War," *Social
Hygiene* 4 (1918): 91–137. C. Parnall, "An Outline of the Present Scope of Public
Health Administration in Cities," *Journal of the Michigan State Medical Society* 17
(1918): 393–96. Hermann Biggs, "Compulsory Notification and Registration of
Tuberculosis. Address before the National Association for the Study and Prevention
of Tuberculosis," *Transactions of the National Tuberculosis Association* 3 (1907): 39–56.
John W. Trask, "A Digest of the Laws and Regulations of the Various States Relating
to the Reporting of Cases of Sickness," *Public Health Bulletin No. 45*, 1911.

32. Hermann Biggs, "The Public Health," *Monthly Bulletin of the Department of
Health of the City of New York* 3 (1913): 150.

33. *San Diego Union-Tribune*, June 22, 2001, B9.

34. Dan E. Beauchamp, "Community: The Neglected Tradition of Public
Health," *Hastings Center Report* 15 (1985): 30.

35. Ibid., 31.

36. William J. Novak, *The People's Welfare: Law and Regulation in Nineteenth-Century
America* (Chapel Hill, NC, 2001).

37. Leroy Parker and Robert H. Worthington, *The Law of Public Health and Safety,
and the Powers and Duties of Boards of Health* (Albany, NY, 1892). This principle was
based on a number of legal cases: *Seavey v. Preble*, 64 Me. 120 (1874); *Labrie v. Man-
chester*, 59 N.H. 120 (1879); *Farmington v. Jones*, 36 N.H. 271 (1858); *Inhabitants of
Kennebunk v. Inhabitants of Alfred*, 19 Me. 221 (1841).

38. Parker and Worthington, *The Law of Public Health*, 134.

39. Tiedemann, *State and Federal Control of Persons and Property*, quoted in G. Seymour, "A Year's Progress in Venereal Disease Control," *Social Hygiene* 5 (1919): 64.

40. Wiebe, *Search for Order*. John Higham, *Strangers in the Land: Patterns of American Nativism, 1850–1925* (New York, 1967). David H. Bennett, *The Party of Fear: From Nativist Movements to the New Right in American History* (New York, 1990). Richard Hofstadter, *The Age of Reform* (New York, 1955).

41. Hermann Biggs, *Preventive Medicine in the City of New York* (New York, 1897), 28.

42. Trask, "Vital Statistics," 5. Lawrence F. Flick, "The Duty of the Government in the Prevention of Tuberculosis," *Journal of the American Medical Association* 17 (1891): 289, 290.

43. "The Compulsory Notification and Isolation of Pulmonary Tuberculosis," *Boston Medical and Surgical Journal* 136 (January 28, 1897): 95. Daniel M. Fox, "Social Policy and City Politics: Tuberculosis Reporting in New York, 1889–1900," *Bulletin of the History of Medicine* 49 (1975): 169–95. On professional rivalry and the resistance of British physicians to becoming "employees of the state" in the context of notification, see Mooney, "Public Health versus Private Practice," 258.

44. The same is true of Great Britain. See Mooney, "Public Health versus Private Practice."

45. Ken Gormley, "One Hundred Years of Privacy," *Wisconsin Law Review*, 1992, 2, 3.

46. Ibid. Gary L. Bostwick, "Comment: A Taxonomy of Privacy: Repose, Sanctuary, and Intimate Decision," *California Law Review* 64 (1976): 1447. Tom Gerety, "Redefining Privacy," *Harvard Civil Rights-Civil Liberties Review* 12 (1977). Lawrence Tribe, *American Constitutional Law*, 2nd ed. (Mineola, NY, 1988), 1302–3.

47. "The Right to Privacy in Nineteenth Century America," *Harvard Law Review* 94 (1980–81): 1905.

48. Charles Rosenberg, "The Therapeutic Revolution," in *The Therapeutic Revolution*, ed. Morris Vogel and Charles Rosenberg (Philadelphia, 1979). Elizabeth Fee, *Disease and Discovery: A History of the Johns Hopkins School of Hygiene and Public Health, 1916–1939* (Baltimore, 1987). Norman D. Jewison, "The Disappearance of the Sick Man from Medical Cosmology: 1770–1870," *Sociology* 10 (1976). Michel Foucault, *Birth of the Clinic: An Archaeology of Medical Perception* (New York, 1973).

49. Martin Pernick, "The Patient's Role in Medical Decisionmaking: A Social History of Informed Consent in Medical Therapy," in the President's Commission for the Study of Ethical Problems in Medicine and Biomedical and Behavioral Research, *Making Health Care Decisions* (Washington, DC, 1982).

50. Bostwick, "Comment," 1456–57. See Brandeis's amplifications of his 1890 article with Warren in *Olmstead v. United States* 277 U.S. 478 (1928).

51. Parker and Worthington, *The Law of Public Health*.

52. Samuel Warren and Louis Brandeis, "The Right to Privacy," *Harvard Law Review* 3 (1890): 214.

53. Carl F. Ameringer, *State Medical Boards and the Politics of Public Protection* (Baltimore, 1999), 22–23, 25. See also John A. Harrington, "The Instrumental Uses of Autonomy: A Review of AIDS Law and Policy in Europe," *Social Science and Medicine* 55 (2002).

54. John Bell and Issac Hays, "Code of Ethics (1847)," in Robert B. Baker et al.,

eds., *The American Medical Ethics Revolution: How the AMA's Code of Ethics Has Transformed Physicians' Relationships to Patients, Professionals, and Society* (Baltimore, 1999), 324.

55. Donald E. Konold, *A History of American Medical Ethics, 1847–1912* (Madison, WI, 1962), 46. See also Ruth Faden and Tom Beauchamp, in collaboration with Nancy M. P. King, *A History and Theory of Informed Consent* (New York, 1986). W. Robertson, *Medical Conduct and Practice: A Guide to the Ethics of Medicine* (London, 1921).

56. Robertson, *Medical Conduct and Practice.* On the relation of servants to the household, see Laslett, "Family as a Public and Private Institution," 484–85.

57. Jay Katz, *The Silent World of Doctor and Patient* (New York, 1984). See also Flaherty, *Privacy in Colonial New England,* 56, 61.

58. American Medical Association, *Principles of Medical Ethics* (1912), in Baker et al., *American Medical Ethics Revolution,* 346. Konold, *History of American Medical Ethics.* Robert M. Gellman, "Prescribing Privacy," *North Carolina Law Review* 62 (1984): 7.

59. Gellman, "Prescribing Privacy," 6.

60. Ibid., 269. See also Mooney, "Public Health versus Private Practice," 256.

61. Likewise in Great Britain, physicians sought to have reporting requirements "apply only to the 'sanitarily dangerous and reckless classes . . . while the respectable artisan and small shopkeeper, as well as the classes above them, would be protected from the annoyance of an inquisitorial surveillance and domiciliary visitation.'" Mooney, "Public Health versus Private Practice," 264.

62. Edwin Emery and Michael C. Emery, *The Press and America: An Interpretive History of the Mass Media,* 3rd ed. (Englewood Cliffs, NJ, 1972), 349–55, Gormley, "One Hundred Years of Privacy," 5–6. Sidney Kobre, *The Yellow Press and Gilded Age Journalism* (Tallahassee, FL, 1964), 1. Frank L. Mott, *American Journalism: A History, 1690–1960,* 3rd ed. (New York, 1962), 25–26, 70–77. "The Right to Privacy in Nineteenth Century America," 1909.

63. Mott, *American Journalism,* 444.

64. Biggs, "Public Health," 150.

65. "In the Matter of the Application of William H. Allen, Appellant, to Examine Certain Records on File in the Department of Health in the City of New York, Respondent," 205 N.Y. 158; 98 N.E 470 (1912).

66. Haven Emerson, *A Monograph on the Epidemic of Poliomyelitis [Infantile Paralysis] in New York City in 1916. Based on the Official Reports of the Bureaus of the Department of Health New York* (New York, 1917). F. Cope, "A Model Municipal Department," *American Journal of Sociology* 9 (1904).

67. Shelby M. Harrison, *Community Action through Surveys* (New York, 1916), 3–4.

68. Harriett M. Bartlett, "The Social Survey and the Charity Organization Movement," *American Journal of Sociology* 34 (1928): 332–33. Morone, *Democratic Wish,* 109.

69. Emerson, *A Monograph on the Epidemic of Poliomyelitis,* 234–35.

70. Naomi Rogers, *Dirt and Disease: Polio before FDR* (New Brunswick, NJ, 1992), 54, 41.

71. *New York Times,* May 20, 1928, 22.

72. *New York Times,* April 10, 1941, 25.

73. *New York Times,* June 3, 1931, 33. *New York Times,* December 2, 1924, 44. See also Judith W. Leavitt, *Typhoid Mary: Captive to the Public's Health* (Boston, 1996).

74. "Importance of Communicable Disease Reports," *Northwest Medical Journal* 17 (1918): 216–17. "What Diseases Should Be Reported," *American Journal of Public Health* 9 (1919): 451. Even so, even diphtheria reporting was difficult to achieve in some locales. "Public Health," *Illinois Medical Journal* 19 (1911): 125.

75. "First Report of the Committee on Municipal Health Department Practice of the American Public Health Association," *American Journal of Public Health* 12 (1922): 7–15.

76. Carl E. McCombs, "Reporting Communicable Diseases: A Physician's Point of View," *American Journal of Public Health* 11 (1921): 624. Walter M. Brunet and Mary S. Edwards, "A Survey of Venereal Disease Prevalence in Detroit," *Social Hygiene* 8 (1927): 206–7. Joseph S. Lawrence, "Administrative Progress in Combating Venereal Disease," *Social Hygiene* 10 (1924): 33–40. "Venereal Disease Reports in Illinois," *Social Hygiene* 11 (1925): 180–81. Disease reporting also varied by the age of the patient, with the likelihood of reporting increasing with the age of the patient. Edgar Sydenstricker, "Completeness of Reporting of Measles, Whooping Cough, and Chicken Pox at Different Ages," *Public Health Reports* 44 (1929): 1537–43.

77. J. L. Bowman, "The Medical Profession and Notifiable Diseases: Why Reports Should Be Made," *Public Health Reports* 35 (1920): 2503.

78. William Edler, "The Reporting of Venereal Diseases by Physicians," *Journal of the American Medical Association* 74 (1920): 1764. See also "The Compulsory Notification of Venereal Diseases," *Journal of the American Medical Association* 31 (1898): 1120.

79. *State v. Pierce,* 87 Vt. 144; 88 A. 740 (1913). See also *Michigan v. Brady,* 90 Mich. 459 (1892), *Michigan v. Shurly,* 131 Mich. 177 (1902), *Johnson v. District of Columbia,* 27 App. D.C. 259 (1906), *Chicago v. Craig,* 172 Ill. App. 126 (1912), and *Pennsylvania Commonwealth v. Evans,* 59 Pa. Super. 607 (1915), described in "Review of Court Decisions Pertaining to Morbidity Reports," *Public Health Reports* 43 (1928): 3369–77.

80. *State v. Wordin,* 56 Conn. 216 (1887), 226.

81. *State v. Boone,* 95 *Northeastern Reporter:* 924 (1911), 925, 927. See also "Notification of Infectious Diseases," *Journal of the American Medical Association* 18 (1899): 399, and George F. Shrady, "The Registration of Contagious Diseases," *Medical Record* 31 (1887): 1.

82. "Notification of Contagious Diseases," *Journal of the American Medical Association* 30 (1898): 385. See also "Voluntary vs. Compulsory Notification of Contagious Disease," *Journal of the American Medical Association* 33 (1899): 490, and Henry B. Baker, "Compulsory Notification of Tuberculosis," *Journal of the American Medical Association* 33 (1899): 742.

83. *Johnson v. District of Columbia,* 27 App. D.C. 259 (1906).

84. *Jones v. Stanko,* 160 N.E. 456 (1928).

85. *Michigan v. Shurly,* 91 N.W. 139 (1902), 14.

86. Hibbert Hill, as quoted in McCombs, "Reporting Communicable Diseases," 624–25.

87. "The Value of Certain Inquiries on Venereal Disease Care Reports: A Study

of 8,413 Case Reports in Indiana," *Public Health Reports* 36 (1921): 2257, 2270. McCombs, "Reporting Communicable Diseases," 624.

88. Quoted in Eric Foner, *Give Me Liberty: An American History* (New York, 2005), 805.

89. Ibid., 784–85.

90. Gary Gerstle, "The Protean Character of American Liberalism," *American Historical Review* 99 (1994): 1053.

91. Gormley, "One Hundred Years of Privacy," 10.

92. *Olmstead et al. v. United States*, 277 U.S. 438 (1928), p. 1 of Brandeis dissent.

93. Ibid., p. 3 of Brandeis dissent.

94. Foner, *Give Me Liberty*, 787.

95. Margaret Marsh, *Surburban Lives* (New Brunswick, NJ, 1990), 131–32.

96. Jerome J. Hanus and Harold C. Reylea, "A Policy Assessment of the Privacy Act of 1974," *American University Law Review* 25 (1976): 563–64.

97. William Douglas, *The Right of the People* (New York, 1958).

98. Ibid., 104. *Frank v. Maryland*, 359 U.S. 360 (1959).

99. *Frank v. Maryland*, 359 U.S. 360.

100. *Watkins v. United States*, 354 U.S. 178 (1957).

101. William Whyte, *The Organization Man* (New York, 1956). C. Wright Mills, *White Collar: The American Middle Classes* (New York, 1951).

102. *Eaton v. Price*, 364 U.S. 263 (1960), 5, quoting *Cooper v. Aaron*, 358 U.S. 1 (1958), 4–5.

103. Alexander D. Langmuir Papers, Box 1, Folder 2, JHU Honorary Degree Folder, Alan Mason Chesney Medical Archives, the Johns Hopkins Medical Institutions, Baltimore.

104. Alexander D. Langmuir, "The Potentialities of Biological Warfare against Man," *Public Health Reports* 66 (1951). Alexander D. Langmuir, "Biological Warfare Defense," *American Journal of Public Health* 42 (1952).

105. Alexander D. Langmuir Papers, Alan Mason Chesney Medical Archives, the Johns Hopkins Medical Institutions, Baltimore, Miscellaneous Materials from CDC Personal.

106. *Camara v. City and County of San Francisco*, 387 U.S. 523 (1967).

107. Hanus and Reylea, "Policy Assessment," 565–66.

108. *Osborne v. United States, Lewis v. United States, Hoffa v. United States*, 385 U.S. 323; 87 S. Ct. 439 (1966).

109. Vance Packard, *The Naked Society* (New York, 1964), 41, 5.

110. Myron Brenton, *The Privacy Invaders* (New York, 1964), 12, 13.

111. Hanus and Reylea, "Policy Assessment," 565, 566.

112. Packard, *Naked Society*. Brenton, *The Privacy Invaders*. Alan Westin, *Privacy and Freedom* (New York, 1967).

113. Priscilla M. Regan, *Legislating Privacy: Technology, Social Values, and Public Policy* (Chapel Hill, NC, 1995), 82.

114. Hanus and Reylea, "Policy Assessment," 567.

115. See also "Project: Government Information and the Rights of Citizens," *Michigan Law Review* 73 (1974–75): 1315.

116. *Wall Street Journal*, June 27, 1975, 1.

117. "Project: Government Information," 1223–24.

118. Ibid., 1224.

119. Westin, *Privacy and Freedom*, 57.

120. Ibid., 382. Packard, *Naked Society*, 94, 145.

121. There was even some indication of concern that too great an emphasis on medical privacy could undermine other important social interests. In 1961, for example, the authoritative legal treatise *On Evidence* argued for retracting the doctrine of medical "privilege." While many states had protected encounters between physician and patient from court proceedings, as they did exchanges between lawyers and their clients, "the practical employment of the privilege has come to mean little but the suppression of useful truth." "Physician-Patient Privilege," in John Henry Wigmore, *Evidence at Trials in Common Law*, 1st rev. ed. (Boston, 1961), 831.

122. William Phillips, Kurt Gorwitz, and Anita K. Bahn, "Electronic Maintenance of Case Registers," *Public Health Reports* 77 (1962): 503–4. See also Samuel Milham, "Congenital Malformation Surveillance System Based on Vital Records," *Public Health Reports* 78 (1963): 448.

123. "Sees No Safety in Glib Use of Indiscriminate Numbers," *Public Health Reports* 78 (1963): 145.

124. Department of Health, Education, and Welfare, "Records, Computers and the Rights of Citizens: Report of the Secretary's Advisory Committee on Automated Personal Data Systems" (Washington, DC, 1973), http://aspe.os.dhhs.gov/datacncl/1973privacy/c3.htm, accessed December 2, 2004.

125. Ibid.

126. Regan, *Legislating Privacy*, 81.

127. "Project: Government Information," 1223, 1293.

128. Tribe, *American Constitutional Law*, 1311.

129. Regan, *Legislating Privacy*, 76. See also 75, 76–77. Hanus and Reylea, "Policy Assessment," 573–74.

130. *Privacy Act of 1974*, sec. p, no. 3, www.usdoj.gov/oip/privstat.htm, accessed December 2, 2004.

131. "Project: Government Information," 1304, 1305. The Privacy Act merely limits data collection to information which is "relevant and necessary to accomplish a purpose of the agency required to be accomplished by statute or by executive order of the President."

132. Ibid., 1293, 1302, 1307.

133. Assistant Secretary for Planning and Evaluation and Secretary of the U.S. Department of Health and Human Services, *Personal Privacy in an Information Society: The Report of the Privacy Protection Study Commission*, chapter 7, "Record-Keeping in the Medical-Care Relationship," July 1977, http://aspe.hhs.gov/datacncl/1977privacy/c7.htm, accessed December 2, 2004.

134. Nancy Tomes, "Patients or Health-Care Consumers? Why the History of Contested Terms Matters," in *Health Care History and Policy in the United States*, ed. Rosemary A. Stevens, Charles E. Rosenberg, and Lawton R. Burns (New Brunswick, NJ, 2006).

135. Boston Women's Health Collective, *Our Bodies, Ourselves* (Boston, 1969), 1.

136. Ibid., 253.

137. David J. Rothman, *Strangers at the Bedside: A History of How Law and Bioethics Transformed Medical Decision Making* (New York, 1991), 144.

138. Tribe, *American Constitutional Law*, 1308–9.

139. David T. Courtwright, *Dark Paradise: A History of Opiate Addiction in America* (Cambridge, MA, 2001), 163.

140. *Roe v. Ingraham*, 403 F. Supp. 931 (1975).

141. *Whalen v. Roe*, 429 U.S. 589; 97 S. Ct. 869; 51 L. Ed. 2d 64 (1977).

142. *Roe v. Ingraham*, 403 F. Supp. 931.

143. Ronald Bayer, "Drug Addiction and Liberal Social Policy: The Limits of Reform" (Ph.D. diss., University of Chicago, 1976), 293–99.

144. *Roe v. Ingraham*, 357 F. Supp. 1217.

145. Ibid.

146. Ibid., 480 F.2d 102.

147. David F. Musto, *The American Disease* (New York, 1987), 258.

148. *Roe v. Ingraham*, 403 F. Supp. 931.

149. Ibid.

150. *Whalen v. Roe*, 429 U.S. 589; 97 S. Ct. 869; 51 L. Ed. 2d 64.

151. Ibid.

152. Nor had the psychiatry section of the New York State Medical Society joined in the suit.

153. *Whalen v. Roe*, 429 U.S. 589; 97 S. Ct. 869; 51 L. Ed. 2d 64.

154. Brennan, concurring opinion, *Whalen v. Roe*, 429 U.S. 589; 97 S. Ct. 869; 51 L. Ed. 2d 64.

CHAPTER 2

1. A noteworthy exception is Susan Craddock, *City of Plagues: Disease, Poverty, and Deviance in San Francisco* (Minneapolis, 2000), 12.

2. Sheila M. Rothman, *Living in the Shadow of Death: Tuberculosis and the Social Experience of Illness in American History* (New York, 1994). Barbara Bates, *Bargaining for Life: A Social History of Tuberculosis, 1876–1938* (Philadelphia, 1992). Linda Bryder, *Below the Magic Mountain: A Social History of Tuberculosis in Twentieth-Century Britain* (Oxford, 1988). Barron Lerner, *Contagion and Confinement: Controlling Tuberculosis along the Skid Road* (Baltimore, 1998).

3. "Tuberculosis and Boards of Health," *New York Medical Journal* 59 (1894): 277.

4. Lawrence F. Flick, "The Duty of the Government in the Prevention of Tuberculosis," *Journal of the American Medical Association* 17 (1891): 287–90.

5. "Special Meeting of the College of Physicians and Surgeons of Philadelphia, Held Jan. 12, 1894, the President, S. Weir Mitchell, MD, Chair, on the Registration of Tuberculosis," *Journal of the American Medical Association* 23 (1894): 263.

6. Ibid., 265.

7. Hermann Biggs, "The Registration of and Preventive Measures against Tuberculosis," *Boston Medical and Surgical Journal* 130 (1894): 322.

8. "Special Meeting," 224.

9. C.-E. A. Winslow, *The Life of Hermann Biggs* (Philadelphia, 1929), 138–39. "Special Meeting," 264, 223–25. Hermann Biggs, "To Rob Consumption of Its Terrors," *Forum*, 1894, 760.

10. "Special Meeting," 223. Similar arguments were proffered in Boston six years later. "Compulsory Notification of Tuberculosis," *Boston Medical and Surgical Journal* 142 (1900): 575–76.

11. "Special Meeting," 225.

12. Ibid., 222. See also Biggs, "Preventive Measures against Tuberculosis," 322.

13. Quoted in S. Knopf, *A History of the National Tuberculosis Association* (New York, 1922), 6.

14. Hermann Biggs and John Henry Huddleston, "The Sanitary Supervision of Tuberculosis as Practised by the New York City Board of Health," *American Journal of Medical Sciences* 109 (1895): 18.

15. Order of the Board of Health, February 13, 1894, as reprinted in ibid., 20.

16. New York City Department of Health, *Annual Report of the Department of Health of the City of New York for the Calendar Year 1894* (New York, 1895), 93.

17. Ibid., 94. Biggs, "Preventive Measures against Tuberculosis," 322.

18. Winslow, *Life of Hermann Biggs*, 134. *New York Times*, March 19, 1894, 9.

19. Hermann Biggs, "Compulsory Notification and Registration of Tuberculosis," address before the National Association for the Study and Prevention of Tuberculosis, *Transactions of the National Tuberculosis Association* 3 (1907): 8–9.

20. Quoted in Winslow, *Life of Hermann Biggs*, 135.

21. Hermann Biggs et al., "Announcements: The Status of Pulmonary Tuberculosis in New York City, and Its Control by the Board of Health," *Medical News* 70 (1897): 126.

22. Ibid.

23. "Tuberculosis and Health Department Regulations at New York," *Journal of the American Medical Association* 28 (1897): 616, citing a report in the *Medical Review* for February of that year.

24. Daniel Fox, "Social Policy and City Politics: Tuberculosis Reporting in New York, 1889–1900," *Bulletin of the History of Medicine* 49 (1975): 169–95.

25. "Importance of Communicable Disease Reports," *Northwest Medical Journal* 17 (1918): 216–17. "What Diseases Should Be Reported," *American Journal of Public Health* 9 (1919): 451. Even so, even diphtheria reporting was difficult to achieve in some locales. "Public Health," *Illinois Medical Journal* 19 (1911): 125.

26. Edward O. Otis, "The Significance of the Tuberculosis Crusade and Its Future," *Journal of Social Science* 42 (1904): 125. Samuel Hopkins Adams, "Tuberculosis: The Real Race Suicide," *McClure's Magazine* 24 (1905): 234.

27. Barbara Gutmann Rosenkrantz, "Dubos and Tuberculosis, Master Teachers," in *The White Plague*, by Rene Dubos and Jean Dubos (New Brunswick, NJ, 1987), xiv–xv n. 1.

28. Rothman, *Living in the Shadow of Death*, 184. In Philadelphia the mortality rate in 1870 was 350 per 100,000 and had dropped to less than 200 per 100,000 by 1910. By 1925 the mortality rate was less than 100 per 100,000. Bates, *Bargaining for Life*, 315, 338.

29. George Fowler, as quoted in Hermann Biggs, "Preventive Medicine in the City of New York," *Medical News* 71 (1897): 323.

30. Lawrence F. Flick, "Registration of Tuberculosis," *Modern Medicine, Surgery and Sanitation* 29 (1900): 49.

31. Biggs, "To Rob Consumption," 761.

32. "Compulsory Reporting of Cases of Pulmonary Tuberculosis," *Medical Record* 51 (1897): 459. See also S. A. Knopf, "The Compulsory Reporting of Tuberculosis," *New York Medical Journal* 70 (1899): 443.

33. Flick, "Registration of Tuberculosis," 49.

34. See physician testimony reported by Knopf, "Compulsory Reporting of Tuberculosis," 443.

35. Hermann Biggs, "Sanitary Measures for the Prevention of Tuberculosis in New York City and Their Results," *Journal of the American Medical Association* 34 (1902): 1635.

36. Hermann Biggs, "Compulsory Notification and Registration of Tuberculosis," *Transactions of the National Tuberculosis Association* 3 (1907): 42 (emphasis added).

37. John Shaw Billings, "Discussion on Compulsory Notification and Registration of Tuberculosis," *Transactions of the National Tuberculosis Association* 3 (1907): 15.

38. George F. Shrady, "The Registration of Contagious Diseases," *Medical Record* 31 (1887): 1. On physician support for the registration of acute infections, see John W. Trask, "Vital Statistics: A Discussion of What They Are and Their Uses in Public Health Administration," *Public Health Reports*, Supplement No. 12 (1914).

39. George F. Shrady, "The Health Board and Compulsory Reports," *Medical Record* 51 (1897): 126. "Regular Meeting of the Philadelphia County Medical Society, November 14, 1900," *Journal of the American Medical Association* 35 (1900): 1426.

40. "Compulsory Reporting of Cases of Pulmonary Tuberculosis," 462.

41. Winslow, *Life of Hermann Biggs*, 146.

42. Ibid.

43. Quoted in ibid, 145–46. "The Registration of Tuberculosis," *Medical News* 77 (1900): 820.

44. Knopf, *A History of the National Tuberculosis Association*, 7–9. Historians disagree about whether this legislative battle was largely fabricated or real. Fox, "Social Policy and City Politics." Elizabeth Fee and Evelyn M. Hammonds, "Science, Politics, and the Art of Persuasion: Promoting the New Scientific Medicine in New York City," in *Hives of Sickness: Public Health and Epidemics in New York City*, ed. David Rosner (New Brunswick, NJ, 1995).

45. "The Compulsory Notification and Isolation of Pulmonary Tuberculosis," *Boston Medical and Surgical Journal* 136 (1897): 318.

46. Cited in Winslow, *Life of Hermann Biggs*, 148.

47. Hermann Biggs, "The Registration of Tuberculosis. Read before the Philadelphia County Medical Society November 14, 1900," *Philadelphia Medical Journal on Tuberculosis* 6 (1900): 1027.

48. Arthur R. Reynolds, "Notification of Tuberculosis," *Journal of the American Medical Association* 35 (1900): 1017–18.

49. John S. Fulton, "Comments of Dr. John S. Fulton, Baltimore, on Hermann M. Biggs, 'Compulsory Notification and Registration of Tuberculosis,' An Address before the National Association for the Study and Prevention of Tuberculosis," *Transactions of the National Tuberculosis Association* 3 (1907): 16.

50. Eugene H. Porter, "Comments of Dr. Eugene H. Porter, Albany, on Hermann M. Biggs, 'Compulsory Notification and Registration of Tuberculosis,' An Address before the National Association for the Study and Prevention of Tuberculosis," *Transactions of the National Tuberculosis Association* 3 (1907): 15.

51. *New York Times*, March 30, 1913, SM10.

52. *New York Times*, January 9 1905, 6.

53. *New York Times,* March 30, 1913, SM10. See also *New York Times,* January 23, 1998, 5, and Adams, "Tuberculosis," 234.

54. *New York Times,* January 26, 1898, 6. *New York Times,* January 23, 1998, 5.

55. *New York Times,* November 28, 1897, 8.

56. Winslow, *Life of Hermann Biggs,* 148.

57. Fulton, "Comments of Fulton," 7. See also "Compulsory Notification of Tuberculosis," *Journal of the American Medical Association* 33 (1899): 742.

58. "Tuberculosis and Boards of Health," 277.

59. W. Baldwin, "Compulsory Reports and Registration of Tuberculosis in the United States," *New York Medical Journal* 84 (1906): 1121. R. Smith, "Municipal Control of Tuberculosis," *Northwest Medicine* 5 (1913): 75–76. "Peoria Begins a Crusade against Tuberculosis," *Illinois Medical Journal* 6 (1904): 397.

60. Sheila Rothman, for example, has focused on the coercive, punitive system of treatment and isolation facilities Biggs created in New York City shortly after the turn of the century. She argues that the institutional organization and philosophy were fundamentally flawed. Those institutions, created to hold recalcitrant, intractable infectious patients by force, were, in her analysis, "too prison-like to be hospitals and too hospital-like to be prisons." Rothman, "The Sanatorium Experience: Myths and Realities," in *The Tuberculosis Revival: Individual Rights and Social Obligations in a Time of AIDS* (New York, 1992), 73. See also Craddock, *City of Plagues,* 245.

61. "Resolution to Medical Societies," in *Transactions of the Second Annual Conference of State and Territorial Health Officers with the United States Public Health and Marine-Hospital Service* (Washington, DC, 1904), 50.

62. *Washington Post,* June 3, 1902, 9.

63. Winslow, *Life of Hermann Biggs,* 134.

64. John Shaw Billings, "The Registration and Sanitary Supervision of Pulmonary Tuberculosis in New York City," *Department of Health of the City of New York Monograph Series* 1 (New York, 1912), 44.

65. Ibid., 39. See also Craddock, *City of Plagues,* 244.

66. Billings, "Registration and Supervision of Tuberculosis," 14, 86.

67. Ibid., 17–18.

68. Ibid., 20.

69. New York City Department of Health, *Annual Report of the Department of Health of the City of New York for the Years 1910–1911* (New York, 1912), 66.

70. Resolutions of the Board of Health, March 30, 1910, as reprinted in Billings, "Registration and Supervision of Tuberculosis." See also pp. 21–22.

71. Ibid. and 21–22. New York City Department of Health, *Annual Report for 1910–1911,* 72.

72. Billings, "Registration and Supervision of Tuberculosis," 22. New York City Department of Health, *Annual Report for 1910–1911,* 72.

73. New York City Department of Health, *Annual Report for 1910–1911,* 72.

74. Hermann Biggs, "The Administrative Control of Tuberculosis," *Medical News* 84 (1904): 341.

75. Biggs and Huddleston, "Sanitary Supervision of Tuberculosis," 26. See also Smith, "Municipal Control of Tuberculosis," 75–76.

76. Frances Perkins, cited in David Rosner, "Commentary: C. E.-A. Winslow: Sci-

entist, Activist, and Theoretician of the American Public Health Movement throughout the First Half of the Twentieth Century," *Journal of Public Health Policy* 19 (1998): 151.

77. Samuel Roberts, *Infectious Fear: Tuberculosis, Public Health, and the Logic of Race and Illness in Baltimore, Maryland, 1880–1930* (Ph.D. diss., Princeton University, 2002), 282–85.

78. Ibid., 232–33.

79. Ibid., 6–8. See also G. Farrar Patton, "Vital Statistics of Tuberculosis in Louisiana," *New Orleans Medical and Surgical Journal* 55 (1902): 235–36.

80. Tera Hunter, *To 'Joy My Freedom: Southern Black Women's Lives and Labors after the Civil War* (Cambridge, MA, 1997), 189–93.

81. Ibid., 204. See also 205–10.

82. Nancy Tomes, *The Gospel of Germs: Men, Women, and the Microbe in American Life* (Cambridge, MA, 1998), 222.

83. Nayan Shah, *Contagious Divides: Epidemics and Race in San Francisco's Chinatown* (Berkeley, CA, 2001), 68–69. Amy Fairchild, *Science at the Borders: Immigrant Medical Inspection and the Shaping of the Modern Industrial Labor Force* (Baltimore, 2003), 32, 180–82, 219–20. As opposed to Shah, Susan Craddock takes a very different though hardly uncritical view of public health and race during late nineteenth and early twentieth centuries, noting that while the Chinese were blamed for many things, TB was not one of them. To be sure, health officials were aware of the high rates of morbidity and mortality among both the Chinese and African American populations in San Francisco. Nonetheless the "tuberculous body," Craddock argues, "was not racialized in social and medical discourses." The city's minority populations were not demonized but ignored: "Little was ever done about this problem in terms of intensified public health intervention, better hospital care, or material assistance." Craddock, *City of Plagues*, 40, 193.

84. Emily Abel, *Tuberculosis and the Politics of Exclusion: A History of Public Health and Migration in Los Angeles* (New Brunswick, NJ, in press).

85. Hermann Biggs, "The Registration of Tuberculosis," *Journal of the American Medical Association* 35 (1900): 1414.

86. Bertram H. Waters, "The Importance of Registration, Special Dispensaries, and Early Diagnosis of Pulmonary Tuberculosis," *New York State Journal of Medicine* 8 (May 1908): 243. Biggs, "Registration of Tuberculosis," 559–60. "Tuberculosis," *Washington Post*, February 4, 1903, 6.

87. "American Medical Association, Committee on Public Health, Resolution to the Officers and Members of State and County Medical Societies," in *Transactions of the Second Conference*, 70.

88. Ibid., 50.

89. "Control of Tuberculosis," *New York State Journal of Medicine* 4 (1904): 358.

90. Billings, "Registration and Supervision of Tuberculosis," 12.

91. Biggs, "Compulsory Notification," address, 7.

92. New York City Department of Health, *Annual Report for 1894*, 93. Biggs and Huddleston, "Sanitary Supervision of Tuberculosis," 25. Biggs, "Compulsory Notification," 43. See also Billings, "Registration and Supervision of Tuberculosis," 11.

93. Fulton, "Comments of Fulton," 16–17.

94. Biggs, "Sanitary Measures," 1636.

95. "Notification of Infectious Diseases," *Boston Medical and Surgical Journal* 166 (1912): 606. See also Eugene J. O'Neill, "The Need and Value of Strict Enforcement of Notification in Cases of Suspected and Diagnosed Pulmonary Tuberculosis," *Illinois Medical Journal* 39 (1921): 24.

96. Billings, "Registration and Supervision of Tuberculosis," 39.

97. Biggs, "Compulsory Notification," address, 9.

98. Ibid., 10. New York City Department of Health, *Annual Report for 1894*, 98–99.

99. Biggs, "Sanitary Measures," 1636.

100. Biggs, "Compulsory Notification," address, 10.

101. Billings, "Registration and Supervision of Tuberculosis," 12.

102. New York City Department of Health, *Annual Report of the Department of Health of the City of New York for the Calendar Year 1918* (New York, 1919), 62–63.

103. Billings, "Registration and Supervision of Tuberculosis," 44, table 4.

104. John Shaw Billings, "Comments of Dr. John S. Billings Jr., New York, on Hermann M. Biggs, 'Compulsory Notification and Registration of Tuberculosis,' An Address before the National Association for the Study and Prevention of Tuberculosis," *Transactions of the National Tuberculosis Association* 3 (1907): 16.

105. New York City Department of Health, *Annual Report for 1918*, 63–64. See also Biggs and Huddleston, "Sanitary Supervision of Tuberculosis," 25, and Biggs, "Compulsory Notification," 16. These indicate the relatively limited information that New York City health officials required physicians to report.

106. Marshall Langton Price, "The Sanitary Control of Tuberculosis with Special Reference to the Maryland System," in *Transactions of the Sixth International Congress on Tuberculosis, Washington, D.C., September 28 through October 5, 1908* (Philadelphia, 1908), 214.

107. Billings, "Registration and Supervision of Tuberculosis," 12. The emphasis on physician rights and noninterference would persist and often be explicitly articulated. George W. Bowles, "The Venereal Problem," *Journal of the National Medical Association* 12 (1920): 14. Edmund G. Zimmer, "Why Report Venereal Disease?" *Journal of Venereal Disease Information* 20 (1939): 229.

108. Craddock, *City of Plagues*, 245.

109. Billings, "Registration and Supervision of Tuberculosis ," 55.

110. New York City Department of Health, *Advice for Patients Suffering from Pulmonary Tuberculosis (Consumption)*, Circular No. 2, reprinted in ibid., 61. On the distribution of circulars, see Biggs, "Preventive Medicine," 94.

111. New York City Department of Health, *Annual Report for 1894*, 94.

112. Biggs, "Registration of Tuberculosis," reprinted in *Philadelphia Medical Journal on Tuberculosis*, 1923, vi.

113. New York State law (May 17, 1913), chap. 559, as reported in *Public Health Reports* 28 (1913): 2261.

114. Fulton, "Comments of Fulton," 16.

115. "First Report of the Committee on Municipal Health Department Practice of the American Public Health Association," *American Journal of Public Health* 12 (1922): 14.

116. Billings, "Registration and Supervision of Tuberculosis," 9.

117. Ibid., 48. See also Biggs, "The Registration of and Preventive Measures against Tuberculosis," 322.

118. Lenore Perky Webster to H. Allen, 1907. Webster's cause was to convince the U.S. Bureau of Vital Statistics to include disabled children in the census. She persuaded Allen to urge the bureau to consent to such registration "entirely apart from the humanitarian reasons in behalf of the crippled children. It seems to be of great importance because authorities agree that from 70 to 90 percent of [these] children are tuberculus." H. Allen to Cressy L. Wilbur, May 26, 1907, Community Service Society (CSS) Archives, Box 37, Folder 19, Butler Library, Columbia University, New York. In New York the Crippled Children's Driving Fund kept a detailed registry of the children with tuberculosis of the bones that it sought to rehabilitate. "Department of Philanthropy, Charity and Social Problems," *Annals of the American Academy of Political and Social Science* 26 (1905): 778–79. See also Henry C. Wright, *Survey of Cripples in New York City* (New York, 1920).

119. Association for the Aid of Crippled Children (AACC), *1910 Annual Report*, inside front cover and p. 10, CSS Archives, Box 37, Folder 197, Butler Library, Columbia University, New York. *AACC Annual Report*, inside cover and pp. 8–9, 21–22, CSS Archives, Box 37, Folder 19, Butler Library, Columbia University, New York.

120. Letter from the Federation of Associations of Cripples (FAC) to major aid societies in New York, April 27, 1914, CSS Archives, Box 37, Folder 19, Butler Library, Columbia University, New York.

121. Harriett M. Bartlett, "The Social Survey and the Charity Organization Movement," *American Journal of Sociology* 34 (1928): 330. Arthur Dunham, "The Development of Child Welfare Programs," *Annals of the American Academy of Political and Social Science* 212 (1940): 216. Henry H. Kessler, *The Crippled and Disabled: Rehabilitation of the Physically Handicapped in the United States* (New York, 1935), 55. Frank Dekker Watson, *The Charity Organization Movement in the United States* (New York, 1971), 118–19. Harry H. Howett, "Who Cares for the Cripple?" *Hospital Social Service* 16 (1927): 545. Lillian Brandt, *The Charity Organization Society of the City of New York: Twenty-fifth Annual Report* (1907).

122. Shelby M. Harrison, *Community Action through Surveys* (New York, 1916), 8.

123. Howett, "Who Cares for the Cripple?" 545.

124. Blaine A. Brownell, "The Commercial-Civic Elite and City Planning in Atlanta, Memphis, and New Orleans in the 1920s," *Journal of Southern History* 41 (August 1975). Roosevelt quoted in Gabriel Kolko, *The Triumph of Conservatism* (New York, 1963), 196. James A. Morone, *The Democratic Wish: Popular Participation and the Limits of American Government* (Princeton, NJ, 1990), 108–15.

125. Howard S. Anders, "The Adaptation of the Public to the Principles and Practices of the Prevention of Tuberculosis," *Medical News* 87 (1905): 1154. Adams, "Tuberculosis," 234.

126. *Washington Post*, October 7, 1908, 4.

127. Billings, "Registration and Supervision of Tuberculosis," table 4, 44.

128. Emily Abel, "Taking the Cure to the Poor: Patients' Responses to New York City's Tuberculosis Program, 1894 to 1918," *American Journal of Public Health* 87, (1997): 1808–15.

129. Brandt, *Charity Organization Society*.

130. As quoted in Morone, *Democratic Wish,* 5.

131. Bartlett, "The Social Survey," 338. Watson, *Charity Organization Movement,* 145–47, 234.

132. Bartlett, "The Social Survey," 339. Watson, *Charity Organization Movement,* 122. Morone, *Democratic Wish,* 109–10.

133. Bartlett, "The Social Survey," 338. Watson, *Charity Organization Movement,* 113, 123–28.

134. New York City, for example, had a less extensive system of tracking charity relief. See Brandt, *Charity Organization Society,* 71–75.

135. Letter from the FAC to major aid societies in New York, April 27, 1914, CSS Archives, Box 37, Folder 19, Butler Library, Columbia University, New York.

136. Eva W. Rorty to the FAC, May 15, 1914, CSS Archives, Box 37, Folder 19, Butler Library, Columbia University, New York.

137. Brandt, *Charity Organization Society,* 75.

138. *New York Times,* October 13, 1912, SM5.

139. Many cities, like Peoria, Illinois, and states explicitly modeled their tuberculosis reporting and control campaigns on New York City. "Peoria Begins a Crusade," 397.

140. Baldwin, "Compulsory Reports and Registration," 1121.

141. Ibid.

142. Isadore Dyer, "The Report of Tuberculosis in New Orleans," *New Orleans Medical and Surgical Journal* 60 (1907): 147–48.

143. Association of State and Territorial Health Officers, "A Model State Law for Morbidity Reports," *Public Health Reports* 27 (1913): 1329.

144. "The Notifiable Diseases: Diseases and Conditions Required to Be Reported in the Several States," *Public Health Reports* 34 (1919): 233–38.

145. Reynolds, "Notification of Tuberculosis," 1017–18.

146. "Report on the Method of Collecting Morbidity Statistics in the State of Pennsylvania," *Public Health Reports* 21 (1906): 1534.

147. Comments of J. N. Hurty on Biggs, "Compulsory Notification," 54–55.

148. Arkansas and Utah were exceptions. Arkansas, Reg. Bd. of H., May 16, 1913, as reported in *Public Health Reports* 28 (1913): 2494. See also Manahoy City, PA, Reg. Bd. of H., July 5, 1912, as reported in *Public Health Reports* 28 (1913): 1475–76, and North Dakota, Act of March 15, 1913, chap. 59, as reported in *Public Health Reports* 28 (1913): 2808. Michigan required the patient to self-report upon receiving a diagnosis if the physician failed to do so (and in Michigan there was also considerable physician resistance to reporting). Henry B. Baker, "Compulsory Notification of Tuberculosis," *Journal of the American Medical Association* 33 (1899): 1452.

149. Ord. 82 N.S., August 21, 1912, as reported in *Public Health Reports* 28 (1913): 2883.

150. Utah, Chap. 68, Act March 9, 1913, as reported in *Public Health Reports* 28 (1913): 2452. Rothman, *Living in the Shadow of Death.*

151. Henry Sewall, "Comments of Dr. Henry Sewall, Denver, on Hermann M. Biggs, 'Compulsory Notification and Registration of Tuberculosis,' An Address before the National Association for the Study and Prevention of Tuberculosis," *Transactions of the National Tuberculosis Association* 3 (1907): 19.

152. Fulton, "Comments of Fulton," 16.

153. "Tuberculosis and Boards of Health," 277.

154. Baldwin, "Compulsory Reports and Registration," 1120.

155. Ibid., 1121.

156. Ibid., 1122.

157. Biggs, "Preventive Medicine," 326. See also *New York Times,* May 12, 1901, 21.

158. Abel, "Taking the Cure."

159. Biggs and Huddleston, "Sanitary Supervision of Tuberculosis," 26. New York City Department of Health, *Annual Report for 1894,* 99.

160. Billings, "Registration and Supervision of Tuberculosis ," 90.

161. Biggs and Huddleston, "Sanitary Supervision of Tuberculosis," 25.

162. Neil M. Cohen and Ruth Schwartz Cohen, *Our Parents' Lives: The Americanization of Eastern European Jews* (New York, 1989), 62–63. See also Chaia Sonia, *A Family's Odyssey Russian Style* (New York, 1980), 229, and Marie Jastrow, *A Time to Remember: Growing Up in New York before the Great War* (New York, 1979), 62–69.

163. Unemployment Committee of the National Federation of Settlements, *Case Studies of Unemployment* (Philadelphia, 1931), 71.

164. Bates, *Bargaining for Life,* 16–18. Georgina D. Feldberg, *Disease and Class: Tuberculosis and the Shaping of Modern North American Society* (New Brunswick, NJ, 1995), 14, 44, 3–5. Rothman, *Living in the Shadow of Death,* 13–15.

165. Rose Cohen, *Out of the Shadow: A Russian Jewish Girlhood on the Lower East Side* (Ithaca, NY, 1995), 186. See also Abraham Koosis, *Child of War and Revolution: The Memoirs of Abe Koosis* (Oakland, CA, 1984), 33, 35; and Alexander Keyssar, *Out of Work: The First Century of Unemployment in Massachusetts* (Cambridge, England, 1986), 47.

166. Cohen, *Out of the Shadow,* 195.

167. Ibid., 231, 233.

168. Billings, "Registration and Supervision of Tuberculosis," 61–64. See also Craddock, *City of Plagues,* 48–52.

CHAPTER 3

1. William Edler, "The Reporting of Venereal Diseases by Physicians," *Journal of the American Medical Association* 74 (1920): 1765.

2. Albert E. Carrier, "Venereal Prophylaxis," *Journal of the Michigan State Medical Society* 4 (1905): 416, 419.

3. Matthias Nicoll, "Recent Factors in the Control of Venereal Diseases in the State of New York," *New York State Journal of Medicine* 18 (1918): 455–56.

4. S. L. Strong, "A Symposium on the Reportability and Control of Venereal Diseases," *Boston Medical and Surgical Journal* 169 (1913): 904–6.

5. Guy L. Kiefer, "Report of the Committee on Control of Venereal Disease by a Municipality," *Journal of the American Medical Association* 57 (1911): 1053.

6. Allan Brandt, *No Magic Bullet: A Social History of Venereal Disease in the United States since 1880* (New York, 1987), 11–19.

7. Prince Morrow, "Health Department Control of Venereal Diseases," *New York Medical Journal* 94 (1911): 130. See also *New York Times,* January 18, 1914, SM10, and *Boston Daily Globe,* October 9, 1915, 3.

8. Morrow, "Health Department Control," 130.

9. Editorial, "Venereal Diseases," *New Orleans Medical and Surgical Journal* 77

(1925): 562. Isadore Dyer, "The Control of Venereal Diseases," *New Orleans Medical and Surgical Journal* 71 (1919): 382.

10. Editorial, "Venereal Diseases an Active Public Health Question," *New Orleans Medical and Surgical Journal* 71 (1918): 4.

11. Harold M. Wilson, "Venereal Control," *New Orleans Medical and Surgical Journal* 72 (1919): 63.

12. P. Johnson, "Social Hygiene and the War," *Social Hygiene* 4 (1918): 95.

13. Hermann Biggs, "The Public Health," *Monthly Bulletin of the Department of Health of the City of New York* 3 (1913): 136.

14. Ibid., 143.

15. Ibid., 150.

16. Ibid. (emphasis added). See also E. H. Marsh, "A Plan for the Prevention of Venereal Diseases in New York State," *New York Medical Journal* 197 (1918): 1178.

17. "The Medical Association of the Greater City of New York, Annual Meeting, Held January 20, 1913," *New York Medical Journal* 97 (1913): 1004. See also "Reporting Venereal and Other Diseases," *New Orleans Medical and Surgical Journal* 76 (1923): 207.

18. Edward L. Keyes, "The Effect of Venereal Disease upon the Public Health," *New York Medical Journal* 91 (1910): 9.

19. Biggs, "Public Health," 143.

20. Ibid., 135.

21. Ibid., 145.

22. Ibid., 143. Hermann Biggs, "Venereal Diseases: The Attitude of the Department of Health in Relation Thereto," *New York Medical Journal* 96 (1913): 1009.

23. Biggs, "Public Health," 144. Thomas B. Shea would also argue "the time has arrived when this disease should be controlled the same as other infectious diseases." Thomas B. Shea, "What the City Should Do to Control Syphilis," *Boston Medical and Surgical Journal* 171 (September 10, 1914): 415.

24. Biggs, "Public Health," 144. See also Biggs, "Venereal Diseases," 1009; Carrier, "Venereal Prophylaxis," 414; and *Chicago Daily Tribune*, April 18, 1922, 1.

25. Frank R. Starkey, "Prophylaxis of Venereal Disease," *Journal of the Michigan State Medical Society* 17 (1918): 84.

26. Biggs, "Venereal Diseases," 1009 (emphasis added). See also Biggs, "Public Health," 13.

27. John Shaw Billings, "The Registration and Sanitary Supervision of Pulmonary Tuberculosis in New York City," *Department of Health of the City of New York Monograph Series* 1 (New York, 1912), 20.

28. Biggs, "Public Health," 144–45.

29. Ibid., 13.

30. Biggs, "Venereal Diseases," 1011.

31. "Medical Association, Annual Meeting," 1004.

32. "The Compulsory Notification of Venereal Diseases," *Journal of the American Medical Association* 31 (1898): 1119–20.

33. Biggs, "Venereal Diseases," 1011.

34. Ibid.

35. Biggs, "Public Health," 149.

36. Ibid.

37. Morrow, "Health Department Control," 132.

38. Biggs, "Public Health," 150.

39. Ibid.

40. Laws of 1901, chap. 466, sec. 1545. See also sec. 1175.

41. "In the Matter of the Application of William H. Allen, Appellant, to Examine Certain Records on File in the Department of Health in the City of New York, Respondent," Opinion of Williard Bartlett, 205 N.Y. 147 (1912).

42. See also ibid., 205 N.Y. 158–160.

43. Ibid., 205 N.Y. 158; 98 N.E. 470.

44. Biggs, "Public Health," 150–51. See also Keyes, "The Effect of Venereal Disease upon the Public Health," 9, and "Medical Association, Annual Meeting," 1004.

45. See also Johnson, "Social Hygiene and the War," 112. Johnson indicates that these fears would persist among physicians.

46. Biggs, "Venereal Diseases," 1010.

47. Biggs, "Public Health," 144.

48. Ibid., 136.

49. New York City Department of Health, *Annual Report of the Department of Health of the City of New York for the Calendar Year 1913* (New York, 1914), 84.

50. New York City Department of Health, *Annual Report of the Department of Health of the City of New York for the Calendar Year 1918* (New York, 1919), 71.

51. New York State Department of Health, *Manual of Laws Relating to Syphilis, Gonorrhea and Chancroid: A Compilation of the Laws and Regulations* (Albany, NY, 1919), 7, 21, 35. New York State Department of Health, *Communicable Diseases: A Compilation of the Laws and Regulations* (Albany, NY, 1919), 21. New York State Department of Health, *Special Rules and Regulations: A Compilation of the Laws and Regulations* (Albany, NY, 1919), 35. Hermann Biggs, "Compulsory Notification and Registration of Tuberculosis," address before the National Association for the Study and Prevention of Tuberculosis *Transactions of the National Tuberculosis Association* 3 (1907): 6–7.

52. Louis I. Harris, "The Venereal Disease Problem," *New York Medical Journal* 109 (1919): 531–32.

53. "Enforcement of Reporting in New York City," *Social Hygiene* 9 (1923): 244.

54. Louis Dublin and Mary August Clark, "A Program for the Statistics of the Venereal Diseases," *Public Health Reports* 36 (1921): 3072. "Venereal Disease Control," *Boston Medical and Surgical Journal* 181 (1919): 187. "Venereal Diseases Regulations Explained: Observance Declared Patriotic Duty," *Illinois Medical Journal* 33 (1918): 342–43.

55. "A Model State Law for Morbidity Reports," *Public Health Reports* 27 (1913): 1323–29.

56. Timothy Newell Pfeiffer, "The Matter and Method of Social Hygiene Legislation," *Journal of Social Hygiene* 3 (1917): 69–72. See also "The Notifiable Diseases: Diseases and Conditions Required to Be Reported in the Several States," *Public Health Reports* 31 (1916): 881.

57. "Legislation to Prevent the Spread of Venereal Diseases," *Social Hygiene* 1 (1915): 635–36.

58. Vermont, act no. 218, February 3, 1913, reported in *Public Health Reports* 28 (1913): 1179.

59. Frank G. Boudreau, "The New Plan of Collecting Vital Statistics in Ohio: How the Physician Can Aid in the Health Campaign," *Ohio State Journal of Medicine*

11 (May 1915): 308. "Amended Venereal Disease Regulations," *Social Hygiene* 11 (1925): 420.

60. Johnson, "Social Hygiene and the War," 95.

61. Gertrude Seymour, "A Year's Progress in Venereal Disease Control," *Social Hygiene* 5 (1919): 61.

62. "Importance of Communicable Disease Reports," *Northwest Medical Journal* 17 (1918): 925 (emphasis added).

63. H. Cole, "How Physicians of Ohio May Aid in the Campaign against Venereal Disease," *Ohio State Journal of Medicine* 15 (1919): 68.

64. William F. Petrie, "Relation of Vital Statistics to Public Health Administration," *American Journal of Public Health* 9 (1919): 71.

65. Isadore Dyer, "Venereal Diseases an Active Public Health Question," *New Orleans Medical and Surgical Journal* 71 (1918): 4.

66. "Reporting of Venereal Diseases," *Northwest Medicine* 17 (1918): 28.

67. H. Moore, "Four Million Dollars for the Fight against Venereal Diseases," *Social Hygiene* 5 (1919): 15–26.

68. American Association for Study and Prevention of Infant Mortality, "Ninth Annual Meeting, Held in Chicago, December 5–7," *New York Medical Journal* 109 (1919): 126.

69. Cole, "How Physicians in Ohio May Aid in the Campaign," 69. "Physicians Indorse Campaign," *Social Hygiene* 5 (1919): 392.

70. "The Control of Venereal Diseases," *Public Health Reports* 33 (1918): 3.

71. Seymour, "Year's Progress," 49–50. In 1918 the PHS suggested coded reporting. See also Johnson, "Social Hygiene and the War," 100, and George E. Worthington, "Developments in Social Hygiene Legislation from 1917 to September 1, 1920," *Social Hygiene* 6 (1920): 566.

72. Seymour, "Year's Progress," 53.

73. Even in six states, including Vermont, that formally opted for name-based reporting, particularly in those that enacted legislation before the war, there was considerable flexibility that affected the nature of notification. By 1921 only seven states required the use of names for reported cases. Dublin and Clark, "Program for Statistics of Venereal Diseases," 3072. See also "The Massachusetts Venereal Disease Program," *Boston Medical and Surgical Journal* 177 (1918): 100.

74. Dublin and Clark, "Program for Statistics of Venereal Diseases," 3072. See also "Massachusetts Venereal Disease Program," 100.

75. "Control of Venereal Disease in Massachusetts," *Journal of the American Medical Association* 70 (1918): 1234. See also "The Western Australia Act for the Control of Venereal Disease," *Social Hygiene* 3 (1917): 148–49.

76. "Notification of Venereal Diseases," *Boston Medical and Surgical Journal* 179 (1918): 748.

77. "New Regulation for Venereal Disease Reports," *California State Journal of Medicine* 16 (1918): 375. Johnson, "Social Hygiene and the War," 127.

78. "Venereal Diseases Regulations Explained," 343. See also G. G. Taylor, "Approved Methods of Venereal Disease Control," *Illinois Medical Journal* 38 (1920): 120. The Illinois plan was still in effect in 1937. *Chicago Daily Tribune,* January 9, 1937, 9. *Chicago Daily Tribune,* January 8, 1937, 17.

79. "Venereal Diseases Regulations Explained," 343–44.

80. American Medical Association, resolution of June 7, 1917, reprinted in Public Health Service, *Venereal Disease Handbook for Community Leaders* (Washington, DC, 1924), 61. Johnson, "Social Hygiene and the War," 99–100.

81. "New Regulation for Venereal Disease Reports," 375. "Venereal Diseases Regulations Explained," 343.

82. H. N. Cole, "Venereal Diseases: Their Diagnosis, Treatment and Control," *Ohio State Medical Journal* 15 (1919): 783–84. See also "Resolutions of the Western Social Hygiene Association, December 10 and 11, 1917, at Tacoma, Washington," *Social Hygiene* 4 (1918): 88.

83. L. Bowman, "The Medical Profession and Notifiable Diseases: Why Reports Should Be Made," *Public Health Reports* 35 (1920): 2506–7. See also John W. Trask, "Morbidity Reports: Their Importance to the Local Health Officer and His Work," *Public Health Reports* 28 (1913): 2526, 2529. Brock C. Hampton, "Collection of Morbidity Data and Other Sanitary Information by the United States Public Health Service," *Public Health Reports* 38 (1923): 2827. Wilson, "Venereal Control," 71.

84. Taylor, "Approved Methods," 119–120, and Moore, "Four Million Dollars," 16. Henry F. Vaughan, "Municipal Control of Venereal Diseases," *Social Hygiene* 14 (1928): 544. "Notification and Control of Venereal Disease," *Social Hygiene* 15 (1929): 237. Lee K. Frankel, "The Interest of Life Insurance Companies in Social Hygiene," *Social Hygiene* 1 (1914): 62. Paul B. Brooks, "The Relation of the General Practitioner to the Prevention of Venereal Disease," *New York State Journal of Medicine* 13 (1913): 101. A similar anti-exceptionalist plea was also articulated for TB reporting: Eugene J. O'Neill, "The Need and Value of Strict Enforcement of Notification in Cases of Suspected and Diagnosed Pulmonary Tuberculosis," *Illinois Medical Journal* 39 (1921): 22.

85. George W. Bowles, "The Venereal Problem," *Journal of the National Medical Association* 12 (1920): 13.

86. J. T. Phillips, "Why Report Communicable Diseases?" *Journal of the National Medical Association* 14 (1922): 74.

87. Ibid.

88. Bowles, "The Venereal Problem," 14.

89. Ibid., 75.

90. Phillips, "Why Report Communicable Diseases?" 74.

91. Millard Knowlton, "Venereal Disease: A Problem of All Races," *Journal of the National Medical Association* 13 (1921): 24, 26–27. Phillips, "Why Report Communicable Diseases?" 74.

92. Bowles, "The Venereal Problem," 12–13.

93. Knowlton, "Venereal Disease," 28.

94. James Jones, *Bad Blood: The Tuskegee Syphilis Experiment* (New York, 1993), 94.

95. Ibid., 178.

96. Ibid., 179.

97. H. L. Dalton, "AIDS in Blackface," *Daedalus* (1989): 205–27.

98. Taylor, "Approved Methods," 120.

99. "The Notifiable Diseases: Diseases and Conditions Required to Be Reported in the Several States," *Public Health Reports* 34 (1919): 233, 238.

100. Vaughan, "Municipal Control of Venereal Diseases," 540.

101. Public Health Service, "Legal Aspects of Venereal Disease Control: Local,

State, and Federal Control," in *Venereal Disease Manual for Social and Corrective Agencies*, VD Bulletin No. 81 (Washington, DC, 1926), 37 (emphasis added).

102. "Notification and Control of Venereal Disease," 237.

103. "The Expansion and Alteration of Existing Treatment Facilities," *Transactions of the Thirty-fourth Annual Conference of State and Territorial Health Officers with the United States Public Health Service* 34 (1936): 32.

104. Charles Walter Clarke and Theodore Rosenthal, "The Private Physician's Role in the New York City Syphilis Control Activities," *Journal of the American Medical Association* 111 (1938): 2289. See also *Chicago Daily Tribune*, March 7, 1938, 11.

105. Clarke and Rosenthal, "Private Physician's Role," 2289–90.

106. H. M. Guilford, "The Wisconsin Venereal Disease Program," *Wisconsin Medical Journal* 36 (1937): 457–61. See also Public Health Service, "Legal Aspects of Venereal Disease Control," in *Venereal Disease Manual,* 38–39.

107. As quoted in Guilford, "Wisconsin Venereal Disease Program," 457–61. See also Public Health Service, "Legal Aspects of Venereal Disease Control," in *Venereal Disease Manual,* 38–39.

108. Gertrude Seymour, "A Summary of New Public Health Measures for Combating Venereal Disease," *Social Hygiene* 4 (1918): 389–94. Vaughan, "Control of Venereal Diseases," 544. John H. Stokes, "Reporting of Syphilis and Gonorrhea," *Journal of Venereal Disease Information* 7 (1926): 387–88. Brandt, *No Magic Bullet,* 88–89.

109. Stokes, "Reporting of Syphilis and Gonorrhea," 387–88. Guilford, "Wisconsin Venereal Disease Program," 457–61. See also Public Health Service, "Legal Aspects of Venereal Disease Control," in *Venereal Disease Manual,* 38–39.

110. Stokes, "Reporting of Syphilis and Gonorrhea," 387–88.

111. H. G. Irvine, "An Efficient State Program against Venereal Diseases," *Social Hygiene* 4 (1918): 457.

112. "Venereal Disease Legislation in New York," *Social Hygiene* 5 (1919): 394.

113. Dublin and Clark, "Program for Statistics of Venereal Diseases," 3075.

114. Thomas Parran, "Statistical and Public Health Research in Syphilis," *Journal of Social Hygiene* 14 (1928): 518.

115. Trask, "Morbidity Reports," 2528.

116. Parran, "Statistical and Public Health Research in Syphilis," 514. See also "A Proposed Automatic System for Tabulating Venereal Disease Morbidity, Clinical, and Epidemiological Reports," *Transactions of the Thirty-sixth Annual Conference of State and Territorial Health Officers with the United States Public Health Service* 36 (1938): 17.

117. Seymour, "Year's Progress," 65. See also Walter M. Brunet, "Venereal Disease Prevalence in the City of New York. I. Richmond County (Staten Island)," *Journal of Venereal Disease Information* 10 (1929): 232; Eugene R. Kelley, "The Massachusetts Venereal Disease Program," *Boston Medical and Surgical Journal* 178 (1918): 101; and Strong, "Symposium," 904.

118. Parran, "Research in Syphilis," 513.

119. Vaughan, "Control of Venereal Diseases," 540.

120. Wade H. Frost, "The Importance of Epidemiology as a Function of Health Departments," *American Journal of Public Health* 13 (1923): 34–35.

121. Parran, "Research in Syphilis," 515. A decade before, Prince Morrow had proposed a similar "census" in which private physicians and hospitals would report

numbers in their care but not the names or addresses of their patients. Morrow, "Health Department Control," 132.

122. Parran, "Research in Syphilis," 521.

123. E. Godfrey, "The New York State Program for Syphilis Control," *Social Hygiene* 23 (1937): 13. B. Johnson, "State Laws and Regulations of State Boards of Health Which Deal with the Venereal Diseases," *Social Hygiene* 24 (1938): 516.

124. *New York State Sanitary Code*, sec. 2.10(b) (1985). Guthrie Birkhead, Personal Communication, June 16, 2003.

125. See, for example, *Washington Post,* July 29, 1948, 11. *Washington Post,* October 8, 1948, B7.

126. Public Health Service, Venereal Disease Branch, *Field Manual* (Atlanta, July 1962), H-2–H-3.

127. W. Clark, "Find the 'Missing Million'—and Help Stamp Out Venereal Disease," *Social Hygiene* 33 (1947): 374. See also F. C. Beelman, "Private Physician Reporting of Syphilis Morbidity," *Journal of Venereal Disease Information* 38 (1947): 119–20.

128. "Change in Reporting Cases of Syphilis, Gonorrhea and Chancroid," *Connecticut Medical Journal* 7 (1943): 787–88. The District of Columbia, however, reverted to name-based reporting as early as 1926. "Reports of Venereal Disease, District of Columbia," *Journal of American Medicine,* 1926, 1842.

129. "Change in Reporting," 787–88. See also "Reports of Venereal Disease," 1842.

130. John W. Trask, "A Digest of the Laws and Regulations of the Various States Relating to the Reporting of Cases of Sickness," *Public Health Bulletin No. 45* (1911): 140.

131. Leona Baumgartner, "Syphilis Eradication—a Plan for Action Now," in *Proceedings of World Forum on Syphilis and Other Treponematoses* (Washington, DC, 1962), 28. In 1940 the death rate for syphilis was 10.7 per 100,000. By 1950 that rate had been cut in half and then halved again by 1955. Brandt, *No Magic Bullet,* 171.

132. W. H. Aufranc, "Are Venereal Diseases Disappearing? Over-all Picture throughout the Country," *American Journal of Syphilis* 35 (1951): 135–37, cited in Brandt, *No Magic Bullet,* 171.

133. Ibid., 176, 178. Baumgartner, "Syphilis Eradication," in *Proceedings of World Forum,* 28.

134. Rudolph H. Kampmeier, "Responsibility of a Physician in a Program for Syphilis Eradication," in *Proceedings of World Forum,* 72. Public Health Service, *Field Manual,* H-3. "World Forum on Syphilis," *Public Health Reports* 78 (1963): 300. Brandt, *No Magic Bullet,* 177.

135. "Tenth Annual Joint Statement of the Association of State and Territorial Health Officers, the American Venereal Disease Association, and the American Social Health Association," 1963, Association of State and Territorial Health Officers Archives, Box 2, American Social Health Association Folder, National Library of Medicine, Bethesda, MD. For somewhat different annual statistics, see http://www.cdc.gov/std/stats/syphilis2.htm#fig24, accessed May 11, 2006.

136. Public Health Service, Venereal Disease Branch chief's statement, "Control of Venereal Diseases," December 1963, p. 1, part 1, Record Group 442, Box 108374, Program Planning Conference Folder, National Archives and Records Administra-

tion, Atlanta. *New York Times,* March 26, 1964, 37. *New York Times,* April 5, 1964, E7. *New York Times,* April 5, 1965, 33.

137. E. Gurney Clark, "Needs for Further Progress in Venereal Disease Control," *The Journal Lancet* 80 (1960): 3.

138. William J. Brown, Thomas F. Sellers, and Evan W. Thomas, "Challenge to the Private Physician in the Epidemiology of Syphilis," *Journal of the American Medical Association* 171 (1959): 389–93.

139. John W. Lentz, "Health Department Responsibilities to Practicing Physicians," in *Proceedings of World Forum,* 55–56.

140. Baumgartner, "Syphilis Eradication," in *Proceedings of World Forum,* 29–30. See also Public Health Service, *The Eradication of Syphilis: Task Force Report of the Surgeon General of the Public Health Service on Syphilis Control in the United States* (Washington, DC, 1962).

141. Baumgartner, "Syphilis Eradication," in *Proceedings of World Forum,* 27.

142. Ibid., 30. See also Clark, "Needs for Further Progress," 3.

143. Public Health Service, "Control of Venereal Diseases," p. 2, part 1, p. 4, part 2. See also Theodore J. Bauer to surgeon and chief, Bureau of State Services, Re: "The Eradication of Syphilis," January 12, 1962, Record Group 442, Box 105232, Eradication of Syphilis Folder, National Archives and Records Administration, Atlanta; and Russell Havlak, e-mail, March 20, 2003. Document in possession of authors.

144. "VD Case Reporting," *Public Health Reports* 78 (1963): 896. "Task Force Reports on Syphilis Control," *Public Health Reports* 77 (1962): 458. "M.D.'s in Solo Practice Remiss in Reporting VD," *Public Health Reports* 78 (1963): 130. William J. Brown, "The Public Health Service Venereal Disease Program," *Archives of Environmental Health* 13 (1966): 373–74. Arthur C. Curtis, "National Survey of Venereal Disease Treatment," *Journal of the American Medical Association* 186 (1963): 373–74. Roy L. Cleere et al., "Physicians' Attitudes toward Venereal Disease Reporting," *Journal of the American Medical Association* 202 (1967): 941–46. "Tenth Annual Joint Statement of the Association of State and Territorial Health Officers, the American Venereal Disease Association, and the American Social Health Association," 1963, Association of State and Territorial Health Officers Archives, pp. 2–3, 6, Box 2, American Social Health Association Folder, National Library of Medicine, Bethesda, MD.

145. Edward F. Tuerk, "Legal Basis for Syphilis Control," in *Proceedings of World Forum,* 86. Suzanne Dandoy and Edward M. McKenna, "Laboratory Reporting of Syphilis Reactors in the Los Angeles Program," *Public Health Reports* 79 (1964): 1016.

146. "World Forum on Syphilis," 303. "APHA Western Branch Report: Venereal Disease Control," *Public Health Reports* 77 (1962): 1000–1.

147. Dandoy and McKenna, "Laboratory Reporting of Syphilis Reactors," 1019. See also Brown, "Venereal Disease Program," 374.

148. Public Health Service, "A Follow-Up Report of the Surgeon General's Task Force on Syphilis Control," Atlanta, June 16–17, 1966, p. 7, Record Group 90, Box 334068, Public Advisory Committee on VD Control Folder, National Archives and Records Administration, Atlanta. See also American Public Health Association et al., "Today's VD Problem," February 1966, p. 33, Record Group 442, Box 318288, VD Program Informational Materials Folder, National Archives and Records Administration, Atlanta; and Alan W. Donaldson to chief, Centers for Disease Control, Washington office, and deputy chief, Communicable Disease Center, Re: Proposal

for State Legislation, March 25, 1964, Record Group 442, Box 108379, Legal 1964, Proposed Legislation Folder, National Archives and Records Administration, Atlanta.

149. Public Health Service, "Follow-Up Report," 1–2, 5–6.

150. Chief, Venereal Diseases Branch, Public Health Service, to assistant chief, Communicable Disease Center, Memorandum, February 27, 1964, and attached California administrative code, Record Group 442, Box 108379, Legal 1964, Proposed Legislation Folder, National Archives and Records Administration, Atlanta. Dandoy and McKenna, "Laboratory Reporting of Syphilis Reactors," 1016.

151. Brown, Sellers, and Thomas, "Challenge to the Private Physician," 389–93. Kampmeier, "Responsibility of a Physician," in *Proceedings of World Forum,* 1096.

152. E. Sunkes, "Health Department Responsibilities to Private and Hospital Laboratories," in *Proceedings of World Forum.* Kampmeier, "Responsibility of a Physician," in *Proceedings of World Forum.*

153. Harry Pariser, A. F. Marino, and Robert Hagler, "Health Department–Physician Partnership in Syphilis Epidemiology," *Public Health Reports* 77 (1962): 573. For similar Los Angeles procedures, see Dandoy and McKenna, "Laboratory Reporting of Syphilis Reactors," 1016–17.

154. "World Forum on Syphilis," 298.

155. Ibid., 297–98. See also American Public Health Association et al., "Today's VD Problem," 39.

156. Susan Craddock, *City of Plagues: Disease, Poverty, and Deviance in San Francisco* (Minneapolis, 2000), 245.

157. Russell Havlak, e-mail, March 25, 2003. Document in possession of authors.

158. W. A. Ketterer to Arthur C. Hollister, Memorandum, Re: Dr. Cockburn's Proposed Paper, April 8, 1963, pp. 1–2, Record Group 442, State and Community Service Division, VD Manuscript Files, Box 70A470, Cockburn, T. Aidan, Folder, National Archives and Records Administration, Atlanta.

159. American Public Health Association et al., "Today's VD Problem," 33.

160. T. Aidan Cockburn, "Comments on the Proposal to Eradicate Syphilis from the USA," transcript of proposed article, February 1963, pp. 506, Record Group 442, VD Manuscript Files, Box 70A470, Cockburn, T. Aidan, Folder, National Archives and Records Administration, Atlanta.

161. American Public Health Association et al., "Today's VD Problem," 34 (emphasis in original). See also Kampmeier, "Responsibility of a Physician," in *Proceedings of World Forum,* 75.

162. Public Health Service, *Field Manual,* PMD-6.

163. Ibid.

164. Public Health Service, "Control of Venereal Diseases," part 1, p. 1.

165. Public Health Service, Venereal Disease Branch, *Report of the Venereal Disease Branch Fiscal Year 1966,* 8, Record Group 90, Box 334069, VD Branch Report, FY 1966 Folder, National Archives and Records Administration, Atlanta.

166. Ibid.

167. Public Health Service, "Follow-Up Report," 1–2, 5–6.

168. "Serology Could Speed Syphilis Control," *Public Health Reports* 79 (1964): 236.

169. Public Health Service, "Follow-Up Report," 1–2.

170. William J. Brown, "Public Health Aspects of Syphilis," *Southern Medical Jour-*

nal 59 (1966): 640. The medical literature of this period was replete with discussions of how difficult it was for physicians, particularly older practitioners, to begin a dialogue with patients regarding their sexual contacts.

171. *New York Times,* April 5, 1965, 33.

172. American Medical Association, Proceedings, House of Delegates, San Francisco, California, June 21–25, 1964, 113th Annual Session, p. 134, American Medical Association Archives, Chicago.

173. *New York Times,* September 2, 1965, 1.

174. American Medical Association, Proceedings, House of Delegates, Chicago, Illinois, June 26–30, 1966, 115th Annual Session, 54–55.

175. American Medical Association, Proceedings, House of Delegates, Atlantic City, NJ, June 20–24, 1971, 120th Annual Session, p. 285, American Medical Association Archives, Chicago. See also American Medical Association, Proceedings, House of Delegates, New Orleans, November 28–December 1, 1971, 25th Clinical Convention, p. 133, American Medical Association Archives, Chicago; American Medical Association, Proceedings, House of Delegates, Cincinnati, November 26–29, 1972, 26th Clinical Convention, p. 287, American Medical Association Archives, Chicago; and American Medical Association, Proceedings, House of Delegates, Anaheim, December 2–5, 1973, 27th Clinical Convention, p. 97, American Medical Association Archives, Chicago.

176. "Eradication of Syphilis: The Missing Element," *Annals of Internal Medicine* 72 (1970): 280. "Reporting Venereal Disease," *Journal of the American Medical Association* 202 (1967): 982.

177. *Wall Street Journal,* April 23, 1965, 1.

178. Cleere et al., "Physicians' Attitudes," 946.

179. *New York Times,* March 17, 1970, 23. Cleere et al., "Physicians' Attitudes."

180. Cleere et al., "Physicians' Attitudes," 946.

181. *New York Times,* March 17, 1970, 23.

182. Ibid.

183. *New York Times,* April 5, 1965, 33.

CHAPTER 4

1. "Uniform Reporting of Accidents and Diseases," *American Labor Legislation Review* 2 (1912): 541.

2. David A. Moss, *Socializing Security: Progressive-Era Economists and the Origins of American Social Policy* (Cambridge, MA, 1996), 59–76 and passim.

3. "Proceedings of the 4th Annual Meeting of the American Association for Labor Legislation: Discussion of Immediate Problems," *American Labor Legislation Review* 1 (1911): 73–75.

4. Ibid., 79–81.

5. John B. Andrews, "The Beginning of Occupational Disease Reports," *American Labor Legislation Review* 1 (1911): 109.

6. John B. Andrews, "Labor Legislation of 1911," *American Labor Legislation Review* 1 (1911): 10.

7. John B. Andrews, "Reports of Occupational Diseases and Accidents," *American Political Science Review* 6 (1912): 240–42.

8. Ibid.

9. Ibid., 241.

10. John B. Andrews, "Labor Legislation of 1912," *American Labor Legislation Review* 10 (1912): 427. "A Model State Law for Morbidity Reports," *Public Health Reports* 28 (1913): 1325.

11. Andrews, "Reports of Occupational Diseases," 241.

12. Andrews, "Labor Legislation of 1912," 10.

13. "Connecticut Law Chap 14, Act of Apr 22, 1913," *Public Health Reports* 28 (1913): 1583 and 1590. "Ohio, Act of May 6 1913," *Public Health Reports* 28 (1913): 1466.

14. W. Gilman Thompson, "Reporting of Occupation Diseases by Physicians," *Business and the Public Welfare* 2 (1912): 28.

15. Cressy L. Wilbur, "Notification of Occupational Diseases," *American Labor Legislation Review* 2 (1912): 339–45.

16. As cited in Henry B. Selleck and Alfred Whittaker, *Occupational Health in America* (Detroit, 1962), 81.

17. Alice Hamilton, *Exploring the Dangerous Trades: The Autobiography of Alice Hamilton, M.D.* (Boston, 1943), 114.

18. David Rosner and Gerald E. Markowitz, *Deadly Dust: Silicosis and the Politics of Occupational Disease in Twentieth-Century America* (Princeton, NJ, 1991), 15–29.

19. Frederick Hoffman, "Mortality from Consumption in Occupations Exposing to Municipal and General Organic Dust," *Bulletin of the Bureau of Labor* 82 (1909): 472.

20. Rosner and Markowitz, *Deadly Dust,* 18–28.

21. Rupert Blue, "Memorandum for the Secretary—January 26," as cited by Christopher C. Sellers, *Hazards of the Job: From Industrial Disease to Environmental Health Science* (Chapel Hill, NC, 1997), 123.

22. Sellers, *Hazards of the Job,* 135–38.

23. Joseph Schereschewsky to J. W. Kerr, as cited in Sellers, *Hazards of the Job,* 136. For other examples of PHS studies that used code numbers rather than names, see J. J. Bloomfield and W. M. Gafafer, "The Public Health Administrator's Responsibility in the Field of Occupational Disease Legislation," *Public Health Reports* 56 (1941): 2033–41.

24. *Muller v. Oregon,* 208 U.S. 412 (1908). For limits to working hours in smelters, see *Holden v. Hardy,* 169 U.S. 366 (1898).

25. *Lochner v. New York,* 198 U.S. 45 (1905).

26. For an analysis of freedom in the progressive era as defined by the relation of the state to corporations, see Eric Foner, *The Story of American Freedom* (New York, 1998), 157–58.

27. Clarence Davey Selby, *Studies of the Medical and Surgical Care of Industrial Workers* (Washington, DC, 1919), 5.

28. Ibid., 15.

29. Angela Nugent, "Fit for Work: The Introduction of Physical Examinations in Industry," *Bulletin of the History of Medicine* 57 (1983): 578–95. See also Selleck and Whittaker, *Occupational Health in America,* 62.

30. On company doctors as "finger wrappers," see Selby, *Studies of Medical and Surgical Care.* For AMA warnings about industrial physicians, see American Medical Association, "Minutes of the House of Delegates" (paper presented at the Sixty-

fourth Annual Session of the American Medical Association, Minneapolis, June 3–6, 1912), 12–15; Editorial, *Journal of the American Medical Association* 94 (1930): 33–34; and Editorial, *Journal of the American Medical Association* 89 (1927): 1891.

31. For other examples of workers as machines, see C. Cowdrick, "Keeping the Human Machinery off the Scrap Pile," *Industrial Management* 63 (1922): 35. W. Fulton, "Records—the Seeing Eye of Industrial Medicine," *Industrial Medicine* 13 (1944): 1–37.

32. James D. Hackett, *Health Maintenance in Industry* (Chicago, 1925), iii.

33. Harlow Brooks, "Inspection in Physical Diagnosis," in *The Relation of Medicine to Industry: Proceedings of the Conference Board of Physicians in Industry—Tenth Anniversary Meeting in New York City, April 4* (New York, 1924), 43–44.

34. The definitive history of the industrial medical exam is found in Nugent, "Fit for Work." For immigrant medical examinations, see Amy Fairchild, *Science at the Borders: Immigrant Medical Inspection and the Shaping of the Modern Industrial Labor Force* (Baltimore, 2003).

35. National Industrial Conference Board, *Medical Care of Industrial Workers* (New York, 1926), 101.

36. Brooks, "Inspection in Physical Diagnosis," in *Relation of Medicine to Industry*, 40.

37. Nugent, "Fit for Work."

38. Samuel Gompers, "Wages and Health," as cited in Nugent, "Fit for Work," 592.

39. *Report of the Proceedings of the Thirty-fourth Annual Convention of the American Federation of Labor, 9–21 November 1914*, as cited in Nugent, "Fit for Work," 590. On steelworkers' demands, see David Brody, *Labor in Crisis: The Steel Strike of 1919* (Philadelphia, 1965).

40. Hamilton, *Exploring the Dangerous Trades*, 198.

41. John B. Andrews, *Labor Problems and Labor Legislation* (New York, 1919), 84.

42. R. Williams, "The United States Public Health Service and Industrial Medicine," in *Relation of Medicine to Industry*, 48.

43. Emery R. Hayhurst, "The Role of the State in Industrial Hygiene," *American Journal of Public Health* 15 (1925): 682.

44. Ibid., 684.

45. Bureau of Labor Statistics, "Occupational Safety and Health Statistics," in *BLS Handbook of Methods* (Washington, DC, 1997), 70–79. Clarence Olds Sappington, *Essentials of Industrial Health* (Philadelphia, 1943).

46. Anthony Bale, "Compensation Crisis: The Value and Meaning of Work-Related Illnesses in the United States, 1842–1932" (Ph.D. diss., Brandeis University, 1986).

47. Rosner and Markowitz, *Deadly Dust*.

48. Benjamin W. Mintz, *OSHA: History, Law, and Policy* (Washington, DC, 1984), 3. David Rosner and Gerald E. Markowitz, "Research and Advocacy: Federal Occupational Safety and Health Policies during the New Deal," in *Dying for Work: Workers' Safety and Health in Twentieth-Century America* (Bloomington, IN, 1987).

49. George Gilbert Davis, Ella Maude Salmonsen, and Joseph Lewis Earlywine, *The Pneumoconioses (Silicosis): Bibliography and Laws* (Chicago, 1934). Gerald E. Markowitz and David Rosner, "Disability Policy: Restoring Socioeconomic Independence," *Milbank Quarterly* 67 (1989): 237.

50. Henry Sayer, Papers of the American Association for Labor Legislation, Cornell University, as cited by Markowitz and Rosner, "Disability Policy," 237.

51. A. G. Kammer, "Contribution of Industrial Medical Records" (paper presented at the Ninety-sixth Annual Section of the American Medical Association, Atlantic City, NJ, June 11, 1947).

52. A stark example of the difficulty in proving a link between disease and occupation is found in *Stevens v. Driggs*, 152 P. 2d 891 (Idaho, 1944), in which a firefighter who developed pleurisy after battling a fire for three hours in subzero weather was denied compensation on the grounds that pleurisy was "ordinary to life."

53. Some in the PHS urged greater engagement in compensation questions. See, for example, Bloomfield and Gafafer, "Public Health Administrator's Responsibility."

54. Sellers, *Hazards of the Job.*

55. Rosner and Markowitz, "Research and Advocacy," in *Dying for Work.*

56. Selleck and Whittaker, *Occupational Health in America*, 396, and Victoria Trasko and J. J. Bloomfield, "An Analysis of Industrial Hygiene Activities in State and Local Health Departments, 1940–1941," *Public Health Reports* 57 (1942): 853–72. For friction between labor and health departments, see Rosner and Markowitz, "Research and Advocacy," in *Dying for Work*, Selleck and Whittaker, *Occupational Health in America*, 396, and Trasko and Bloomfield, "Analysis of Industrial Hygiene."

57. Morris Fishbein cites World War II as a high point for industrial medicine. Morris Fishbein, *A History of the American Medical Association, 1847 to 1947* (Philadelphia, 1947).

58. T. Lyle Hazlett, "Address to the American Association of Industrial Physicians and Surgeons, 1942," as cited in Selleck and Whittaker, *Occupational Health in America*, 309.

59. Fulton, "Records."

60. George Schwabe, as quoted in David Rosner and Gerald E. Markowitz, "More Than Economism: The Politics of Workers' Safety and Health, 1932–1947," *Milbank Quarterly* 64 (1986): 349.

61. Ewan Clague, oral history dictated to the Truman Library, March 4 and 5, 1964, http://www.trumanlibrary.org/oralhist/clague.htm, accessed May 15, 2005.

62. J. Page and M. O'Brien, *Bitter Wages: Ralph Nader's Study Group Report on Disease and Injury on the Job* (New York, 1973), 69–113.

63. Ibid., 108–13.

64. Paul Starr, *The Social Transformation of American Medicine* (New York, 1982), 282.

65. Paul Brodeur, *Expendable Americans* (New York, 1974), 45, 81. D. Kotelchuck, "History of the Coal Worker Health Movement," in *Dying for Work*. M. Neufeld, "The Historical Relationship of Liberals and Intellectuals to Organized Labor in the United States," *Annals of the American Academy of Political and Social Sciences* 350 (1963): 116. Page and O'Brien, *Bitter Wages.*

66. Victoria Trasko, "Occupational Disease Reporting," *Public Health Reports* 68 (1953): 946.

67. Ibid.

68. For opposition to early occupational health and safety legislation, see Nicholas Askounes Ashford and Ford Foundation, *Crisis in the Workplace: Occupational*

Disease and Injury: A Report to the Ford Foundation (Cambridge, MA, 1976), and "Life or Death for Your Business: Labor Secretary Wants the Power to Shut You Down in the Name of Health and Safety," *Nation's Business,* April 1968, 37.

69. *New York Times,* January 2, 1970, 17.

70. Brodeur, *Expendable Americans.* Curtis Seltzer, "Moral Dimensions of Occupational Health: The Case of the 1969 Coal Mine Health and Safety Act," in *The Health and Safety of Workers,* ed. Ronald Bayer (New York, 1988), 242–70.

71. U.S. Congress, House Committee on Education and Labor, *Federal Coal Mine Health and Safety Act. Report No. 91–7161* (Washington, DC, 1969).

72. Page and O'Brien, *Bitter Wages,* 123.

73. Michael Pollack, "Occupational Health—a Must for '70," *Textile Labor,* February 1971, 3.

74. Page and O'Brien, *Bitter Wages,* 128.

75. For changes in the environmental movement, see Hal Rothman, Gerald D. Nash, and Richard W. Etulain, *The Greening of a Nation? Environmentalism in the United States since 1945* (Fort Worth, 1998).

76. Anthony Mazzochi, as cited in Gerald E. Markowitz and David Rosner, *Deceit and Denial: The Deadly Politics of Industrial Pollution* (Berkeley, CA, 2002), 158.

77. Peter Bommarito, "It's a Life and Death Matter!" *United Rubber Worker,* March 1970, 3.

78. *United Rubber, Cork, Linoleum and Plastic Workers of America, AFL-CIO, CLC,* June 4, 1973, 8–9. *United Rubber Worker,* September 1972.

79. Jeanne Mager Stellman and Susan M. Daum, *Work Is Dangerous to Your Health: A Handbook of Health Hazards in the Workplace and What You Can Do about Them* (New York, 1973).

80. Ibid., 344–59. Sales information from Jeanne Mager Stellman, Interview, October 10, 2004.

81. Brodeur's series, Annals of Industry, would be published as a book: Brodeur, *Expendable Americans.*

82. *New York Times,* September 14, 1971, 19. Eric Frumin, Interview, May 5, 2005.

83. Lawrence S. Bacow, *Bargaining for Job Safety and Health* (Cambridge, MA, 1980), 69–70.

84. A. Hosey and L. Ede, "A Review of State Occupational Health Legislation," *Journal of the American Industrial Hygiene Association* 31 (1972): 30–43.

85. Hearings before the Senate Subcommittee on Labor, as cited in Page and O'Brien, *Bitter Wages,* 153. For the AMA hopes that their registry would succeed where government efforts had not, see *Newsletter of the National Safety Council of Chicago,* July 1968, 1.

86. C. O. Dernehl, "Lessons from the AMA Registry on Adverse Reactions Due to Occupational Exposures" (paper presented at the AMA Occupational Health Conference, Chicago, September 11–12, 1972).

87. S. Pell, M. O'Berg, and B. Karrh, "Cancer Epidemiologic Surveillance in the DuPont Company," *Journal of Occupational Medicine* 20 (1978): 725.

88. Bruce Karrh, as cited in "Lost in the Workplace: Is There an Occupational Disease Epidemic?" (Seminar for the News Media, Washington, DC, September 13–14, 1979), 75–82. DuPont's claim that they released information to employees

exposed would be challenged with the finding that some of their employees had been exposed to asbestos but not notified of their risk.

89. Markowitz and Rosner, *Deceit and Denial.*

90. See, for example, David P. McCaffrey, *OSHA and the Politics of Health Regulation* (New York, 1982), Page and O'Brien, *Bitter Wages,* and Robert Stewart Smith, *The Occupational Safety and Health Act: Its Goals and Its Achievements* (Washington, DC, 1976).

91. *Occupational Safety and Health Act of 1970* (29 USC 651) and 29 CFR Part 1904, §8(c)2.

92. Ibid.

93. Ibid., §6(b)7.

94. For BLS rationale for keeping the survey anonymous, see Earl S. Pollack, Deborah Gellerman Keimig, and U.S. National Research Council Panel on Occupational Safety and Health Statistics, *Counting Injuries and Illnesses in the Workplace: Proposals for a Better System* (Washington, DC, 1987), 18.

95. When Dr. Bingham became head of OSHA in 1977, this comment would be used by the lead industry to charge that she was prejudiced in favor of wage guarantees. See Mintz, *OSHA,* 143.

96. Bureau of National Affairs, August 7, 1975, as cited in McCaffrey, *OSHA and Politics,* 89.

97. FR 41: 46742 (October 22, 1976); FR 42: 23601 (May 10, 1977); FR 43: 19584 (May 5, 1978). Unlike the vinyl chloride standard, the coke oven and arsenic standards did not require removal of high-risk employees. The cotton dust standard required removal of employees unable to wear respirators. See also Mintz, *OSHA,* 142–61.

98. *Occupational Safety and Health Act of 1970,* §6(b)7.

99. FR 37: 11318–319 (June 7, 1972). Workers had sought protections similar to those extended to coal miners: medical exams performed by independent doctors, with the records stored at NIOSH. See Brodeur, *Expendable Americans,* 124.

100. *Industrial Union Department v. Hodgson,* 499 F.2d 467 (D.C. Cir. 1974).

101. FR 43: 31019–21 (July 19, 1978).

102. As cited in R. Bayer, "Biological Monitoring in the Workplace: Ethical Issues," *Journal of Occupational Medicine* 28 (1986): 937.

103. "Lost in the Workplace," 85. See also AFL-CIO testimony in favor of the ruling, as cited in Bayer, "Biological Monitoring."

104. Alan Westin, "Confidentiality of Medical Records," in *Occupational Safety and Health Symposia 1978,* U.S. Department of Health, Education, and Welfare, Division of Technical Services, National Institute for Occupational Safety and Health (Cincinnati, 1979).

105. To protect confidentiality, access to the records had to be authorized in writing by the employee. FR 45: 35214 (May 23, 1980).

106. See *Louisiana Chemical Association v. Bingham,* 550 F. Supp. 1136 (W.D. La. 1982), and Mintz, *OSHA,* 161. In hopes of securing a ruling in its favor, industry sued in the same court that had struck down OSHA's benzene standard in 1980.

107. D. P. Discher, *Pilot Study for Development of an Occupational Disease Surveillance Method,* U.S. Department of Health, Education, and Welfare (Washington, DC, 1975).

108. See, for example, Bureau of Labor Statistics, "Occupational Safety and Health Statistics." Office of the President of the United States, U.S. Department of

Labor, and U.S. Department of Health Education and Welfare, *The President's Report on Occupational Safety and Health* (Washington, DC, 1982).

109. National Institute for Occupational Safety and Health, *The Right to Know: Practical Problems and Policy Issues Arising from Exposures to Hazardous Chemical and Physical Agents in the Workplace* (Washington, DC, 1977), 9–14.

110. As quoted in McCaffrey, *OSHA and Politics*, 52. Similar arguments would be used to object to OSHA requirements that warning signs be posted for hazardous materials.

111. *General Motors v. Finklea*, 459 F. Supp. 235 (D.C. Ohio 1978).

112. *E. I. DuPont de Nemours and Co. v. Director of NIOSH*, 442 F. Supp. 821 (S.C. W.Va. 1977).

113. Brief on Behalf of Appellant, Westinghouse Electric Corporation, in the U.S. Court of Appeals for the Third Circuit, No. 80–1269, *United States v. Westinghouse Electric Corporation*, received and filed March 31, 1980, 39.

114. Ibid., 13.

115. Ibid., i, 5, 9, 15–16.

116. Ibid., 24.

117. Ibid., 23. See also *United States v. Westinghouse Electric Corporation*, 638 F.2d 570 (1980). The Third Circuit Court also acknowledged the risk posed by computers in this case.

118. Ibid., 5.

119. Brief for the Appellee, in the U.S. Court of Appeals for the Third Circuit, No. 80–1269, *United States v. Westinghouse Electric Corporation*, received and filed April 30, 1980, 15–16, 38 (emphasis added).

120. Ibid., 33, 36–37.

121. Ibid., 47 n. 16.

122. Rosenberg noted that the General Motors case had not, in fact, turned on the right of privacy but rather more narrowly on Ohio law. *United States v. Westinghouse Electrical Corporation*, 483 F. Supp. 1265.

123. Ibid.

124. Reply Brief on Behalf of Appellant, Westinghouse Electric Corporation, in the U.S. Court of Appeals for the Third Circuit, No. 80–1269, *United States v. Westinghouse Electric Corporation*, received and filed May 14, 1980, 6–7.

125. Ibid., 3.

126. Ibid., 11.

127. *United States v. Westinghouse Electric Corporation*, 638 F.2d 570. Cases cited by the court included *Planned Parenthood of Missouri v. Danforth* (1976), in which the court upheld the state's right to require reporting regarding abortions, and *Schacter v. Whalen* (1978), a Court of Appeals for the Second Circuit decision allowing the New York State Department of Health to subpoena physician medical records. That security measures need not be "foolproof" was a precedent established in *Schacter v. Whalen*.

128. *United States v. Westinghouse Electric Corporation*, 638 F.2d 570.

129. Testimony of John Finklea, as cited in McCaffrey, *OSHA and Politics*, 142.

130. National Institute for Occupational Safety and Health, *The Right to Know* (1977).

131. As quoted in R. Bayer, "Notifying Workers at Risk: The Politics of the Right-to-Know," *American Journal of Public Health* 76 (1986): 1353.

132. Eula Bingham, as quoted by McCaffrey, *OSHA and Politics*, 140.

133. Anthony Robbins, Interview, March 3, 2005.

134. Ibid.

135. *Washington Post*, August 24, 1981, 1.

136. As quoted in Bayer, "Notifying Workers at Risk," 1354.

137. Ibid., 1352−56.

138. As cited in ibid. See also P. A. Schulte, "Ethical Issues in the Communication of Results," *Journal of Clinical Epidemiology* 44 (1991): 57S−61S.

139. "If NIOSH does not notify workers of their risks," the Ethics Committee noted, "no one else can and will." Centers for Disease Control and Prevention, "Deliberations: Right to Know and Worker Notification," as cited in Schulte, "Ethical Issues," 58S.

140. *Washington Post*, October 23, 1984, A17.

141. See, for example, *High Risk Occupational Disease Notification and Prevention Act* (H.R. 1190), 102nd Cong., 1st sess., February 28, 1991; U.S. Congress, Hearings of House Committee on Education and Labor on *High Risk Occupational Disease Notification and Prevention Act of 1985*, 99th Cong., 1st and 2nd sess., Congressional Information Service No. 86-H341−96; M. Bolle, "High Risk Occupational Disease Notification and Prevention Act: Side-By-Side Comparison of H.R. 162 and S79," Congressional Research Service (Washington, DC, 1988). See also Bayer, "Notifying Workers at Risk."

142. See Judson MacLaury, "The Thorne Auchter Administration, 1981−1984: Oh, What a (Regulatory) Relief," in *The Occupational Safety and Health Administration: A History of Its First Thirteen Years, 1971−1984*, www.dol.gov/oasam/programs/history/osha13auchter.htm, accessed March 15, 2005.

143. Ibid., and Robbins, Interview. See also Eric Frumin, Testimony before the Manpower Subcommittee of the House Committee on Government Operations, June 9, 1984, Microfiche, U.S. Government Document Repository, Lehman Social Services Library, Columbia University.

144. See Frumin, Testimony before the Manpower Subcommittee.

145. "The name of your agency is OSHA, not OSA," Representative Barney Frank, chair of the subcommittee, told Thorne Auchter. *Boston Globe*, November 13, 1983, 1.

146. *Occupational Illness Data Collection: Fragmented, Unreliable, and Seventy Years Behind Communicable Disease Surveillance* (Washington, DC, 1984).

147. Donald J. Millar, Janet Norwood, and Patrick Tyson, Testimony before the Manpower Subcommittee of the House Committee on Government Operations, June 9, 1984. Document in possession of authors.

148. The estimate was based on figures provided by Donald Millar. Millar, Testimony before the Manpower Subcommittee, 20−25.

149. U.S. Congress, House Committee on Government Operations, *Occupational Health Hazard Surveillance: 72 Years Behind and Counting: Sixty-first Report* (Washington, DC, 1986), 5, 28.

150. Ibid., 5, 21.

151. Keystone Center, *Keystone National Policy Dialogue on Work-Related Illness and Injury Recordkeeping* (Keystone, CO, 1989). Pollack, Keimig, and U.S. National Research Council Panel, *Counting Injuries and Illnesses*. Additional reports on prob-

lems in occupational disease surveillance were detailed in General Accounting Office, "Options for Improving Safety and Health in the Workplace" (Washington, DC, 1990), as well as in news reports of widespread injury and record tampering in industry. See, for example, *Washington Post,* March 20, 1987, A4.

152. Testimony of Philip Landrigan, as cited in Committee on Government Operations, *Occupation Illness Data Collection: Fragmented, Unreliable, and Seventy Years Behind Communicable Disease Surveillance* (Washington, DC, 1984), 3.

153. D. D. Rutstein et al., "Sentinel Health Events (Occupational): A Basis for Physician Recognition and Public Health Surveillance," *American Journal of Public Health* 73 (1983): 1054–62.

154. In 1980 NIOSH had awarded four states—Maine, New York, Rhode Island, and Utah—funds to contribute data to a national system on occupational morbidity and mortality. T. M. Frazier, "Developing a National Occupational Health Surveillance System in the United States," *Scandinavian Journal of Work, Environment and Health* 7 (1981): 129. Joann Muldoon et al., "Occupational Disease Surveillance Data Sources, 1985," *American Journal of Public Health* 77 (1987): 1006–8.

155. Edward Baker, "Sentinel Event Notification System for Occupational Risks (SENSOR): The Concept," *American Journal of Public Health* 79 (1989): 19.

156. Massachusetts, where SENSOR was a joint project of the Department of Public Health and the state equivalent of the Department of Labor, was the exception. Massachusetts SENSOR Program, "Mandatory Reporting of Occupational Disease: A Discussion Paper" (Boston, August 1990). Document in possession of authors.

157. B. Levy et al., *Evaluation of the Sentinel Event Notification System for Occupational Risks (SENSOR)* (Atlanta, 1992). Edward Baker and Thomas Matte, "Surveillance of Occupational Illness and Injury," in *Public Health Surveillance,* ed. William Halperin, Edward L. Baker, and Richard R. Monson (New York, 1992), 178.

158. Langmuir, who served on a special CDC committee on occupational disease surveillance from 1976 to 1978, recalled, "We tried valiantly to get something started in surveillance of occupational disease but I struck out. The little problem of definition baffled me." Langmuir to Phillip Landrigan, November 17, 1987, Alexander D. Langmuir Papers, Box 6, Alan Mason Chesney Medical Archives, the Johns Hopkins Medical Institutions, Baltimore.

159. Thomas D. Matte, Edward L. Baker, and Patricia A. Honchar, "The Selection and Definition of Targeted Work-Related Conditions for Surveillance under SENSOR," *American Journal of Public Health* 79 (1989): 21–25.

160. Centers for Disease Control and Prevention, "Occupational Disease Surveillance: Occupational Asthma," *Morbidity and Mortality Weekly Report* 39 (1990): 119. Letitia Davis, Interview, December 3, 2004.

161. Asthma reporting in Michigan, for example, increased from 18 cases in 1984–86 to 101 cases in 1988–89. Centers for Disease Control and Prevention, "Occupational Disease Surveillance."

162. John Sestito, Interview, November 21, 2004. Davis, Interview. Ken Rosenman, Interview, April 21, 2005.

163. Massachusetts SENSOR Program, "Mandatory Reporting."

164. Letitia Davis to Peter Torkildsen, Memorandum, December 1991, from the Files of Letitia Davis.

165. Difficulties in collaboration between labor and health departments were

also identified in the 1992 evaluation of SENSOR. See Levy et al., "Evaluation of SENSOR," 13.

166. Davis to Torkildsen, Memorandum.

167. Michigan would at times notify doctors that failure to report was a misdemeanor or threaten a small fine but did not actively seek to levy penalties. Rosenman, Interview.

168. Levy et al., "Evaluation of SENSOR," 25.

169. J. Gittleman, "Surveillance Activities: Meeting Notes" (unpublished notebooks, 1990–98, provided by J. Gittleman), February 15, 1991–May 13, 1998.

170. James Melius, Interview, May 10, 2005. Davis, Interview.

171. Sestito, Interview.

172. For assessment of data collection on occupational mortality, see L. A. Layne, "Occupational Injury Mortality Surveillance in the United States: An Examination of Census Counts from Two Different Surveillance Systems, 1992–1997," *American Journal of Industrial Medicine* 45 (2004): 1–13.

173. Markowitz and Rosner, *Deceit and Denial.* Christian Warren, *Brush with Death: A Social History of Lead Poisoning* (Baltimore, 2000).

174. M. E. Baser, "The Development of Registries for Surveillance of Adult Lead Exposure, 1981 to 1992," *American Journal of Public Health* 82 (1992): 1113–18. C. Druschel, M. Sharpe-Stimac, and P. Cross, "Process of and Problems in Changing a Birth Defects Registry Reporting System," *Teratology* 64 (2001): S30–36.

175. Baser, "Development of Registries," 1115. M. Goldberg et al., *Occupational Blood Lead Surveillance of Construction Workers—Health Programs in Twelve States* (Washington, DC, 1996), 2.

176. Robert Roscoe, Interview, May 3, 2005.

177. Department of Health and Human Services, *Worker Health Chartbook 2004* (Cincinnati, 2004), 291.

178. James Melius, Interview, May 9, 2005.

179. Roscoe, Interview.

180. Depending on the severity of the case and the resources of the state, followup includes phone contact with physician, employee, and employer; industrial hygiene inspection; or referral to state or federal OSHA for inspection. See Goldberg et al., *Occupational Blood Lead Surveillance,* 8.

181. "Controlling Lead Toxicity in Bridge Workers—Connecticut, 1991–1994," *Morbidity and Mortality Weekly Report* 44 (1995): 76–79. B. L. Materna et al., "Results of an Intervention to Improve Lead Safety among Painting Contractors and Their Employees," *American Journal of Industrial Medicine* 41 (2002): 119–30.

182. J. Gittleman, Interview, December 20, 2005.

183. California Health and Safety Code (1991, 1996), sec. 105185–95, www.dhs.ca.gov/ohb/OLPPP/hs105185.htm, accessed May 15, 2005.

184. Warren, *Brush with Death,* 221.

185. Centers for Disease Control and Prevention, "Elevated Blood Lead Levels in Adults—United States, Second Quarter, 1992," *Morbidity and Mortality Weekly Report* 41 (1992): 715–16. Since 2002 reports of adult blood lead levels have been published annually, rather than quarterly, in the *Morbidity and Mortality Weekly Report.* Roscoe, Interview.

186. The number of states participating in ABLES fluctuated between 1991 and

2001 and had risen as high as twenty-seven in 1998. Between 1998 and 2001, twenty-one states had reported lead levels for two or more years. Robert Roscoe et al., "Adult Blood Lead Epidemiology and Surveillance—United States, 1998–2001," *Morbidity and Mortality Weekly Report Surveillance Summary* 51 (2002): 1.

187. Roscoe, Interview.

188. Institute of Medicine, "Employers and Business," in *The Future of the Public's Health in the 21st Century* (Washington, DC, 2003), 268–306.

189. For an overview of key issues raised by genetic screening, see K. Rothenberg et al., "Genetic Information and the Workplace: Legislative Approaches and Policy Changes," *Science* 275 (1997): 1755–57, and M. A. Rothstein, "Genetic Testing: Employability, Insurability, and Health Reform," *Journal of the National Cancer Institute Monograph* 17 (1995): 87–90.

CHAPTER 5

1. Victor A. Triolo and Michael B. Shimkin, "The American Cancer Society and Cancer Research Origins and Organization, 1913–1943," *Cancer Research* 29 (1969): 1615–40.

2. History of Cancer Control Project, *A History of Cancer Control in the United States, 1946–1971* (Washington, DC, 1979), 1:107.

3. Nicholas L. Petrakis, "Historic Milestones in Cancer Epidemiology," *Seminars in Oncology* 6 (1979): 433–43.

4. Massachusetts Department of Public Health, Committee on Cancer, *Cancer Control: The What, Whither, How* (Boston, 1944).

5. George W. Stephenson, "The Commission on Cancer: An Historical Review," *Bulletin of the American College of Surgeons* 64 (1979): 7–13.

6. Bruce V. Lewenstein, "Industrial Life Insurance, Public Health Campaigns, and Public Communication of Science, 1908–1951," *Public Understanding of Science* 1 (1992): 347–65. William G. Rothstein, *Public Health and the Risk Factor: A History of an Uneven Medical Revolution* (Rochester, 2003), 146–75.

7. Frederick L. Hoffman to Forrest Dryden, May 20, 1914, Hoffman Papers, Box 4, Folder 15, Columbia University, New York.

8. Frederick L. Hoffman to Forrest Dryden, January 6, 1915, Hoffman Papers, Box 4, Folder 17, Columbia University, New York.

9. Frederick L. Hoffman to Forrest Dryden, April 27, 1915, Hoffman Papers, Box 4, Folder 17, Columbia University, New York.

10. Frederick L. Hoffman, "Cancer and Civilization" Typescript, 1913, Hoffman Papers, Box 16, Folder 81.

11. Frederick L. Hoffman, "Discussion," *American Journal of Public Health* 20 (1930): 19–20.

12. Public Health Service, "A Model State Law for Morbidity Reports," *Public Health Reports* 27 (1913): 1323–29.

13. John W. Trask, "Public Health Administration: Its Dependence upon Reports of Cases of Sickness," *Public Health Reports* 28 (1913): 1.

14. Judith W. Leavitt, *Typhoid Mary: Captive to the Public's Health* (Boston, 1996).

15. James T. Patterson, *The Dread Disease: Cancer and Modern American Culture* (Cambridge, MA, 1987).

16. W. S. Bainbridge, "The Cancer Patient's Dilemma," *New York Medical Journal,* July 3, 1915.

17. Committee on Cancer, "What Official Public Health Agencies Should Do about Cancer," *American Journal of Public Health* 17 (1927): 1135–41.

18. Ibid.

19. Patterson, *Dread Disease.*

20. W. F. Willcox, "The Alleged Increase of Cancer," *Journal of Cancer Research* 2 (1917): 267–365.

21. Wendell M. Strong, "Is Cancer Mortality Really Increasing?" *Journal of Cancer Research* 6 (1922): 251–56.

22. J. W. Schereschewsky, "The Course of Cancer Mortality in the Ten Original Registration States for the 21-Year Period, 1900–1920," in *Public Health Bulletin No. 155* (Washington, DC, 1925).

23. Louis Dublin, "Cancer Situation Far from Alarming," *Scientific American,* July 1937, 32.

24. Francis Carter Wood, "Need for Cancer Morbidity Statistics," *American Journal of Public Health* 20 (1930): 11.

25. Ibid., 18.

26. Ernest A. Codman, "The Registry of Cases of Bone Sarcoma," *Surgery, Gynecology and Obstetrics* 34 (1922): 335–43.

27. Ernest A. Codman, "The Method of Procedure of the Registry of Bone Sarcoma," *Surgery, Gynecology and Obstetrics* 38 (1924): 714.

28. Codman, "Registry of Cases," 343.

29. Edward F. McCarthy, "The Registry of Bone Sarcoma: A History," *Iowa Orthopedic Journal* 15 (1995): 74–78.

30. Codman, "Method of Registry."

31. Nathaniel W. Faxon, "Vital Statistics That Hospitals Should Collect and Publish," *Modern Hospital* 18 (1922): 155.

32. Eleanor J. MacDonald, "The Evolution of Cancer Control in Massachusetts," *Medical Woman's Journal* 45 (1938): 264–70.

33. Henry Chadwick and Herbert Lombard, "A State Cancer Program," *American Journal of Public Health* 28 (1938): 15.

34. Interdepartmental Committee to Coordinate Health and Welfare Activities, *Toward Better National Health* (Washington, DC, 1939).

35. Chadwick and Lombard, "State Cancer Program."

36. Hoffman, "Discussion."

37. Eleanor J. MacDonald, "The Evolution of Cancer Control in Massachusetts," in *History of Cancer Control,* 3:542.

38. M. C. MacDonald, "The Contribution of Yale University School of Medicine to the Connecticut Cancer Program," *Connecticut State Medical Journal* 11 (1947): 347–51.

39. Matthew Griswold, "The Cancer Program in Connecticut," *Journal of the American Medical Association* 110 (1938): 221B.

40. Ibid.

41. Eleanor J. MacDonald, "The State-wide Cancer Registry in Connecticut," *Medical Woman's Journal* 51 (1944): 26–29, 35.

42. Ibid.

43. Patterson, *Dread Disease,* 114–36.

44. Harold F. Dorn, "Illness from Cancer in the United States," *Public Health Reports* 59 (1944): 34.

45. Ibid.

46. Ibid.

47. "National Cancer Survey," *Journal of the American Medical Association* 110 (1938): 1291.

48. Harold F. Dorn, "The Use of Statistics in Cancer Control Programs," *American Journal of Public Health* 39 (1949): 602–6.

49. Morton L. Levin and Russell S. Ferguson, "Summary of Report of the New York State Legislative Cancer Survey Commission," *New York State Journal of Medicine* 39 (1939): 731.

50. *History of Cancer Control,* 3:756–58.

51. Proceedings, 36th Meeting, National Advisory Cancer Council, December 11–12, 1947, vol. 1, p. 66, Record Group 443, National Advisory Cancer Council Transcripts of Meetings; November 6–8, 1952, Box 11, National Archives and Records Administration, College Park, MD.

52. Ibid., 416.

53. Austin V. Diebert, "A Half Century of State Cancer Legislation," *Public Health Reports* 63 (1948): 1128–35.

54. Patterson, *Dread Disease,* 131–35.

55. National Advisory Cancer Council, November 9, 1937, Record Group 443, Box 6, Transcripts of Meetings, 1937–38, National Archives and Records Administration, College Park, MD.

56. National Advisory Cancer Council, Minutes, March 31, 1941, p. 79, Record Group 443, Box 8, Proceedings 15, 15, 17, 18th Mtg. 1941, National Archives and Records Administration, College Park, MD (emphasis added).

57. Ibid., 80.

58. Ibid.

59. Eleanor J. MacDonald, "Accuracy of the Cancer Death Records," *American Journal of Public Health* 28 (1938): 818–24.

60. Proceedings, 36th Meeting, National Advisory Cancer Council, vol. 2, p. 416; November 6–8, 1952, Record Group 443, National Advisory Cancer Council Transcripts of Meetings, November 6–8, 1952, Box 11, National Archives and Records Administrations, College Park, MD.

61. Minutes, October 3, 1938, p. 11, Record Group 443, Box 6, National Advisory Cancer Council Transcripts of Meetings, 1937–38, National Archives and Records Administration, College Park, MD.

62. MacDonald, "Accuracy of Death Records," 818–24. Harold F. Dorn and Joseph I. Horn, "The Reliability of Certificates of Deaths from Cancer," *American Journal of Hygiene* 34 (1941): 12–23.

63. Patterson, *Dread Disease.*

64. MacDonald, "Accuracy of Death Records."

65. Fifth Meeting of the National Advisory Cancer Council, April 28, 1938, pp. 658–59, Record Group 443, Box 6, National Advisory Cancer Council Transcripts of Meetings, 1937–38, National Archives and Records Administration, College Park, MD.

66. Patterson, *Dread Disease,* 171–72.

67. National Advisory Cancer Council, Proceedings, 36th Meeting, December 11–12, 1947, vol. 1, p. 416, Record Group 443, National Advisory Cancer Council Transcripts of Meetings, 1947; November 6–8, 1952, Box 11, National Archives and Records Administration, College Park, MD.

68. Gastric Cancer Committee, Minutes, September 28–29, 1950, Record Group 443, National Advisory Cancer Council Transcripts of Meetings, 1947–June 1951, Box 13, National Archives and Records Administration, College Park, MD.

69. Gerald M. Oppenheimer, "Becoming the Framingham Study, 1947–1950," *American Journal of Public Health* 95 (2005): 602–10.

70. History of Cancer Control Project, *History of Cancer Control,* 3:541–44.

71. Dorn, "Use of Statistics," 603.

72. Minutes, October 21–29, 1950, p. 16, Record Group 443, National Advisory Cancer Council Transcripts of Meetings, 1947–June 1951, Box 13, National Archives and Records Administration, College Park, MD.

73. Patterson, *Dread Disease,* 188.

74. Dorn, "Use of Statistics," 603.

75. Evelyn A. Potter and Mildred R. Tully, "The Statistical Approach to the Cancer Problem in Massachusetts," *American Journal of Public Health* 35 (1945): 487.

76. Richard Doll, "Tobacco: A Medical History," *Journal of Urban Health* 75 (1999): 289–313.

77. Alexander G. Gilliam, "Opportunities for Application of Epidemiologic Method to Study of Cancer," *American Journal of Public Health* 43 (1953): 1252.

78. Stephenson, "Commission on Cancer."

79. "End Results," *Journal of the National Cancer Institute* 19 (1957): 285. B. Aubrey Schneider, "Progress in Cancer Control through Cancer Registries," *CA: A Cancer Journal for Clinicians* 8 (1958): 207–10.

80. John Laszlo, Edwin Cox, and Carole Angle, "The Hospital Tumor Registry: Present Status and Future Prospects," *Cancer* 38 (1976): 395.

81. Charles R. Smart, "The Physician and Tumor Registries," *Rocky Mountain Medical Journal* 67 (1970): 51.

82. History of Cancer Control Project, *History of Cancer Control,* 4:52.

83. Ibid., 3:542.

84. Harold F. Dorn and Sidney J. Cutler, *Morbidity from Cancer in the United States,* Public Health Monograph No. 56 (Washington, DC, 1959), 3.

85. History of Cancer Control Project, *History of Cancer Control,* 1:52–53.

86. Amy L. Fairchild and James Colgrove, "Out of the Ashes: The Life, Death, and Rebirth of the 'Safer' Cigarette in the United States," *American Journal of Public Health* 94 (2004): 192–204.

87. Richard A. Rettig, *Cancer Crusade: The Story of the National Cancer Act of 1971* (Princeton, NJ, 1977). Patterson, *Dread Disease,* 247–54. History of Cancer Control Project, *History of Cancer Control,* 2:703–23.

88. History of Cancer Control Project, *History of Cancer Control,* 2:711.

89. Carol Hahn Johnson, "The Surveillance, Epidemiology, and End Results Program," in *Cancer Registry Management: Principles and Practice,* by Carol L. Hutchison et al. (Alexandria, VA, 2005).

90. *New York Times,* May 28, 1970, 27.

91. Tom Reynolds, "National Statistics Source Reaches 20th Anniversary," *Journal of the National Cancer Institute* 85 (1993): 1899.

92. Johnson, "Surveillance, Epidemiology, and End Results Program," in *Cancer Registry Management*.

93. Phil Brown, "Popular Epidemiology and Toxic Waste Contamination: Lay and Professional Ways of Knowing," *Journal of Health and Social Behavior* 33 (1992): 267–81.

94. Steven P. Schwartz, Paul E. White, and Robert G. Hughes, "Environmental Threats, Communities, and Hysteria," *Journal of Public Health Policy* 6 (1985): 58–77.

95. Harold C. Barnett, "Crimes against the Environment: Superfund Enforcement at Last," *Annals of the American Academy of Political Science* 525 (1993): 119–33.

96. Phyllis Wingo, Interview, September 8, 2005.

97. John P. Enterline et al., "United States Cancer Reporting Laws: Structure and Utility," *American Journal of Public Health* 74 (1984): 449–52. Holly Howe, Interview, August 11, 2005.

98. *New York Times*, January 1, 1977, 23.

99. *New York Times*, June 12, 1976, 51. *New York Times*, February 20, 1978, 11.

100. *New York Times*, June 12, 1976, 51.

101. Raymond L. Powell and Robin J. Dietrich, "A Statewide Cancer Registry: The Pennsylvania Experience," *Topics in Healthcare Records Management* 11 (1990): 74–81.

102. Allen Kraut et al., "Completeness of Case Ascertainment of the State Cancer Registry," *New Jersey Medicine* 89 (1992): 772–73.

103. *Idaho Falls Post Register,* February 20, 1997, A1.

104. Dwight T. Janerich, William S. Burnett, and Gerald Feck, "Cancer Incidence in the Love Canal Area," *Science* 212 (1981): 1404–7.

105. Helen I. Meissner, Lawrence Bergner, and Katherine M. Marconi, "Developing Cancer Control Capacity in State and Local Public Health Agencies," *Public Health Reports* 107 (1992): 15–23.

106. Steven G. Epstein, *Impure Science: AIDS, Activism, and the Politics of Knowledge* (Berkeley, CA, 1996).

107. Barron H. Lerner, *The Breast Cancer Wars: Hope, Fear, and the Pursuit of a Cure in Twentieth-Century America* (New York, 2001).

108. Ibid.

109. Judith Swan et al., "Cancer Surveillance in the U.S.: Can We Have a National System?" *Cancer* 83 (1998): 1282–91.

110. Bernie Sanders, Testimony, 102nd Cong., 2nd sess., *Congressional Record* 138, February 25, 1992, 422.

111. Nancy Bruning, "One in Nine: Lies, Damn Lies, and Statistics?" *Breast Cancer Action Newsletter* 13 (June 1992) (emphasis in original).

112. John Healey, "The Cancer Weapon America Needs Most," *Reader's Digest* (June 1992): 72.

113. Mary D. Hutton and Gayle Greer Clutter, "The National Program of Cancer Registries," in *Cancer Registry Management: Principles and Practice*.

114. *Cancer Registries Amendment Act of 1992*, Public Law 102–515, *U.S. Statutes at Large* 106 (1992).

115. "State Cancer Registries: Status of Authorizing Legislation and Enabling

Regulations—United States, October 1993," *Morbidity and Mortality Weekly Report* 43 (1994): 71–75.

116. "Legislative Alerts—Federal," www.braintumor.org/pservices/legislative fed1.asp, accessed September 13, 2005.

117. Raising Health Awareness through Examining Benign Brain Tumor, Alpha One, and Breast Implant Issues, Hearing before the Subcommittee on Health of the Committee on Energy and Commerce, 107th Cong., 1st sess., November 15, 2001 (Washington, DC, 2002).

118. Http://thomas.loc.gov/cgi-bin/query/C?r107:./temp/~r107wqk706, accessed January 15, 2007.

119. *State Journal-Register* (Springfield), May 16, 2000, 11.

120. *May v. Central Illinois Public Service Co.*, 260 Ill. App. 3d 41 (1994), 45.

121. Ibid. (emphasis added).

122. *State Journal-Register* (Springfield), January 12, 1998, 1.

123. *Southern Illinoisan v. Department of Public Health*, 319 Ill. App. 3d 979 (2001).

124. *Southern Illinoisan v. Department of Public Health*, No. 5–02–0836 (2004), www.state.il.us/court/opinions/appelatecourt/2004, accessed December 2, 2004. *Southern Illinoisan v. the Department of Public Health*, 319 Ill. App. 3d 979.

125. *Southern Illinoisan v. Department of Public Health*, 349 Ill. App. 3d 431 (2004), 435.

126. *Southern Illinoisan v. Department of Public Health*, No. 5–02–0836.

127. *Southern Illinoisan v. Illinois Department of Public Health*, 218 Ill. 2d 390 (2006).

128. Associated Press State and Local Wire, February 3, 2006.

129. *Hassig v. New York State Department of Health*, 294 A.D.2d 781 (2002).

130. Trust for America's Health, *Improving Cancer Tracking Today Saves Live Tomorrow: Do States Make the Grade?* (Washington, DC, 2003).

131. Amy L. Fairchild, "Dealing with Humpty Dumpty: Research, Practice, and the Ethics of Public Health Surveillance," *Journal of Law, Medicine, and Ethics* 31 (2003): 615–23.

132. Jeremy Sugarman et al., "Ethical Ramifications of Alternative Means of Recruiting Research Participants from Cancer Registries," *Cancer* 86 (1999): 647–51.

133. Laura M. Beskow, Robert S. Sandler, and Morris Weinberger, "Research Recruitment through U.S. Central Cancer Registries: Balancing Privacy and Scientific Issues," *American Journal of Public Health* 96 (2006): 1920–6.

134. Transcript of the January 29, 1998, Roundtable Discussion Held by the Subcommittee on Privacy and Confidentiality, National Committee on Vital and Health Statistics, www.ncvhs.hhs.gov/980129tr.htm, accessed November 1, 2005.

135. Wingo, Interview.

136. Transcript of the January 29, 1998, Roundtable Discussion.

137. *Cancer Registry Study Pursuant to HJR 524 and SB 942*, House Document No. 73 (Richmond, VA, 2000).

138. Julie R. Ingelfinger and Jeffrey M. Drazen, "Registry Research and Medical Privacy," *New England Journal of Medicine* 350 (2004): 1452.

139. "House Passes Nixon Bill Aimed at Disclosure for Cancer Patients," hrc.leg .wa.gov/members/Nixon/newsreleases/021904.htm, accessed August 15, 2005.

140. Howe, Interview.

141. David B. Thomas, "Alternatives to a National System of Population-Based State Cancer Registries," *American Journal of Public Health* 92 (2002): 1065.

CHAPTER 6

1. Amy Louise Hunter and William C. Keettel, "Supplemental Birth Certification Information Used in Planning Crippled Children and Maternal and Child Health Programs," *American Journal of Public Health* 33 (1943): 660. John W. Trask, "The Practicing Physician: What He Should Know about the Registration of Births and Deaths and the Reporting of Sickness," *Public Health Reports* 31 (1916): 50–51. Ruth Tartakoff, "Social Aspects of Medical Care for Crippled Children," *Bulletin of the American Association of Medical Social Workers* 11 (1938): 31. Henry H. Kessler, *The Crippled and Disabled: Rehabilitation of the Physically Handicapped in the United States* (New York, 1935), 61–65.

2. Harry H. Howett, "Who Cares for the Cripple?" *Hospital Social Service* 16 (1927): 545, 556.

3. Ibid.

4. Neal Nathanson and John R. Martin, "The Epidemiology of Poliomyelitis: Enigmas Surrounding Its Appearance, Epidemicity, and Disappearance," *American Journal of Epidemiology* 110 (1979): 672–92.

5. Karen M. Farizo, Stephen L. Cochi, and Peter Patriarca, "Poliomyelitis in the United States: A Historical Perspective and Current Vaccination Policy," *Clinical Review* 39 (1990). John Paul, *A History of Poliomyelitis* (New Haven, CT, 1971), 79.

6. National Conference on Recommended Practices for the Control of Polio-myelitis, "Recommended Practices for the Control of Poliomyelitis," Ann Arbor, MI, June 1949, p. 8, Medical Program Records, Series 15, Box 16, Poliomyelitis, State Health, and Welfare Agencies, 1940–49, Folder, March of Dimes, White Plains, NY.

7. California, Resolution of the Board of Health, September 7, 1912, as reported in *Public Health Reports* 28 (1913): 2009. See also legislation for New Castle, Pennsylvania, Regulations, Board of Health, October 3, 1912, as reported in *Public Health Reports* 28 (1913): 1592.

8. "The Notifiable Diseases: Diseases and Conditions Required to Be Reported in the Several States," *Public Health Reports* 34 (1919).

9. Howett, "Who Cares for the Cripple?" 556.

10. State of New Jersey, *Report of the New Jersey State Temporary Commission for Inquiry Relating to the Distribution and Condition of Crippled Children* (Trenton, NJ, 1928), 18. See also Charles R. Gardipee, "The Handicapped Child," *Annals of the American Academy of Political and Social Science* 355 (1964): 124–25. Richard Arthur Bolt, "Progress in Saving Maternal and Child Life," *Annals of the American Academy of Political and Social Science* 212 (1940): 102.

11. *Chicago Daily Tribune,* March 28, 1932, 19.

12. Nathanson and Martin, "Epidemiology of Poliomyelitis," 672–85.

13. Paul, *History of Poliomyelitis,* 4.

14. C. W. Areson and H. W. Hopkirk, "Child Welfare Programs of Churches and Fraternal Orders," *Annals of the American Academy of Political and Social Science* 121 (1925): 94.

15. Ibid., 85–88. Matthew P. Adams, Emma C. Puschner, and Pauline V. Young,

"Fraternal Social Work and Its Relation to Professional Social Work," *Social Forces* 8 (1929): 255–56.

16. Areson and Hopkirk, "Child Welfare Programs," 90. Adams, Puschner, and Young, "Fraternal Social Work," 257–58. Kessler, *Crippled and Disabled*, 58–59. Tartakoff, "Social Aspects of Medical Care," 31. Howett, "Who Cares for the Cripple?" 546.

17. Mansel G. Blackford, "The Lost Dream: Businessmen and City Planning in Portland, Oregon, 1903–1914," *Western Historical Quarterly* 15 (1984): 49–50, 53. Sol Cohen, "The Industrial Education Movement, 1906–17," *American Quarterly* 20 (1968).

18. Kenneth L. Kusmer, "The Functions of Organized Charity in the Progressive Era: Chicago as a Case Study," *Journal of American History* 60 (1973): 672–73.

19. John Collier, "Community Councils—Democracy Every Day: Plans for Community Councils in the Great Cities," *Survey* 40 (1918). Robert Fisher, "Community Organizing and Citizen Participation: The Efforts of the People's Institute in New York City, 1910–1920," *Social Service Review* (1977).

20. Howett, "Who Cares for the Cripple?" 546. For a thorough and incisive analysis of the ways in which the New Jersey Crippled Children's Commission illuminates an understanding of business associationalism, see also Marian Jones, "Extending the Antlers of Protection" (master's thesis, Columbia University, 2004). Jones provided extensive research support for this chapter and then thoroughly explored the ways in which the New Jersey story informs the history of associationalism, as well as theories of social capital.

21. Joseph Brandes, *Herbert Hoover and Economic Diplomacy: Department of Commerce Policy, 1921–1928* (Pittsburgh, 1962).

22. Alan Brinkley, *The Unfinished Nation: A Concise History of the American People* (Boston, 2004), 2:645–46.

23. J. Joseph Huthmacher and Warren I. Susman, introduction to *Herbert Hoover and the Crisis of American Capitalism: Essays and Rejoinders by Ellis W. Hawley, Murray N. Rothbard, Robert F. Himmelberg, and Gerald D. Nash* (Cambridge, MA, 1973), viii. Ellis W. Hawley, "Herbert Hoover and American Capitalism," in *Herbert Hoover*, 5–6.

24. Howett, "Who Cares for the Cripple?" 546. Brinkley, *Unfinished Nation*, 2:645.

25. Joanne G. Hogan, "The Michigan Birth Defects Registry: Development and Operation," *Journal of American Health Information Management Association* 65 (1994): 38–40.

26. Charles Edward Ellis, *An Authentic History of the Benevolent and Protective Order of Elks* (Chicago, 1910), 24.

27. Sheila Rothman, *Woman's Proper Place: A History of Changing Ideals and Practices, 1870 to the Present* (New York, 1978), 135–42. Blanche Wiesen Cook, *Eleanor Roosevelt* (New York, 1992), 290, 362. Gardipee, "Handicapped Child," 123. Arthur Dunham, "The Development of Child Welfare Programs," *Annals of the American Academy of Political and Social Science* 212 (1940): 219. Katharine F. Lenroot, "Child Welfare, 1930–40," *Annals of the American Academy of Political and Social Science* 212 (1940).

28. State of New Jersey, *Report of the New Jersey State Crippled Children's Commission* (Trenton, NJ, 1932), 9. Bolt, "Progress in Saving Maternal and Child Life," 97, 102.

29. State of New Jersey, *Report of the New Jersey State Temporary Commission for Inquiry Relating to the Distribution and Condition of Crippled Children* (Trenton, NJ, 1930). The first public-at-large representative was a former governor. The function

was apparently filled by community members with experience with disability over time. In 1935, for example, the public representative was a community member whose daughter had contracted polio. State of New Jersey, *Report of the New Jersey State Crippled Children's Commission* (Trenton, NJ, 1936), 36.

30. Other communities undertook similar surveys. For example, the New York Committee on After Care of Infantile Paralysis Cases registered and began providing services to children paralyzed during the 1916 polio epidemic. But despite their calls to create a central agency that would continuously register and provide services to crippled children, their efforts remained limited to assisting only those children affected in 1916. Henry C. Wright, *Survey of Cripples in New York City* (New York, 1920).

31. New Jersey, *Report of the New Jersey State Temporary Commission* (1928), 25.

32. Alvin J. Schmidt, *Fraternal Organizations* (Westport, CT, 1980), 102–3.

33. There is some evidence that national efforts, spearheaded by the National Foundation for Infantile Paralysis, were likewise limited by race, particularly in the Jim Crow South. See David M. Oshinsky, *Polio: An American Story* (Oxford, 2005), 65–67. For contemporary data comparing orthopedic impairments in black and white children, see Dorothy F. Holland and George St. J. Perrott, "Health of the Negro," *Milbank Memorial Fund Quarterly* 16 (1938).

34. New Jersey, *Report of the Temporary Commission* (1928), 28.

35. State of New Jersey, *Report of the New Jersey State Temporary Commission for Inquiry Relating to the Distribution and Condition of Crippled Children* (Trenton, NJ, 1929), 6.

36. New Jersey, *Report of the New Jersey State Temporary Commission* (1930), 6.

37. State of New Jersey, *Report of the New Jersey State Crippled Children's Commission* (Trenton, NJ, 1935), 21.

38. Adams, Puschner, and Young, "Fraternal Social Work."

39. New Jersey, *Report of the Temporary Commission* (1928), 37.

40. Collier, "Community Councils," 711.

41. New Jersey, *Report of the Crippled Children's Commission* (1932), 22.

42. State of New Jersey, *Report of the New Jersey State Temporary Commission for Inquiry Relating to the Distribution and Condition of Crippled Children* (Trenton, NJ, 1931), 5. See also New Jersey, *Report of the Crippled Children's Commission* (1932), 7.

43. Tartakoff, "Social Aspects of Medical Care," 31.

44. New Jersey, *Report of the Crippled Children's Commission* (1932), 10.

45. New Jersey, *Report of the Temporary Commission* (1929), 4, 5.

46. New Jersey, *Report of the Temporary Commission* (1930), 15.

47. New Jersey, *Report of the Crippled Children's Commission* (1935), 28.

48. New Jersey, *Report of the Temporary Commission* (1931), 15. State of New Jersey, *Report of the Crippled Children's Commission* (1932), 21.

49. New Jersey, *Report of the Crippled Children's Commission* (1932), 20.

50. State of New Jersey, *Report of the New Jersey State Crippled Children's Commission* (Trenton, NJ, 1933), 12.

51. State of New Jersey, *Report of the Temporary Commission* (Trenton, NJ, 1930), 15.

52. New Jersey, *Report of the Crippled Children's Commission* (1932), 15.

53. Gardipee, "Handicapped Child," 121, 126. Kessler, *Crippled and Disabled.* New Jersey, *Report of the Temporary Commission* (1928), 6, 17, 21, 24, 31.

54. New Jersey, *Report of the Crippled Children's Commission* (1932), 17.

55. New Jersey, *Report of the Temporary Commission* (1928), 6, 17, 21, 24, 31.

56. New Jersey, *Report of the Crippled Children's Commission* (1933), 14.

57. New Jersey, *Report of the Temporary Commission* (1931), 5.

58. New Jersey, *Report of the Crippled Children's Commission* (1933), 12. See also *Report of the Crippled Children's Commission* (1935), 19.

59. New Jersey, *Report of the Crippled Children's Commission* (1933), 21.

60. Dunham, "Development of Child Welfare Programs," 216, 218.

61. New Jersey, *Report of the Crippled Children's Commission* (1935), 25, 27.

62. "Final Report: White House Conference on Children in a Democracy" (Washington, DC, 1940), 10, 127, 129.

63. Eric Foner, *The Story of American Freedom* (New York, 1998), 197. In the New Deal era, the language of self-sufficiency was recast. The challenge was to remediate the problem of unequal opportunities for full participation in a democracy: "To bring [a disadvantaged] child as nearly as possible up to par with other children in having access to the fruits of civilization is therefore of the very essence of democratic purpose." "Final Report," 254, 3, 8–9, 10. With advances in surgical techniques, physical and social restoration also became important themes. Tartakoff, "Social Aspects of Medical Care."

64. Lenroot, "Child Welfare," 9. National concern would soon extend to "orthopedic impairments" affecting the entire population. See Bernard D. Karpinos, "The Physically Handicapped," *Public Health Reports* 58 (1943).

65. "Final Report," 258.

66. Ibid., 258, 267.

67. Ibid., xx–xxi.

68. Ibid., 258 (emphasis added), 267–69.

69. Gardipee, "Handicapped Child," 123. Dunham, "Development of Child Welfare Programs," 220. "Final Report," 276–77.

70. "Final Report." The White House Conference report estimated that the true number of crippled children was more than half a million.

71. State of New Jersey, "Calendar Year—1940: Summary of Activities, the New Jersey State Crippled Children's Commission," p. 4, New Jersey State Archives, Trenton, NJ.

72. Ibid. State of New Jersey, *Report of the New Jersey State Crippled Children's Commission* (Trenton, NJ, 1947).

73. J. Thomas McIntire, *New Jersey State Cerebral Palsy Program* (Trenton, NJ, 1943). Winthrop M. Phelps, "The New Jersey State Project for Cerebral Palsy," *Journal of the Medical Society of New Jersey* 34 (1937).

74. National Volunteer Agencies Caring for Crippled Children and Adults to Basil O'Connor, Memorandum, Re: Agencies Operating Countywise in the Crippled Children and Adult Field, June 8, 1943; National Volunteer Agencies Caring for Crippled Children and Adults to Basil O'Connor, Memorandum, June 5, 1943, Medical Program Records, Series 15, Box 16, Poliomyelitis, State Health, and Welfare Agencies, 1940–49, Folder, March of Dimes, White Plains, NY.

75. Jane Smith, *Patenting the Sun: Polio and the Salk Vaccine* (New York, 1990), 82. Oshinsky, *Polio*, 41–60.

76. Dr. Van Riper to Mr. O'Connor, Memorandum, Re: Conference with State

Crippled Children's Directors, Children's Bureau, and National Foundation for Infantile Paralysis, May 11–12, 1949, Medical Program Records, Series 15, Box 16, Poliomyelitis, State Health, and Welfare Agencies, 1940–49, Folder, March of Dimes, White Plains, NY.

77. National Foundation for Infantile Paralysis to physicians, July 26, 1940, Medical Program Records, Series 15, Box 16, Poliomyelitis, State Health and Welfare Agencies, 1940–49, Folder, March of Dimes, White Plains, NY.

78. P. J. A. C. to Basil O'Connor, Memorandum, Re: New Polio Cases, July 26, 1940, Medical Program Records, Series 15, Box 16, Poliomyelitis, State Health, and Welfare Agencies, 1940–49, Folder, March of Dimes, White Plains, NY.

79. D. W. Gudakunst to state health officers and directors of Crippled Children's Services (copy), June 29, 1944, Medical Program Records, Series 15, Box 16, Poliomyelitis, State Health, and Welfare Agencies, 1940–49, Folder, March of Dimes, White Plains, NY.

80. Ibid.

81. Ibid. (emphasis in original).

82. Van Riper to O'Connor (emphasis added).

83. Joe W. Savage to state representatives, Memorandum, Re: State Level Agreements with Crippled Children's Service, July 25, 1949, Medical Program Records, Series 15, Box 16, Poliomyelitis, State Health, and Welfare Agencies, 1940–49, Folder, March of Dimes, White Plains, NY.

84. West J. Altenburg to Savage, Memorandum, Re: Medical Care Program, June 16, 1949, p. 1, Medical Program Records, Series 15, Box 16, Poliomyelitis, State Health, and Welfare Agencies, 1940–49, Folder, March of Dimes, White Plains, NY.

85. Federal Security Agency et al., "Coordinated State Planning to Combat Poliomyelitis: A Suggested Guide for Use by State Poliomyelitis Planning Committees," May 23, 1949, Medical Program Records, Series 15, Box 16, Poliomyelitis, State Health, and Welfare Agencies, 1940–49, Folder, March of Dimes, White Plains, NY.

86. Altenburg to Savage.

87. "Some of the Problems Facing the National Foundation for Infantile Paralysis, under Study by Polio Planning Committees in Arizona, California, Colorado, New Mexico, Oregon, Washington, Wyoming, to Be Presented at Planning Meetings in Idaho, Nevada, Utah," August 21, 1950, Medical Program Records, Series 15, Box 16, Poliomyelitis, State Health, and Welfare Agencies, 1950–52, Folder, March of Dimes, White Plains, NY.

88. Medical Program Records, Series 15, Box 16, Poliomyelitis, State Health, and Welfare Agencies, 1953–54, 1954, 1955, 1956–68, Folders, March of Dimes, White Plains, NY.

89. *Washington Post*, April 28, 1968, A1. *Los Angeles Times*, September 30, 1961, 8. *New York Times*, April 18, 1959, 1.

90. *Washington Post*, April 28, 1968, A6.

91. National Foundation for Infantile Paralysis to Board of Trustees, Confidential Memorandum, Re: Proposal for an Expanded Program for the National Foundation for Infantile Paralysis, May 20, 1958, p. 20, Medical Program Records, Series 3, Box 6, Series 3, Expanded Program, March of Dimes, White Plains, NY.

92. Public Relations Department, "The National Foundation—March of Dimes,

Program of Action against Birth Defects," c. 1962, Medical Program Records, Series 3, Box 4, Birth Defects, Thalidomide, 1962–70, March of Dimes, White Plains, NY.

93. National Foundation for Infantile Paralysis to Board of Trustees, Re: Proposal for an Expanded Program, p. 4 (emphasis in original).

94. Ibid.

95. *New York Times*, April 29, 1973, 33–34.

96. Ibid.

97. Ibid.

98. "Biology, Medicine, and Birth Defects, 1965," News Release, December 1965, p. 2, Medical Program Records, Series 3, Box 3, Birth Defects, March of Dimes, White Plains, NY.

99. Larry D. Edmonds et al., "Congenital Malformations Surveillance: Two American Systems," *International Journal of Epidemiology* 10 (1981): 247.

100. See, for example, *Washington Post*, August 16, 1962, D1.

101. Catherine Law et al., "Characteristics Influencing Informed Consent on a Congenital Malformations Registry," *American Journal of Public Health* 78 (1988): 573.

102. Larry Edmonds, Interview, November 18, 2004.

103. *New York Times*, July 30, 1962, 21. *New York Times*, April 18, 1959, 1.

104. *New York Times*, May 1, 1967, 41.

105. Elizabeth M. Armstrong, *Conceiving Risk, Bearing Responsibility: Fetal Alcohol Syndrome and the Diagnosis of Moral Disorder* (Baltimore, 2003), 193.

106. Janet Golden, *Message in a Bottle: The Making of Fetal Alcohol Syndrome* (Cambridge, MA, 2005). Armstrong, *Conceiving Risk, Bearing Responsibility*.

107. Armstrong, *Conceiving Risk, Bearing Responsibility*, 193. A. Asch, "Prenatal Diagnosis and Selective Abortion: A Challenge to Practice and Policy," *American Journal of Public Health* 89 (1999): 1649–57.

108. Alexandra Minna Stern, *Eugenic Nation: Faults and Frontiers of Better Breeding in Modern America* (Berkeley, CA, 2005).

109. Virginia Apgar to Joseph F. Nee, Memorandum, August 11, 1965, Medical Program Records, Box 3, Series 3, Birth Defects Folder, Birth Defects Registries (Apgar), 1965–69, March of Dimes, White Plains, NY.

110. Virginia Apgar and Gabriel Stickle, "Birth Defects: Their Significance As a Public Problem" (paper presented at the meeting of the American Medical Association, June 21, 1967), pp. 2–3, 6, Virginia Apgar, Box 2, Typescripts, Congenital Abnormalities and Birth Defects, 1967–70, March of Dimes, White Plains, NY. She references "Hospitalization and Surgical Care of Children," *Statistical Bulletin of the Metropolitan Life Insurance Company*, December 1963–October 1964.

111. Apgar to Nee.

112. Gardipee, "Handicapped Child," 127.

113. Apgar and Stickle, "Birth Defects," 7, 8.

114. David Sarnoff, "Electronic Medical Files," *Public Health Reports* 80 (1965): 778. William Phillips, Kurt Gorwitz, and Anita K. Bahn, "Electronic Maintenance of Case Registers," *Public Health Reports* 77 (1962): 503–4. See also Samuel Milham, "Congenital Malformation Surveillance System Based on Vital Records," *Public Health Reports* 78 (1963): 448.

115. Bioethics Advisory Committee Meeting, Minutes, October 14, 1977, Bioethics Committee Records, Box 1, March of Dimes, White Plains, NY.

116. Ibid.

117. Jose. F. Condero, "Registries of Birth Defects and Genetic Disorders," *Pediatric Clinics of North America* 39 (1992): 65. Edmonds et al., "Congenital Malformations Surveillance," 247. Joann Petrini, Karla Damus, and Richard B. Johnston, "An Overview of Infant Mortality and Birth Defects in the United States," *Teratology* 56 (1997): 8.

118. Larry D. Edmonds, "Birth Defect Surveillance at the State and Local Level," *Teratology* 56 (1997): 5. Bengt Kallen, *Epidemiology of Human Reproduction* (Boca Raton, FL, 1988), 76–77. Milham, "Congenital Malformation Surveillance System," 448–50.

119. Armstrong, *Conceiving Risk, Bearing Responsibility,* 5, 157–61.

120. Public Relations Department, March of Dimes, "Hopeful Research in Birth Defects Inspires March of Dimes Workers," News Release, December 27, 1965, Medical Program Records, Series 3, Box 3, Birth Defects Registries (Apgar), 1965–69, March of Dimes, White Plains, NY. Virginia Apgar, "Science's War on Birth Defects," Typescript, c. 1960, March of Dimes, White Plains, NY. Virginia Apgar, "Prospective Studies in Human Teratogenesis" (paper presented at the Third Scientific Session of the Irish and American Paediatric Society, Moyne Institute, Dublin, Ireland, June 26, 1970), p. 5. S. M. Kane, "Administrative Significance of Computerized Medical Studies," *Circulation Research* 11 (1962): 647–49, Virginia Apgar, Box 2 of 3, Typescripts, Congenital Abnormalities and Birth Defects, 1967–1970, March of Dimes, White Plains, New York.

121. Fluoridation, Medical Program Records, Series 3, Box 3, Birth Defects, Chemicals, Fluoridation, 1959–64; Herbicides, Medical Program Records, Series 3, Box 3, Birth Defects, Chemicals, Herbicide 2–4–5–T; Lead Paint, Medical Program Records, Series 3, Box 3, Birth Defects, Chemicals, Lead Paint, 1970, Folder. Apgar, March of Dimes, White Plains, NY. *Los Angeles Times,* August 29, 1972, A1. *New York Times,* January 28, 1971, 32.

122. Gerald Markowitz and David Rosner, *Deceit and Denial: The Deadly Politics of Industrial Pollution* (Berkeley, CA, 2002), 168–208.

123. Ibid., 208–9.

124. Although it would not come to light until the 1980s, two communities in the area of Plaquemine, Louisiana, discovered "that a growing number of their water wells were polluted with chemicals used in the production of vinyl chloride." Ibid., 242. See also 243–45.

125. *Los Angeles Times,* February 18, 1978, A1. *Los Angeles Times,* June 14, 1979, B21. *Los Angeles Times,* September 5, 1979, B3. *Washington Post,* November 9, 1979, A12. *New York Times,* March 22, 1980, 6. *Wall Street Journal,* March 5, 1980, 8. *Washington Post,* July 26, 1980, A21. *New York Times,* April 9, 1983.

126. *New York Times,* March 5, 1976, 61.

127. *New York Times,* April 9, 1983, 1.

128. Sara Tjossem, Personal Communication, November 15, 2006.

129. Executive Office of the President, Office of Management and Budget, "Statement of Administrative Policy" on *Children's Health Act of 2000,* May 9, 2000, p. 2. Jo Merrill, Interview, November 4, 2005.

130. Edmonds, Interview.

131. Http://www.cbdmp.org/spd_history.htm, accessed September 10, 2005.

132. Medical Program Records, Series 3, Box 3, Birth Defects, California Birth Defects Monitoring Program, Scientific Accomplishments, 1990–91, March of Dimes, White Plains, NY.

133. Http://www.cbdmp.org/, accessed September 10, 2005.

134. Http://www.cbdmp.org/spd_community_intro.htm, accessed September 10, 2005.

135. Edmonds, "Birth Defect Surveillance," 5. Kallen, *Epidemiology of Human Reproduction,* 76–77.

136. Kay A. Johnson, "Birth Defects and Infant Mortality," Infant Mortality Report Series, Vol. 1, No. 2 (March of Dimes Birth Defects Foundation, December 1991): 4, 79, Medical Program Records, Series 3, Box 3, Birth Defects, Birth Defects and Infant Mortality, Report, 1991, March of Dimes, White Plains, NY.

137. *Houston Chronicle,* September 2, 1991, 1. *Houston Chronicle,* August 2, 1992. *Houston Post,* July 11, 1993.

138. David Smith, Interview, July 16, 2002.

139. Bill Mongelluzzo, "Twin Plants Shine On in Mexico," *Journal of Commerce,* May 18, 1987, 4A.

140. *New York Times,* September 23, 1992, C12. Smith, Interview.

141. *Houston Chronicle,* June 16, 1993, 22.

142. *Houston Post,* July 11, 1993, A1.

143. *Houston Post,* February 4, 1993, 25.

144. *St. Petersburg Times,* November 18, 1996, 1B. *Houston Post,* July 11, 1993. See also Phil Brown, "Popular Epidemiology: Community Response to Toxic Waste–Induced Disease in Woburn, Massachusetts," *Science, Technology and Human Values* 12 (1987).

145. *Houston Chronicle,* August 2, 1992, State p. 1.

146. *Houston Post,* July 11, 1993, A1.

147. *Houston Chronicle,* June 16, 1993, 22.

148. *Houston Post,* July 11, 1993, A1.

149. Melanie Lockhart, Interview, November 9, 2005.

150. *Houston Chronicle,* March 12, 1993, A23. *Houston Chronicle,* February 21, 2002, A26. *Houston Chronicle,* January 31, 1995, A12.

151. *Houston Chronicle,* August 2, 1992, A1. *New York Times,* September 23, 1992, C12.

152. *Houston Chronicle,* February 21, 2002, A26. *Houston Chronicle,* January 31, 1995, A12.

153. Centers for Disease Control and Prevention, "Temporal Trends in the Incidence of Birth Defects—United States," *Morbidity and Mortality Weekly Report* 46 (1997): 1175. Centers for Disease Control and Prevention, "Spina Bifida and Anencephaly before and after Folic Acid Mandate—United States, 1995–1996 and 1999–2000," *Morbidity and Mortality Weekly Report* 53 (2004): 362.

154. Centers for Disease Control and Prevention, "Spina Bifida and Anencephaly," 364, 362. Janet D. Cragan et al., "Surveillance for Anencephaly and Spina Bifida and the Impact of Prenatal Diagnosis—United States, 1985–1994," *Morbidity and Mortality Weekly Report* 44 (1995): 12–13.

155. David F. Musto, *The American Disease* (New York, 1987), 258.

156. *Planned Parenthood of Central Missouri et al. v. Danforth,* 428 U.S. 52 (1976). Writing for the court, Justice Blackmun added that confidentiality requirements that limited use of the records to health officials and specified that they must be kept only for seven years "assist and persuade us in our determination of the constitutional limits. As so regarded, we see no legally significant impact or consequence on the abortion decision or on the physician-patient relationship."

157. Martin Pernick, *The Black Stork: Eugenics and the Death of "Defective" Babies in American Medicine and Motion Pictures since 1915* (New York, 1996), 48–51, 148.

158. Jesse L. Steinfeld, "Women and Children Last? Attitudes toward Cigarette Smoking and Nonsmokers' Rights," *New York State Medical Journal* 19 (1971): 1257.

159. Armstrong, *Conceiving Risk, Bearing Responsibility,* 71, 90. Golden, *Message in a Bottle,* 35–36.

160. Golden, *Message in a Bottle,* 87, 5, 75.

161. Ibid., 74, 47–48, 97.

162. "Pesticides and Birth Defects: A Minnesota Study," *Pesticide Action Network North America,* June 1996.

163. Alan Brinkley, *Voices of Protest: Huey Long, Father Coughlin and the Great Depression* (New York, 1982), 226–28. Eric Foner, *Give Me Liberty: An American History* (New York, 2005), 835.

164. Aggie Leitheiser, Interview, November 17, 2005. Lockhart, Interview.

165. Twila Brase, Testimony on Unique Patient Identifiers before the Subcommittee on Standards and Security, Hearings on Unique Health Identifiers for Individuals, James R. Thompson Center, Chicago, http://www.nchs.hhs.gov/980721t1.htm, accessed September 10, 2005.

166. Twila Brase, Speech before the National Press Club, June 8, 1999, www.cchconline.org/privacy/spchihf.php3, accessed September 10, 2005. See also Twila Brase, Testimony on Minnesota Department of Health Rule 4653, House Health and Human Services Policy Committee, January 22, 2003, http://www.cchconline.org/testimony/to12203.php, accessed September 10, 2005.

167. Leitheiser, Interview.

168. Twila Brase, "Public Health Rails against Patient Privacy," originally published in the *Texas Society for Psychiatric Physicians Newsletter,* December/January 2001, http://www.cchconline.org/publications/privphart.php3, accessed September 10, 2005.

169. "Health Policy Group Alarmed That Nevada Legislation Poised to Track 'Defective' Kids May Be Start of National Database," April 20, 1999, http://www.cchconline.org/pr/pro42099.php3, accessed September 10, 2005.

170. Asch, "Prenatal Diagnosis and Selective Abortion."

171. Stern, *Eugenic Nation.*

172. *New York Times,* March 13, 1983, p. NJ1. *New York Times,* April 19, 1996, B5.

173. Cragan et al., "Surveillance for Anencephaly and Spina Bifida," 2. Armstrong, *Conceiving Risk, Bearing Responsibility,* 194.

174. *New York Times,* March 13, 1983, p. NJ1. *New York Times,* April 19, 1996, B5.

175. Stern, *Eugenic Nation.*

176. *New York Times,* March 13, 1983, p. NJ1. *New York Times,* April 19, 1996, B5.

177. Birth Defects Work Group, minutes, Minnesota Department of Health, May 29, 2002, and February 26, 2003, http://www.health.state.mn.us/divs/eh/birth defects/workgroup/index.html, accessed September 10, 2005.

178. Leitheiser, Interview. Twila Brase, Testimony before the Minnesota House Health and Human Services Committee, Hearing on Patient Consent and Medical Privacy, February 20, 2001, http://www.cchconline.org/testimony/t022001.php3.

179. Lockhart, Interview.

180. Birth Defects Work Group, minutes, February 26, 2003.

181. *Star Tribune* (Minnesota), June 4, 2004, 1B.

182. Birth Defects Work Group, Minutes, May 29, 2002, and February 26, 2004.

183. Birth Defects Work Group, minutes, May 29, 2002.

184. Birth Defects Prevention and Services Subgroup, minutes, August 13, 2002, http://www.health.state.mn.us/divs/eh/birthdefects/workgroup/index.html.

185. Birth Defects Work Group, minutes, February 26, 2004.

186. Leitheiser, Interview. Birth Defects Prevention and Services Subgroup, minutes. Birth Defects Work Group, minutes, February 26, 2003, and February 26, 2004. March of Dimes, Minnesota Chapter, "Birth Defects Information System (BDIS) APPROVED: March of Dimes Applauds Legislation to Implement New System," News Release, www.marchofdimes.com/minnesota/7256.asp, accessed September 10, 2005.

187. Birth Defects Prevention and Services Subgroup, minutes.

188. Birth Defects Work Group, minutes, May 29, 2002.

189. Birth Defects Work Group, minutes, February 26, 2003.

190. 144.2216, Subd. 4. Minnesota Birth Defects Information System, http://www.health.state.mn.us/divs/eh/birthdefects/statute.html, accessed September 10, 2005.

191. 144.2215, Subd. 2. Minnesota Birth Defects Information System, http://www.health.state.mn.us/divs/eh/birthdefects/statute.html, accessed September 10, 2005.

192. Sarah Wyatt, "Senate Passes Bill Creating Registry of Children with Birth Defects," *Associated Press*, March 7, 2000. "Thompson Signs List of Bills," *Associated Press*, May 8, 2000. Elizabeth Oftedahl et al., "Wisconsin Birth Defects Registry Collecting Data," *Wisconsin Medical Journal* 103 (2004). Carole M. Doeppers, "Data Surveillance: Cause for Concern," ACLU of Wisconsin Data Privacy Project, December 23, 1999, www.aclu-wi.org. Doeppers's editorial was picked up by at least two local papers as well as the *Wisconsin State Medical Journal*. See also Carole M. Doeppers, "Data Surveillance: A Citizen's Guide to Government Registries and Reporting Systems," ACLU of Wisconsin Data Privacy Project, March 2001. Also available on the Wisconsin-ACLU website, www.aclu-wi.org, accessed September 10, 2005.

193. Wyatt, "Senate Passes Bill."

194. National Birth Defects Prevention Network, "Guidelines for Conducting Birth Defects Surveillance National Birth Defects Prevention Network," http://nbdpn.org/current/resources/sgm/NBDPN_Guidelines.pdf, accessed May 11, 2006.

195. Lockhart, Interview.

196. Merrill, Interview. See also Jo Merrill, "Birth Defects Prevention Act Becomes Law," *National Birth Defects Prevention Network Newsletter* 2 (1998): 3.

197. "Birth Defects Prevention Act: Legislative History," Office of Government Affairs, March of Dimes. Document in possession of authors.

198. Merrill, Interview. Merrill, "Birth Defects Prevention Act Becomes Law." Solomon P. Ortiz and Henry Bonilla, "Ortiz, Bonilla Announce Birth Defects Registry Bill," February 22, 1995, Office of Government Affairs, March of Dimes. Document in possession of authors.

199. "Birth Defects Prevention Act of 1993: Statement of Need," p. 1, Office of Government Affairs, March of Dimes. Document in possession of authors. See also "Birth Defects Prevention Act Passed by Congress," News Release, March 10, 1998, March of Dimes, White Plains, NY, and Ortiz and Bonilla, News Release.

200. Http://www.cwfa.org/about.asp, accessed November 16, 2005.

201. Centers for Disease Control and Prevention, Testimony to the National Committee on Vital Health Statistics, Subcommittee on Privacy and Confidentiality, on Health Insurance Portability and Accountability Act Privacy Rule and the Family Educational Rights and Privacy Act Impact on Public Health Practice, prepared by Beverly J. Dozier, February 19, 2004, 3. Document in possession of authors.

202. United Press International, "Capital Comment for April 2, 2003," http://www.upi.com/inc/view.php?StoryID = 20030401–051650–9778r, accessed November 16, 2005.

203. Beverly Dozier-Peeples, "Family Education Rights and Privacy Act of 1974 (20 U.S.C. 1232g) (FERPA)," Powerpoint presentation, November 17, 2005, www.cdc.gov/nceh/tracking/webinars/mar05/dozier.pdf, accessed May 19, 2006.

204. Department of Health and Human Services, Centers for Disease Control and Prevention, "CDC's Strategy for the National Environmental Public Health Tracking Program, Fiscal Years 2005–2010," pp. 14–15, http://www.cdc.gov/nceh/tracking/pdfs/strategy.pdf, accessed November 17, 2005.

205. Dozier-Peeples, "Family Education Rights and Privacy Act."

206. "CDC Obtains Children's Confidential Records without Parental Consent for Autism Study, Says NAA," March 1, 2006, http://news.findlaw.com/prenewswire/20060301/01mar20061456.html, accessed May 17, 2006.

207. F. John Meaney, "Introduction: Birth Defects Surveillance in the United States," *Teratology* 64 (2001).

208. Http://www.cdc.gov/ncbddd/bd/state.htm, accessed November 16, 2005. See also "Birth Defects Surveillance Cooperative Agreements," *National Birth Defects Prevention Network Newsletter* 5 (June 2001): 2, and Naomi Bromberg Bar-Yam, "Birth Defects Surveillance Registries in the United States and Europe," *International Journal of Childbirth Education* 14 (1999): 30.

209. Http://www.cdc.gov/ncbddd/bd/nbdps.htm#states, accessed November 16, 2005.

210. Ibid.

211. Anita M. Farel et al., "Registry to Referral: A Promising Means for Identifying and Referring Infants and Toddlers for Early Intervention Services," *Infants and Young Children* 16 (2003): 104.

212. Lockhart, Interview.

213. Edmonds, Interview.

214. D. K. Walker, "Integrating Birth Defects Surveillance in Maternal and Child Health at the State Level," *Teratology* 61 (2000): 5 (emphasis added). See also

Lorenzo D. Botto et al., "Fostering International Collaboration in Birth Defects Research and Prevention: A Perspective from the International Clearinghouse for Birth Defects Surveillance and Research," *American Journal of Public Health* 96 (2006).

CHAPTER 7

1. "Pneumocystis Pneumonia—Los Angeles," *Morbidity and Mortality Weekly Report* 30 (1981): 250−52.

2. Ibid.

3. "Kaposi's Sarcoma and Pneumocystis Pneumonia among Homosexual Men—New York City and California," *Morbidity and Mortality Weekly Report* 30 (1981): 305−8.

4. American Association of Physicians for Human Rights, *Newsletter,* July 1983, as cited in Ronald Bayer, *Private Acts, Social Consequences: AIDS and the Politics of Public Health* (New York, 1989).

5. William H. Foege, Memorandum, Re: Nondisclosure Agreement, September 28, 1983. Document in possession of authors.

6. Simson L. Garfinkel, "AIDS and the Soundex Code," *IRB* 10 (1988), 8.

7. James O. Mason, Memorandum, Re: Confidentiality of AIDS Surveillance Data, July 6, 1984. Document in possession of authors.

8. Ibid.

9. James R. Allen, Memorandum, Re: Reasons for Reporting Names of AIDS Patients to CDC, July 14, 1983. Document in possession of authors.

10. *American Medical News,* October 7, 1983, as cited in Bayer, *Private Acts.*

11. Ibid.

12. Jeffrey Levi and Christopher J. Collins to James R. Allen, April 25,1984. Document in possession of authors.

13. Ibid.

14. Ibid.

15. James R. Allen to Jeffrey Levi, July 5, 1984. Document in possession of authors.

16. *Bowers v. Hardwick et al.,* 478 U.S. 186 (1986).

17. *New York Native,* June 3−16, 1985, 17, as cited in Bayer, *Private Acts.*

18. United States Conference of Local Health Officers to Ronald Altman, May 8, 1985, as cited in Bayer, *Private Acts.*

19. *New York Native,* June 3−16, 1985, 17, as cited in Bayer, *Private Acts.*

20. Ibid.

21. Ibid., 18.

22. Bayer, *Private Acts.*

23. Thomas Vernon, Interview, 1986, as cited in Bayer, *Private Acts.*

24. "Amendment to the Rules and Regulations Pertaining to Communicable Disease Control to Require Reporting of HTLVIII Antibody Tests," August 21, 1985, as cited in Bayer, *Private Acts.*

25. Colorado Board of Health, Minutes, August 21, 1985, as cited in Bayer, *Private Acts.*

26. Vernon, Interview, 1986.

27. Colorado Board of Health, Minutes, September 18, 1985, as cited in Bayer, *Private Acts.*

28. *Rocky Mountain News*, October 13, 1985, 55.

29. Julian Rush, Interview, November 14, 1986, as cited in Bayer, *Private Acts.*

30. Vernon, Interview.

31. Thomas Vernon, "Remarks," in *AIDS: Impact on Public Policy*, ed. Robert F. Hummel et al. (New York, 1986), 26.

32. Rush, Interview.

33. Ibid.

34. James Mason to State and Territorial Health Officers, December 6, 1985, as cited in Bayer, *Private Acts.*

35. "Additional Recommendations to Reduce Sexual and Drug Abuse–Related Transmission of Human T-lymphotropic Virus Type III/Lymphadenopathy-Associated Virus," *Morbidity and Mortality Weekly Report* 35 (1986): 154.

36. U.S. Conference of Mayors, "AIDS Information Exchange," February 1986, as cited in Bayer, *Private Acts.*

37. Christopher Collins to Kathleen Hoerner, March 24, 1986, as cited in Bayer, *Private Acts.*

38. Khrusho Ghandhi and Brian Lantz to the attorney general of California, October 23, 1985, as cited in Bayer, *Private Acts.*

39. *San Francisco Chronicle*, June 25, 1986, 7, as cited in Bayer, *Private Acts.*

40. *Washington Post*, October 9, 1985, C5, as cited in Bayer, *Private Acts.*

41. Bayer, *Private Acts*, 147.

42. "Initiative Measure to Be Submitted Directly to the Voters," 1985, as cited in Bayer, *Private Acts.*

43. *Wall Street Journal*, August 11, 1986, 38, as cited in Bayer, *Private Acts.*

44. "Rebuttal Argument against Proposition 64," 1986, as cited in Bayer, *Private Acts.*

45. No on 64, "Campaign Report," November 30, 1986, 26, as cited in Bayer, *Private Acts.*

46. Joan K. Leavitt, John Harkess, and Gregory R. Istre, "HIV Reporting in Oklahoma: Guidelines for Physicians and Answers to Common Questions," *Journal of the Oklahoma State Medical Association* 81 (1988): 522.

47. Presidential Commission on the Human Immunodeficiency Virus Epidemic, "Report," June 1988. Document in possession of authors.

48. Stephen C. Joseph, "A Bridge to Treatment: The Needle Exchange Pilot Program in New York City," *AIDS Education and Prevention* 1 (1989): 340–45.

49. *American Medical News*, May 18, 1990, 3, as cited in Ronald Bayer, "The Dependent Center: The First Decade of the AIDS Epidemic in New York City," *Hives of Sickness: Public Health and Epidemics in New York City*, ed. David Rosner (New Brunswick, NJ, 1995).

50. Ibid.

51. *American Medical News*, July 8, 1988, 4.

52. William N. Jones, "The System Works if You Are Willing to Work the System," *Journal of the Arkansas Medical Society* 86 (1990): 349.

53. Ibid., 347.

54. American Medical Association Board of Trustees, "AMA·1990 HIV Policies," December 1990. Document in possession of authors.

55. "HIV Infection Reporting—United States," *Morbidity and Mortality Weekly Report* 38 (1989): 496–99.

56. *New York Native*, October 1, 1990. Document in possession of authors.

57. Ruth L. Berkelman to Wilma Johnson, Memorandum, Re: OMB Approval: Infection with Human Immunodeficiency Disease Report Form, October 25, 1989. Document in possession of authors.

58. Council of State and Territorial Epidemiologists, "Position Statement, 1989–2: HIV Infection Reporting," 1989. Document in possession of authors.

59. Ronald Bayer, L. H. Lumey, and Lourdes Wan, "The American, British and Dutch Responses to Unlinked Anonymous HIV Seroprevalence Studies: An International Comparison," *AIDS* 4 (1990): 283–90.

60. Centers for Disease Control and Prevention, "HIV Seroprevalence Survey of Childbearing Women: Testing Neonatal Dried Blood Specimens on Filter Paper for HIV Antibody," Atlanta, CDC, draft, August 8, 1988, as cited in Bayer, Lumey, and Wan, "American, British and Dutch Responses."

61. Intergovernmental Health Policy Project, George Washington University, "Results from the 1992 AIDS Policy Center HIV Reporting Survey," *Intergovernmental AIDS Reports*, October 1992, 3–5. Document in possession of authors.

62. Carl H. Campbell Jr. and Gary R. West to Ronald O. Valdiserri, Memorandum, Re: Trip Report: AIDS Action Council Consultant Meeting on HIV Reporting and Partner Notification, October 9, 1992. Document in possession of authors.

63. Jeffrey Levi to William Parra, October 7, 1992. Document in possession of authors.

64. Centers for Disease Control and Prevention, "Consultation on Developing Guidelines for HIV Surveillance," January 26–27, 1993, 9. Document in possession of authors.

65. Ibid.

66. Ibid., 17.

67. Ibid., 13.

68. U.S. Congress, *Office of Technology Assessment, The CDC's Case Definition of AIDS: Implications of the Proposed Revisions—Background Paper,* OTA-BP-H-89 (Washington, DC, 1992).

69. Council of State and Territorial Epidemiologists, "Position Statement 2A: Surveillance of HIV Infection and Disease," 1991. Document in possession of authors.

70. "CDC's Expanded AIDS Case Definition Sparks Controversy," *AIDS Alert* 7 (1992): 65–71.

71. Theresa McGovern, "Consensus Statement on the U.S. AIDS Surveillance Definition" (paper presented at the Eighth International Conference on AIDS, Amsterdam, 1992). Document in possession of authors.

72. U.S. Department of Health and Human Services, "Resource Packet for Implementation of the 1993 Expanded Surveillance Case Definition for Acquired Immunodeficiency Syndrome (AIDS)," December 1992. Document in possession of authors.

73. Paul DiDonato and Elizabeth B. Cooper, Memorandum, Re: CONFIDEN-

TIALITY ALERT: The New AIDS Surveillance Definition—Reporting Mechanisms, December 17, 1992 (emphasis in original). Document in possession of authors.

74. Ibid.

75. Stephen Shapiro to David Hansell, July 20, 1993. Document in possession of authors.

76. Liza Solomon, Interview, February 25, 2003.

77. Ibid.

78. Nelson Sabatini to William Roper, May 14, 1992. Document in possession of authors.

79. William Roper to Nelson Sabatini, June 24, 1992. Document in possession of authors.

80. Department of Health and Mental Hygiene, "Development of a Unique Patient Identifying Number System (HB 460, 1992)," December 1992. Document in possession of authors.

81. Solomon, Interview.

82. Planned Parenthood of Metropolitan Washington, DC, Inc., "Comments on Proposed Section 10.52.09 of the Code of Maryland Regulations (COMAR) Pertaining to HIV/CD4$^+$ Lymphocyte Count Reporting by Unique Patient Identifying Number," October 19, 1993. Document in possession of authors.

83. Baltimore Department of Health and Mental Hygiene, *Hearing in the Matter of: Proposal of Adoption of Regulations of Title 10, Sub-title 52, Chapter 9, HIV/CD4$^+$ Lymphocyte Count Reporting by Unique Patient Identifying Number,* October 20, 1993. Document in possession of authors.

84. Joseph Snyder, Testimony of the President of the Medical and Chirurgical Faculty of Maryland, October 26, 1993. Document in possession of authors.

85. Kathleen F. Edwards to P. Gregory Rausch, July 7, 1994. Document in possession of authors.

86. Centers for Disease Control and Prevention, "Consultation on the Future Direction and Practice of HIV Infection and AIDS Case Surveillance in the United States: The Role of (Non-Name) Unique Identifiers in Case Surveillance," May 21–22, 1997, 1. Document in possession of authors.

87. Michael Adams, "The Maryland Lesson: Conducting Effective HIV Surveillance with Unique Identifiers," December 1997, 7. Document in possession of authors.

88. Solomon, Interview.

89. David Smith, Interview, July 16, 2002. Solomon, Interview.

90. Smith, Interview. Solomon, Interview.

91. "Evaluation of HIV Case Surveillance through the Use of Non-name Unique Identifiers—Maryland and Texas, 1994–1996," *Morbidity and Mortality Weekly Report* 46 (1998): 1254.

92. Kevin M. Kramer, "A National Epidemic, a National Conversation, a National Law: In Support of Unique Identifier Reporting for HIV Surveillance," *Journal of Contemporary Health Law and Policy* 16 (1999): 173–209.

93. Liza Solomon et al., "Evaluation of a Statewide Non–Name-Based HIV Surveillance System," *Journal of Acquired Immune Deficiency Syndromes* 22 (1999): 272–79.

94. E. M. Connor et al., "Reduction of Maternal-Infant Transmission of Human Immunodeficiency Virus Type 1 with Zidovudine Treatment," *New England Journal of Medicine* 331 (1994): 1173–80.

95. "HIV and AIDS—United States, 1981–2000," *Morbidity and Mortality Weekly Report* 50 (2001): 430–34.

96. *American Medical News* 31 (1996). Document in possession of authors.

97. Helene D. Gayle, Testimony before the House Committee on Commerce, Subcommittee on Health and the Environment, May 11, 1995. Document in possession of authors.

98. Joseph M. Posid to Andrea Spillars, November 14, 1996, 1. Document in possession of authors.

99. Lawrence O. Gostin, James G. Hodge, and Ronald O. Valdiserri, "Informational Privacy and the Public's Health: The Model State Public Health Privacy Act," *American Journal of Public Health* 91 (2001): 1389.

100. Centers for Disease Control and Prevention to AIDS surveillance coordinators, "Alleged Breach in Confidentiality of AIDS Surveillance Data, State of Florida," September 20, 1996. Document in possession of authors.

101. *Tampa Tribune,* September 20, 1996. *St. Petersburg Times,* September 20, 1996. In possession of authors.

102. Florida Department of Health and Rehabilitative Services, "State Launches Criminal Investigation into AIDS Confidentiality Breach," News Release, September 19, 1996. Document in possession of authors.

103. "Status of CDC Review of State of Florida's Policies and Procedures for Ensuring Confidentiality of AIDS Surveillance Data," October 3, 1996, 1. Document in possession of authors.

104. "Consultation on the Future Direction and Practice of HIV Infection and AIDS Case Surveillance in the United States," n.d. Document in possession of authors.

105. Ibid.

106. Ibid.

107. Cory SerVaas, "Dr. Tom Coburn's Bill Would Bring Back Public Health Measures," *Saturday Evening Post* 270 (1998): 60–67. *HIV Prevention Act of 1997,* HR 1062, 105th Cong., 1st sess., *Congressional Record* 143 (March 13, 1997).

108. Council of State and Territorial Epidemiologists, "Position Statement 1997-ID-4, National HIV Surveillance: Addition to the National Public Health Surveillance System," 1997. Document in possession of authors.

109. "Update: Trends in AIDS Incidence—United States, 1996," *Morbidity and Mortality Weekly Report* 46 (1997): 861–67.

110. *New York Times,* September 11, 1997, A27.

111. Lawrence O. Gostin, John W. Ward, and A. Cornelius Baker, "National HIV Case Reporting for the United States—a Defining Moment in the History of the Epidemic," *New England Journal of Medicine* 337 (1997): 1162–63.

112. Matthew Coles, Michael Adams, and Jennifer Middleton, "HIV Surveillance and Name Reporting: A Public Health Case for Protecting Civil Liberties," October 1997, 11. Document in possession of authors.

113. Kevin DeCock, Interview, July 18, 2002.

114. Ibid.

115. "Security Standards for the Protection of HIV/AIDS Surveillance Information and Data Draft 11," October 30, 1997. Document in possession of authors.

116. Centers for Disease Control and Prevention, "Communication to Surveillance Coordinators," 1998. Document in possession of authors.

117. Dennis H. Osmond et al., "Name-Based Surveillance and Public Health Interventions for Persons with HIV Infection," *Annals of Internal Medicine* 131 (1999): 775–79.

118. Frederick M. Hecht et al., "Does HIV Reporting by Name Deter Testing?" *AIDS* 14 (2000): 1801.

119. Patricia L. Fleming to Ulder J. Tillman, July 27, 1999. Document in possession of authors.

120. *New York Times,* January 23, 1998, B1.

121. New York State AIDS Advisory Council HIV Surveillance Workgroup, Findings, April 1998. Document in possession of authors.

122. AIDS Advisory Council of New York State, "A Minority Report, Workgroup on HIV Surveillance," March 31, 1998. Document in possession of authors.

123. *New York Times,* June 19, 1998, A1.

124. *Boston Globe,* February 24, 1998, B4.

125. Robert W. Wood et al., "The Washington State 'Name-to-Code' HIV Reporting System: A Public Health Perspective," *Journal of Public Health Management and Practice* 8 (2002): 2.

126. *Seattle Times,* January 16, 1999, A1.

127. "CDC Draft Guidelines for Improved Data on U.S. HIV Epidemic; New System Urgently Needed to Guide Prevention Efforts," News Release, n.d. Document in possession of authors.

128. "Review of Comments on CDC Draft Guidelines," Typescript, n.d. Document in possession of authors.

129. Ibid.

130. Ibid.

131. Patricia L. Fleming et al., "Guidelines for National Human Immunodeficiency Virus Case Surveillance, Including Monitoring for Human Immunodeficiency Virus Infection and Acquired Immunodeficiency Syndrome," *Morbidity and Mortality Weekly Report* 48 (1999): 1–28.

132. Committee on Commerce, *Hearing before the Subcommittee on Health and the Environment on H.R. 4807,* 106th Cong., 2nd sess., 2000, 3.

133. Ibid., 2.

134. Institute of Medicine, *Measuring What Matters: Allocation, Planning, and Quality Assessment for the Ryan White CARE Act* (Washington, DC, 2004), 30.

135. *San Francisco Examiner,* October 1, 1998, A8.

136. Institute of Medicine, *No Time to Lose: Getting More from HIV Prevention* (Washington, DC, 2001), 14–25.

137. Institute of Medicine, *Measuring What Matters,* 126.

CHAPTER 8

1. See, for example, Opinion Research Corporation, *Public Attitudes toward Immunization: August 1977 and February 1978* (Princeton, NJ, 1978).

2. Samuel W. Abbott, "Legislation with Reference to Smallpox and Vaccination," *Boston Medical and Surgical Journal* 147 (1902): 268.

3. See, for example, Walter R. Coles to John L. Rice, October 1, 1940, Box 141511, Smallpox Folder, New York City Department of Health Archives, New York.

4. Jeffrey P. Baker, "Immunization and the American Way: 4 Childhood Vaccines," *American Journal of Public Health* 90 (2000): 199–207.

5. On the increasing influence of medical experts on child rearing, see Sydney A. Halpern, *American Pediatrics: The Social Dynamics of Professionalism, 1880–1980* (Berkeley, CA, 1988), 90–98; and Charles R. King, *Children's Health in America: A History* (New York, 1993), 124–42.

6. Susan L. Plotkin and Stanley A. Plotkin, "A Short History of Vaccination," in *Vaccines*, 4th ed., ed. Stanley A. Plotkin and Walter Orenstein (Philadelphia, 2004).

7. F. Robert Freckleton, "Preschool Diphtheria Immunization Status of a New York State Community," *American Journal of Public Health* 39 (1949): 1439–40.

8. A. W. Hedrich, "The Corrected Average Attack Rate from Measles among City Children," *American Journal of Hygiene* 11 (1930): 576–600.

9. Edward S. Godfrey, "Practical Uses of Diphtheria Immunization Records," *American Journal of Public Health* 23 (1933): 810.

10. William J. Meyer, "Determination of Immunization Status of School Children in New York State," *New York State Journal of Medicine* 60 (1960): 2870.

11. Robert E. Serfling, R. G. Cornell, and Ida L. Sherman, "The CDC Quota Sampling Technic with Results of 1959 Poliomyelitis Vaccination Surveys," *American Journal of Public Health* 50 (1960): 1847–57.

12. Theodore J. Bauer to Luther Terry, August 2, 1961, Record Group 442, Box 105229, Associations, Committees, Etc., 1961, Folder, National Archives and Records Administration, College Park, MD.

13. James L. Goddard, "Future Goals of Immunization Programs," in *2nd Immunization Conference Proceedings* (Atlanta, 1965), 10–11.

14. Ibid.

15. Shirley W. Wynne to Arthur W. Proctor, October 22, 1932, Box 141380, Diphtheria Folder, New York City Department of Health Archives, New York.

16. "Immunization Activities Project: First City-wide Mailing of Birth Certificates Follow-Up Program," *Bulletin to Professors of Preventive Medicine*, February 1967, 2. *New York Times*, March 2, 1967, 37. Department of Health (New York), "Health Services General Project Grant," Typescript, September 10, 1968, Box 142241, Preventable Disease Folder, New York City Department of Health Archives, New York.

17. Earl B. Byrne et al., "Infant Immunization Surveillance: Cost vs. Effect," *Journal of the American Medical Association* 212 (1970): 772.

18. Frank L. Lewis, "Application of Childhood Immunization Follow-Up System," in *14th Immunization Conference Proceedings* (Atlanta, 1979).

19. Ibid.

20. Byrne, "Infant Immunization Surveillance."

21. Robert A. Ford to Edward O'Rourke, April 28, 1967, Box 142024, 1967 Folder, New York City Department of Health Archives, New York.

22. Lewis, "Application of Childhood Immunization System," in *14th Immunization Conference Proceedings*.

23. Elizabeth Craven, "CIFS and the Private Provider," in *14th Immunization Conference Proceedings*.

24. Patrick M. Vivier, "National Policies for Childhood Immunization in the United States: A Historical Perspective" (Ph.D. diss., Johns Hopkins University, 1996).

25. Walter Orenstein, Interview, September 25, 2003.

26. Kay A. Johnson, Alice Sardell, and B. Richards, "Federal Immunization Policy and Funding: A History of Responding to Crises," *American Journal of Preventive Medicine* 19 (2000): 99–112.

27. Richard E. Neustadt and Harvey V. Fineberg, *The Epidemic That Never Was: Policy-Making and the Swine Flu Affair* (New York, 1982).

28. Vivier, "National Policies for Childhood Immunization," 166–69.

29. Louise L. Liang, "Overview of Childhood Immunization Follow-Up Systems," in *14th Immunization Conference Proceedings*, 57.

30. John P. Fanning, "Privacy Issues in the Childhood Immunization Follow-Up System," in *14th Immunization Conference Proceedings*, 30.

31. Max R. Pesses, "Five Steps for Maintaining Immunization Levels," in *15th Immunization Conference Proceedings* (Atlanta, 1980), 58.

32. Walton L. Ector, "Immunization Levels of Children in Private Practice," in *15th Immunization Conference Proceedings*.

33. Hugh L. Blumen, "A Comprehensive Immunization Data System," in *15th Immunization Conference Proceedings*.

34. Gordon H. DeFriese et al., "Developing Child Immunization Registries," in *To Improve Health and Health Care 1997*, ed. Stephen L. Isaacs and James R. Knickman (Princeton, NJ, 1997).

35. *Washington Post*, December 31, 1987, A17.

36. *Washington Post*, January 1, 1988, A18.

37. Kay A. Johnson, Interview, November 15, 2004.

38. Walter A. Orenstein et al. "The Elusiveness of Measles Elimination: Ten Years and Still Counting," in *23rd National Immunization Conference Proceedings* (Atlanta, 1989).

39. National Vaccine Advisory Committee, "The Measles Epidemic: The Problems, Barriers, and Recommendations," *Journal of the American Medical Association* 266 (1991): 1547–52.

40. Felicity T. Cutts, Walter A. Orenstein, and Roger H. Bernier, "Causes of Low Preschool Immunization Coverage in the United States," *Annual Review of Public Health* 13 (1992): 395.

41. Gary L. Freed, W. Clayton Bordley, and Gordon H. DeFriese, "Childhood Immunization Programs: An Analysis of Policy Issues," *Milbank Memorial Fund Quarterly* 71 (1993): 65–96.

42. Allison Kempe et al., "The Regional Immunization Registry as a Public Health Tool for Improving Clinical Practice and Guiding Immunization Delivery Policy," *American Journal of Public Health* 94 (2004): 967–72. Alan Hinman, Interview, October 1, 2003.

43. Walter A. Orenstein, "Building the Immunization Superhighway: Childhood Immunization Initiative as the Framework," in *28th National Immunization Conference Proceedings* (Atlanta, 1994).

44. Johnson, Interview.

45. William C. Watson et al., "The All Kids Count National Program: A Robert Wood Johnson Foundation Initiative to Develop Immunization Registries," *American Journal of Preventive Medicine* 13 (1997): 3–6.

46. Johnson, Interview.

47. Kay A. Johnson, "Proposal for a National Vaccination Registry," in *25th National Immunization Conference Proceedings* (Atlanta, 1991).

48. Watson et al., "The All Kids Count National Program," 3–6.

49. Shirley Girouard, Interview, September 22, 2003.

50. Johnson, Interview.

51. Amy Zimmerman-Levitan, Interview, October 22, 2003.

52. Daniel Yankelovich, "The Debate That Wasn't: The Public and the Clinton Plan," *Health Affairs* 14 (1995): 7–22.

53. Kay Johnson, Interview.

54. Ibid.

55. Roy Vagelos and Louis Galambos, *Medicine, Science and Merck* (New York, 2004).

56. Committee on Labor and Human Resources, *Comprehensive Child Immunization Act of 1993: Joint Hearing before the Committee on Labor and Human Resources, United States Senate, and the Subcommittee on Health and the Environment of the Committee on Energy and Commerce,* 103rd Cong., 1st sess., April 21, 1993, 46.

57. Ibid., 4.

58. Ibid., 80, 86, and passim.

59. *Washington Times,* June 17, 1993, A5.

60. Victoria A. Freeman and Gordon H. DeFriese, "The Challenge and Potential of Childhood Immunization Registries," *Annual Review of Public Health* 24 (2003): 227–46.

61. Hinman, Interview.

62. Philip R. Horne, Kristin N. Sarlaas, and Alan R. Hinman, "Costs of Immunization Registries: Experiences from the All Kids Count II Projects," *American Journal of Preventive Medicine* 19 (2000): 94–98.

63. Martin Kaufman, "The American Anti-vaccinationists and Their Arguments," *Bulletin of the History of Medicine* 41 (1967): 463–78.

64. James Colgrove, "Science in a Democracy: The Contested Status of Vaccination in the Progressive Era and the 1920s," *Isis* 96 (2005): 167–91.

65. M. Kulenkampff, J. S. Schwartzman, and J. Wilson, "Neurologic Complications of Pertussis Inoculation," *Archives of Diseases in Childhood* 49 (1974): 46–49.

66. Robert D. Johnston, "Contemporary Anti-vaccination Movements in Historical Perspective," in *The Politics of Healing: Histories of Alternative Medicine in Twentieth-Century North America,* ed. Robert D. Johnston (New York, 2004).

67. Robert T. Chen, Robert L. Davis, and Kristine M. Sheedy, "Safety of Immunizations," in *Vaccines.*

68. Johnston, "Contemporary Anti-vaccination Movements," in *The Politics of Healing.*

69. Girouard, Interview.

70. *Comprehensive Child Immunization Act of 1993, Joint Hearing,* 30.

71. Caroline Breese Hall and Harold Margolis, "Hepatitis B Immunization: Premonitions and Perceptions of Pediatricians," *Pediatrics* 91 (1993): 841–43.

72. Robert M. Wolfe, Lisa K. Sharpe, and Martin S. Lipsky, "Content and Design Attributes of Antivaccination Web Sites," *Journal of the American Medical Association* 287 (2002): 3245–48. P. Davies, S. Chapman, and J. Leask, "Antivaccination Activists on the World Wide Web," *Archives of Diseases of Childhood* 87 (2002): 22–25.

73. *In re Christine M.,* 157 Misc. 2d 4 (1992).

74. Barbara Loe Fisher, "Statement: Immunization Registries Workgroup on Privacy and Confidentiality," www.909shot.com/Loe_Fisher/blf51498tracking.html, accessed September 17, 2003.

75. Www.909shot.com, accessed September 13, 2003.

76. Lawrence O. Gostin, James G. Hodge, and Ronald O. Valdiserri, "Informational Privacy and the Public's Health: The Model State Public Health Privacy Act," *American Journal of Public Health* 91 (2001): 1388−92.

77. David Wood et al., "Immunization Registries in the United States: Implications for the Practice of Public Health in a Changing Health Care System," *Annual Review of Public Health* 20 (1999): 231−55.

78. Zimmerman-Levitan, Interview.

79. "Confidentiality," chap. 2 of *Community Immunization Registries Manual,* http://www.cdc.gov/nip/registry/cir-manual.htm#ch2, accessed June 10, 2004.

80. "Testimony on Immunization Registries," www.cchconline.org/testimony/to71698.php3, accessed June 6, 2005.

81. Centers for Disease Control and Prevention, "Findings of Focus Group Research," 19.

82. Centers for Disease Control and Prevention, "Findings of Focus Group Research on Immunization Registries," www.cdc.gov/nip/registry/fg/fg01.pdf, accessed January 12, 2004.

83. Wood et al., "Immunization Registries in the United States."

84. Johnston, "Contemporary Anti-vaccination Movements," in *The Politics of Healing.*

85. *Austin American-Statesman,* April 25, 1998, A1.

86. David Smith, Interview, July 16, 2002.

87. "Maintenance and Operation of Texas Department of Health's Immunization Registry," February 2003, www.tdh.state.tx.us/immunize/immtrac.htm, accessed October 1, 2004.

88. "The Texas Immunization Registry Controversy," www.Vaccineinfo.net/issues/tracking/txregistry, accessed October 11, 2004.

89. George Isham and Jim Nordin, Interview, December 16, 2004.

90. Aggie Leitheiser, Interview, June 21, 2005.

91. Ibid.

92. Ibid.

93. Dimitri A. Christakis, Laurie Stewart, and David Bibus, "Providers' Perceptions of an Immunization Registry," *American Journal of Preventive Medicine* 17 (1999): 150.

94. Amy Metroka, Interview, October 21, 2003.

95. American Academy of Pediatrics, Committee on Practice and Ambulatory Medicine, "Policy on the Development of Immunization Tracking Systems," *Pediatrics* 97 (1996): 927.

96. Orenstein, "Building the Immunization Superhighway," in *28th National Immunization Conference Proceedings.*

97. Lawrence O. Gostin and Zita Lazzarini, "Childhood Immunization Registries: A National Review of Public Health Information Systems and the Protection of Privacy," *Journal of the American Medical Association* 274 (1995): 1793−99.

98. Zimmerman-Levitan, Interview.

99. *State Journal Register (Springfield, IL),* July 31, 1997, p. 1.

100. Www.idph.state.il.us/health/infect/totsfs.htm, accessed June 15, 2005.

101. Hinman, Interview.

102. Kristin N. Sarlaas et al., "All Kids Count 1991–2004: Developing Information Systems to Improve Child Health and the Delivery of Immunizations and Preventive Services," *Journal of Public Health Management and Practice* 10 (2004): S12.

103. Ibid., S5.

104. "Immunization Information System Progress—United States, 2003," *Morbidity and Mortality Weekly Report* 54 (2005): 722–24.

CHAPTER 9

1. Centers for Disease Control and Prevention, Minutes of Conference Call, February 25, 1998. Document in possession of authors.

2. Model State Public Health Privacy Act, first draft, section 2–101. Document in possession of authors.

3. Meeting of Privacy Law Advisory Committee (PLAC) on the Public Health Privacy Act, July 9, 1998, tape 2, Gostin Files.

4. Ibid.

5. Ibid.

6. Privacy Law Advisory Committee, Minutes, July 9, 1998, p. 12. See also first draft of Model State Public Health Privacy Act, p. 14. Documents in possession of authors.

7. Julio C. Abreu, Christopher E. Anders, and Stephen Scarborough to Lawrence O. Gostin, July 8, 1998. Document in possession of authors.

8. Ibid.

9. Ibid.

10. Stephen Scarborough to Lawrence O. Gostin, Memorandum, November 4, 1998. Document in possession of authors.

11. Model State Public Health Privacy Act, PLAC meeting.

12. Guthrie Birkhead to James Hodge, e-mail, November 25, 1998. See also comments of Verla Neslund, Model State Public Health Privacy Act, meeting, and the comments of Scott Burris to James Hodge, September 28, 1998. Document in possession of authors.

13. Timothy Westmoreland, Model State Public Health Privacy Act, PLAC meeting. See also the comments of Stephen Scarborough and Christopher E. Anders on these tapes.

14. Model State Public Health Privacy Act, second draft, 19. Document in possession of authors.

15. Ibid., 21.

16. Robert Gellman, comments on Model State Public Health Privacy Act, second draft, November 11, 1998.

17. Model State Public Health Privacy Act, second draft, 26.

18. Code of Federal Regulations, Title 45, Public Welfare, Department of Health and Human Services, National Institutes of Health, Office for Protection from Research Risks, Part 46, Protection of Human Subjects (45 CFR 46).

19. Stephen Scarborough to Lawrence O. Gostin, December 30, 1998. Document in possession of authors.

20. Model State Public Health Privacy Act, final draft, 18. Document in possession of authors.

21. Lawrence O. Gostin, James G. Hodge, and Ronald O. Valdiseri, "Informational Privacy and the Public's Health: The Model State Public Health Privacy Act," *American Journal of Public Health* 91 (2001): 1388–92.

22. Comments on Model State Public Health Privacy Act, second draft, November 11, 1998.

23. Joy Pritts, Janlori Goldman, Zoe Hudson, Aimee Berenson, and Elizabeth Harldey, "The State of Health Privacy: An Uneven Terrain," Health Privacy Project, 1999.

24. *Health Insurance Portability and Accountability Act of 1996,* Public Law 104–91 (1996): 1178b.

25. Confidentiality of Individually Identifiable Health Information: Recommendations of the Secretary of Health and Human Services, Pursuant to Section 264 of the Health Insurance Portability and Accountability Act of 1996, Submitted to the Committee on Labor and Human Resources et al., September 11, 1997, 3, 4, 49. Document in possession of authors.

26. Janlori Goldman, Director, Health Privacy Project, Georgetown University, Testimony before the House Committee on Ways and Means, March 24, 1998, http://www.healthprivacy.org/usr_doc/33816%2Epdf, accessed April 18, 2006.

27. Ronald Weich and Catherine Weiss, comments on the proposed rule of the U.S. Department of Health and Human Services regarding standards for privacy of individually identifiable health information, February 17, 2000, 49. Document in possession of authors.

28. Catherine Hanssens, comments on Notice of Proposed Rulemaking: standards for privacy of individually identifiable health information, use, and disclosures for public health activities, comment no. 18176, February 17, 2000, http://erm.hhs.gov/hipaa/erm_comment.process_options?user_id=&rule_id=290&num_comm=41&sort_order=DATE&comm_to_display=39, accessed April 18, 2006.

29. Janlori Goldman, Personal Communication, April 18, 2006.

30. Heather Dominique, comments on Notice of Proposed Rulemaking: standards for privacy of individually identifiable health information, use, and disclosures for public health activities, comment no. 18087, February 17, 2000. Document in possession of authors.

31. Martin Weiss, comments on Notice of Proposed Rulemaking: standards for privacy of individually identifiable health information, use, and disclosures for public health activities, comment no. 17685, February 17, 2000. Document in possession of authors.

32. Janlori Goldman, Testimony before the House Committee on Energy and Commerce, Subcommittee on Health, *Assessing HIPAA: How Federal Medical Record Privacy Regulations Can Be Improved,* March 22, 2001, http://energycommerce.house.gov/reparchives/107/hearings/03222001Hearing134/Goldman182.htm, accessed April 18, 2006.

33. National Committee on Vital and Health Statistics, Subcommittee on Privacy

and Confidentiality, November 19, 2003, http://ncvhs.hhs.gov/031119tr.htm, accessed October 1, 2005.

34. Ibid.

35. *San Francisco Chronicle*, September 26, 2004, A4. *San Francisco Chronicle*, December 7, 2004, B1.

36. Ruth Berkelman and Phyllis Freeman, "Emerging Infections and the CDC Response," in *Emerging Illness and Society: Negotiating the Public Health Agenda*, ed. Randall Packard et al. (Baltimore, 2004), 366.

37. Ruth Berkelman et al., "Infectious Disease Surveillance: A Crumbling Foundation," *Science* 264 (1994): 368.

38. Michael T. Osterholm, Guthrie S. Birkhead, and Rebecca A. Meriwether, "Impediments to Public Health Surveillance in the 1990s: The Lack of Resources and the Need for Priorities," *Journal of Public Health Management Practices* 2 (1996): 11.

39. Raymond Baxter et al., *Assessing Core Capacity for Infectious Diseases Surveillance. Final Report to the Office of the Assistant Secretary for Planning and Evaluation*, November 1, 2000, 2, http://www.lewin.com/NR/rdonlyres/70517B3C-202F-4E23-9F64-A5 D38CDAAD69/0/808.pdf, accessed October 1, 2005.

40. Council of State and Territorial Epidemiologists, *2004 National Assessment of Epidemiologic Capacity: Findings and Recommendations*, 2004, 4, http://www.cste.org/Assessment/ECA/pdffiles/ECAfinal05.pdf, accessed October 1, 2005.

41. Berkelman and Freeman, "Emerging Infections and the CDC Response," in *Emerging Illness and Society*, 367.

42. Osterholm, Birkhead, and Meriwether, "Impediments to Public Health Surveillance."

43. Timothy J. Doyle, M. Kathleen Glynn, and Samuel L. Groseclose, "Completeness of Notifiable Infectious Disease Reporting in the United States: An Analytical Literature Review," *American Journal of Epidemiology* 155 (2002): 871.

44. Pew Environmental Health Commission, Johns Hopkins University School of Public Health, *America's Environmental Health Gap: Why the Country Needs a Nationwide Health Tracking Network* (Baltimore, 2000), 6, http://healthyamericans.org/reports/files/healthgap.pdf, accessed October 1, 2005.

45. Trust for America's Health, *Improving Cancer Tracking Today Saves Live Tomorrow: Do States Make the Grade?* (Washington, DC, 2003).

46. *Columbus Dispatch*, March 14, 1999, 2B.

47. Trust for America's Health, "Birth Defects Tracking and Prevention One Year Later: One Step Forward, Two Steps Back?" April 2003, www.healthyamericans.org/reports/. Pew Environmental Health Commission, *America's Environmental Health Gap*.

48. Trust for America's Health, "Birth Defects Tracking and Prevention."

49. Minnesota Department of Health, Birth Defects Work Group, Minutes, October 3, 2002, http://www.health.state.mn.us/divs/eh/birthdefects/, accessed May 11, 2006.

50. *Columbus Dispatch*, March 1, 2002, 12A. *Plain Dealer* (Cleveland), February 21, 2002, B1. *Columbus Dispatch*, September 25, 2004, 1A. National Birth Defects Prevention Network, "Guidelines for Conducting Birth Defects Surveillance," www.nbdpn.org/current/resources/bdsurveillance.html, accessed May 11, 2006.

51. Pew Environmental Health Commission, Johns Hopkins University School of Public Health, "Transition Report to the New Administration: Strengthening Our Public Health Defenses against Environmental Threats," January 2001, http:// healthyamericans.org/reports/files/transition.pdf, accessed May 11, 2006. See also National Center on Birth Defects and Developmental Disabilities, Centers for Disease Control and Prevention, *State Birth Defects Surveillance Program Directory*, 2004, http://www.nbdpn.org/archives/2004/report2004/10_state_directory.pdf, accessed May 11, 2006.

52. John Sestito, Interview, November 21, 2004. For data on musculoskeletal disorders, see assistant secretary for planning and evaluation and secretary of the U.S. Department of Health and Human Services, "Recommendation 10, Personal Privacy in an Information Society, Chapter 7, Record-Keeping in the Medical-Care Relationship" (paper presented at the Privacy Protection Study Commission, June 1977), 64.

53. Council of State and Territorial Epidemiologists, *2004 National Assessment of Epidemiologic Capacity*.

54. David Sarnoff, "Electronic Medical Files," *Public Health Reports* 80 (1965): 778.

55. Rebecca Meriwether, "Blueprint for a National Public Health Surveillance System for the 21st Century," *Journal of Public Health Management Practice* 2 (1996): 17.

56. Council of State and Territorial Epidemiologists, "A Guide to the Implementation of the National Electronic Disease Surveillance System (NEDSS) in State Public Health Agencies," http://www.cste.org/pdffiles/NEDSS_book_final.pdf, accessed January 31, 2007.

57. General Accounting Office, *Emerging Infectious Diseases: Review of State and Federal Disease Surveillance Efforts*, September 2004, 33, http://www.gao.gov/new.items/d04877.pdf, accessed May 11, 2006.

58. *San Diego Union-Tribune*, June 22, 2001, B9.

59. Michael A. McGeehin, Judith R. Qualters, and Amanda Sue Niskar, "National Environmental Public Health Tracking Program: Bridging the Information Gap," *Environmental Health Perspectives* 112 (2004): 1409–13.

60. Trust for America's Health, "Birth Defects and Developmental Disabilities: The Search for Causes and Cures, Issue Report," July 2005, www.healthyamericans .org/reports/birthdefects05/BirthDefects05.pdf, accessed May 11, 2006.

61. Alan R. Hinman et al., "Integrating Child Health Information Systems," *American Journal of Public Health* 95 (2005): 1923–27. Melanie Lockhart, Interview, November 9, 2005.

62. Deborah Linzer et al., "Evolution of a Child Health Profile Initiative," *Journal of Public Health Management and Practice* 10 (2004): S16–S23.

63. S. Nicole Fehrenbach, Janet C. R. Kelly, and Christie Vu, "Integration of Child Health Information Systems: Current State and Local Health Department Efforts," *Journal of Public Health Management and Practice* 10 (2004): S30–S35.

64. Hinman et al., "Integrating Child Health Information Systems," 1923–27.

65. R. N. Kleinfield and Marc Santora, "Health: Diabetes in New York: Part I, the Problem" *New York Times*, http://video.on.nytimes.com/ifr_main.jsp?nsid=b-bb1 b39f:11079231e40:24a9&fr_story=d3e0a4832728fcd9e54219912e142e4033fd27e

5&st=1170265741796&mp=WMP&cpf=true&fvn=9&fr+013107_125413_wbb1b39f
x11079231e40x24aa&rdm+968416.6962273171, accessed January 9, 2006.

66. *Washington Post,* January 11, 2005, A03. Diana K. Berger, Personal Communication, January 27, 2006.

67. Department of Health and Mental Hygiene, Board of Health, Notice of Intent to Amend Article 13 of the New York City Health Code, 2005, p. 2, www.nyc.gov/html/doh/downloads/pdf/public/notice-intention-art-13.pdf, accessed January 31, 2006. Lynn D. Silver and Diana K. Berger, "Improving Diabetes Care for All New York," http://www.nyc.gov/html/doh/downloads/pdf/diabetes/diabetes-presentation-a1c-registry.pdf, accessed January 3, 2006.

68. Berger, Personal Communication.

69. Ibid.

70. Department of Health and Mental Hygiene, Notice of Intent to Amend Article 13, pp. 3–4.

71. Silver and Berger, "Improving Diabetes Care."

72. *New York Sun,* http://nysun.com/article/17570, accessed December 19, 2005. Letter from Peter M. Kazon, August 16, 2005, Comments presented at a Public Hearing. This letter and the ones that follow are available from the New York City Department of Health and Mental Hygiene.

73. Andrew Schlafly to New York City Department of Health and Mental Hygiene, August 17, 2005.

74. Letters to New York City Department of Health and Mental Hygiene, August 12, 14, and 15, 2005.

75. Letter to New York City Department of Health and Mental Hygiene, August 12, 2005.

76. E-mail to New York City Department of Health and Mental Hygiene, August 15, 2005, available from the New York City Department of Health and Mental Hygiene.

77. *New York Sun,* http://nysun.com/article/17570. Www.medpagetoday.com/Endocrinology/Diabetes/tb1/1422, accessed December 19, 2005.

78. Robin Kaigh, Public Hearing on Intention to Amend Article 13 of the New York City Health Code, August 16, 2005, p. 40, available from the New York City Department of Health and Mental Hygiene.

79. Ibid., 38.

80. Letter to New York City Department of Health and Mental Hygiene, July 27, 2005.

81. Nathaniel Clark, Personal Communication, February 6, 2006.

82. *New York Times,* February 2, 2006, B1. New York City Department of Health and Mental Hygiene, "Stopping the HIV/AIDS Epidemic in New York," February 21, 2006, 14, available from the Office of the Commissioner of Health, New York City Department of Health and Mental Hygiene.

83. Thomas Frieden, Personal Communication, March 6, 2006.

84. *New York Times,* February 2, 2006, B1.

85. Ibid.

86. Frieden, Personal Communication. New York City Department of Health and Mental Hygiene, "NYC Health Department Proposals: Helping HIV-Positive

People Get Optimal Care," circular, March 7, 2006, available from the Office of the Commissioner of Health, New York City Department of Health and Mental Hygiene.

87. *New York Times,* February 6, 2006, 22.

88. *New York Blade,* February 13, 2006, http://www.newyorkblade.com, accessed February 13, 2006.

89. Ibid.

90. Robert Cordero, "Public Comment to the Presidential Advisory Council on HIV/AIDS: Regarding New York City Health Commissioner Dr. Thomas Frieden's Proposals on HIV Testing and Medical Privacy," March 17, 2006, 1, http://www.hw advocacy.com/update/CorderoPACHAprez.pdf, accessed March 27, 2006.

91. Derrick Chandler, Testimony Regarding Thomas Frieden's Proposals on HIV Testing, March 17, 2006, www.hwadvocacy.com/update/downloads/frieden _plan_5_HWtestimony.pdf, accessed March 27, 2006. See also New York AIDS Coalition, "Proposed Changes to Article 27-F, the AIDS Confidentiality Law: Considerations in the Debate," http://www.nyaidscoalition.org/binary-data/NYAC_PDF/pdf/126-1.pdf, accessed March 27, 2006.

92. Testimony Regarding Thomas Frieden's Proposals on HIV Testing.

93. Thomas Frieden to community members, March 6, 2006 (italics in original).

94. Rosemary Stevens, *In Sickness and in Wealth: American Hospitals in the Twentieth Century* (Baltimore, 1989).

95. *Star Tribune* (Minneapolis), June 3, 1998, 6A.

96. Ibid.

97. Institute of Medicine and National Research Council, *Chemical and Biological Terrorism: Research and Development to Improve Civilian Medical Response* (Washington, DC, 1999).

98. Margaret A. Hamburg, "Addressing Bioterrorist Threats: Where Do We Go from Here?" *Emerging Infectious Diseases* 5 (1999): 564.

99. Victor W. Sidel, Robert M. Gould, and Hillel W. Cohen, "Bioterrorism Preparedness: Cooptation of Public Health?" *Medicine and Global Survival* 7 (2001/2002): 82.

100. Centers for Disease Control and Prevention, "Biological and Chemical Terrorism: Strategic Plan for Preparedness and Response: Recommendations of the CDC Strategic Planning Workgroup," *Morbidity and Mortality Weekly Report* 49 (2000): 11. Jeffrey Koplan, "CDC's Strategic Plan for Bioterrorism Preparedness and Response," *Public Health Reports* 116 (2001): 9–16.

101. Centers for Disease Control and Prevention, "Biological and Chemical Terrorism," 9.

102. John A. Jernigan et al., "Bioterrorism-Related Inhalation Anthrax: The First Ten Cases Reported in the United States," *Emerging Infectious Diseases* 7 (2001): 933–44.

103. *New York Times,* September 10, 2002, F1.

104. Government Accounting Office, *Infectious Diseases: Gaps Remain in Surveillance Capabilities of State and Local Agencies,* 108th Cong., 1st sess., September 24, 2003, p. 1.

105. *Washington Post,* February 1, 2002, B1. *Columbus Dispatch,* February 1, 2002, 14A. *Boston Globe,* October 3, 2002, 1, http://www.bt.cdc.gov/surveillance/ears/, accessed May 19, 2006.

106. *Washington Post,* November 24, 2001, A1.

107. *New York Times,* February 6, 2002, A11.

108. *Pittsburgh Post-Gazette,* February 6, 2002, A7.

109. *New York Times,* February 6, 2002.

110. General Accounting Office, *Emerging Infectious Diseases: Review of State and Federal Disease Surveillance Efforts, Report to the Chairman, Permanent Subcommittee on Investigations, Committee on Governmental Affairs, U.S. Senate* (Washington, DC, 2004), 27.

111. *Washington Post,* November 23, 2003, A17.

112. *New York Times,* November 9, 2002, A12.

113. *New York Times,* November 18, 2002, 18.

114. Lawrence O. Gostin et al., "The Model State Emergency Health Powers Act: Planning for and Response to Bioterrorism and Naturally Occurring Infectious Diseases," *Journal of the American Medical Association* 288 (2002): 624.

115. Ibid., 626.

116. George Annas to James Hodge, November 1, 2001. In possession of authors.

117. Bob Barr, "A Fearsome Power Grab by the CDC and State Governors," http://hillsource.house.gov/barr/newsdescr.asp?N = 20020215170247, accessed March 13, 2002.

118. Barbara Loe Fisher, "Editorial: Vaccinating America at Gunpoint," www.909shot.com/History/Newsletters/spsmallpox.htm, accessed March 13, 2002.

119. Janlori Goldman, "Balancing in a Crisis? Bioterrorism, Public Health, and Privacy," in *Lost Liberties: Ashcroft and the Assault on Personal Freedom,* ed. Cynthia Brown (New York, 2003), 170.

120. Ibid., 165.

121. Centers for Disease Control and Prevention, "BioSense: Implementation of a National Early Event Detection and Situational Awareness System," http://www.cdc.gov/mmwr/preview/mmwrhtml/su5401a4.htm, accessed May 11, 2006. Centers for Disease Control and Prevention, "Practice and Experience Deciphering Data Anomalies in BioSense," http://www.cdc.gov/mmwr/preview/mmwrhtml/su5401a21.htm, accessed March 13, 2002. Centers for Disease Control and Prevention, "Data Sources: Implementation of Laboratory Order Data in BioSense Early Event Detection and Situation Awareness System," http://www.cdc.gov/mmwr/preview/mmwrhtml/su5401a6.htm, accessed May 12, 2006.

CONCLUSION

1. Alan Westin, *Privacy and Freedom* (New York, 1967), 32–39. Lawrence Tribe, *American Constitutional Law,* 2nd ed. (Mineola, NY, 1988), 1304.

2. Gary L. Bostwick, "Comment: A Taxonomy of Privacy: Repose, Sanctuary, and Intimate Decision," *California Law Review* 1447 (1976): 1456.

3. Quoted in Tribe, *American Constitutional Law,* 1302.

4. David H. Flaherty, *Privacy in Colonial New England* (Charlottesville, VA, 1972), 21.

5. Quoted in Arthur J. Viseltear, "Emergence of the Medical Care Section of the American Public Health Association, 1926–1948," *American Journal of Public Health* 63 (1973): 991.

6. Allan M. Brandt and Martha Gardner, "Antagonism and Accommodation:

Interpreting the Relationship between Public Health and Medicine in the United States during the 20th Century," *American Journal of Public Health* 90 (2000): 707–15. Elizabeth Fee, *Disease and Discovery: A History of the Johns Hopkins School of Hygiene and Public Health, 1916–1939* (Baltimore, 1987), 227–36. James Colgrove, "Reform and Its Discontents: Public Health in New York City during the Great Society Era," *Journal of Policy History* 19 (2007): 3–25.

7. New York State Department of Health, AIDS Institute, Memorandum, Re: Proposals to Extend Surveillance and Intervention. Document in possession of authors.

8. Janlori Goldman, "Balancing in a Crisis? Bioterrorism, Public Health, and Privacy," *Journal of Health Law* 38 (2005): 526–27.

9. Julie R. Ingelfinger and Jeffrey M. Drazen, "Registry Research and Medical Privacy," *New England Journal of Medicine* 350 (2004): 1452–53. Matthew T. McKenna, Phyllis Wingo, and James Jerry Gibson, letter to the editor, *New England Journal of Medicine* 351 (2004): 613.

10. *Los Angeles Times,* January 18, 2006, B3.

11. Tribe, *American Constitutional Law.*

Text:	10/12 Baskerville
Display:	Baskerville
Compositor:	BookMatters, Berkeley
Indexer:	Ruth Elwell
Printer and binder:	Sheridan Books, Inc.